Second Edition

Health Care Delivery
in the United States

Steven Jonas received his M.D. from Harvard and his M.P.H. from Yale. He is an associate professor in the Department of Community and Preventive Medicine, School of Medicine, State University of New York at Stony Brook.

David Banta received his M.D. from Duke and his M.P.H. and M.S. Hyg. from Harvard. He is the Manager of the Health Program of the Office of Technology Assessment of the United States Congress, Washington, D.C.

Nancy Barhydt-Wezenaar received her M.S. from Albany Medical College and her Dr.P.H. from Columbia University, School of Public Health. She is the Director, Bureau of Health Maintenance Organizations and Home Health Services, New York State Department of Health, Office of Health Systems Management, Albany, New York.

Michael Enright received his M.B.A. in Health Care Administration from George Washington University. He is Director, A. P. Noyes Division, Saint Elizabeths Hospital, Washington, D.C. He is a faculty associate in the Department of Community Medicine, Georgetown University School of Medicine, Washington, D.C.

Ruth S. Hanft received her M.A. from Hunter College. She is Deputy Assistant Secretary for Health Research, Statistics, and Technology, United States Department of Health and Human Services, Washington D.C.

Lorrin M. Koran received his M.D. from Harvard. He is an associate professor in the Department of Psychiatry and Behavioral Sciences, Stanford Medical Center, Palo Alto, California.

Carol McCarthy received her M.S. from the State University of New York at Stony Brook and her Ph.D. from New York University. She is President of the Delaware Valley Hospital Council located in Philadelphia, Pennsylvania.

David A. Pearson received his Ph.D. from Yale University and his M.P.H. from the University of Michigan. He is Associate Dean for Public Health, Department of Epidemiology and Public Health, Yale University School of Medicine, New Haven, Connecticut.

Terrie T. Wetle received her Ph.D. in Urban Studies from Portland State University. She is director of the Program in Long Term Care and assistant professor in the Department of Epidemiology and Public Health, Yale University School of Medicine, New Haven, Connecticut.

Second Edition

Health Care Delivery in the United States

Steven Jonas
and contributors

with a Foreword by
Milton I. Roemer

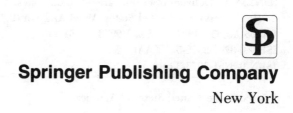

Springer Publishing Company
New York

Springer Publishing Company, Inc.
200 Park Avenue South
New York, N.Y. 10003

82 83 84 85 / 10 9 8 7 6 5 4 3

For purposes of citation of copyrighted sources,
the credits of pp. xvii-xviii constitute an extension
of this copyright page.

First edition, l977

Library of Congress Cataloging in Publication Data

Jonas, Steven.
  Health care delivery in the United States.

  Includes bibliographies and index.
  1. Medical care—United States.   I. Title.
[DNLM: 1. Delivery of health care—United States.
2. Health services—United States. W 84 AA1 J7h (P)]
RA395.A3J65   1981   362.1'0973   81-148
ISBN 0-8261-2072-5   AACR2
ISBN 0-8261-2073-3 (pbk.)

Printed in the United States of America

To Linda F. Jonas, Sandra S. Banta, Richard W. Besdine, Josephine Enright, Herbert Hanft, Stephanie Koran, Michael P. McCarthy, Jo-Ann D. Pearson, Fritz Wezenaar, and to the memory of E. Richard Weinerman

Contents

Foreword to the Second Edition

The term or concept of health care *delivery* was not used in the United States or elsewhere before the mid-1960s. What accounts for the emergence of this idea—describing so well, as it does, the content of this book?

Issues relating to medical care in the United States became prominent in the massive economic Depression of the 1930s. The most dramatic of those issues was the *cost* of medical service—the "cash barrier," as it was usually called, between the people needing services and the nation's increasingly capable scientific resources for providing them. Moreover, it seemed that the greatest problem lay not in a sheer lack of money or "purchasing power" for medical care, but rather in a failure to mobilize collectively the funds that were available.

The rational response was to do in the United States what had been done decades earlier to cope with the same problem in Europe; this was to apply the mechanism of insurance to pay for medical care. Periodic prepayment of small contributions by a number of people into a common fund could assure money to cope with the risk of sickness, unpredictable in any individual but relatively easy to estimate in a population group. Hence the idea of health insurance (or what the Europeans called "sickness insurance") expanded rapidly in the United States from a practice applied to small groups of workers in isolated industries to a movement affecting millions of people everywhere in the nation. The major shortcoming of the robust "voluntary health insurance" movement was deficient coverage of the aged and the poor—a weakness substantially though not wholly remedied by governmental enactment of Medicare and Medicaid in 1965.

In the meantime, for many reasons explored in this book, the demands for and utilization of medical care steadily increased. This was due not only to the strengthened economic support for services—from insurance and also greater public spending—but also to ever-expanding medical technology, aging of the population (with more chronic disease), urbanization, and higher educational levels. The "rising costs of medical care" became a more and more prominent issue; an enlarging percentage of national wealth was required, in spite of the buffering of those costs through insurance and taxation mechanisms.

The insight rapidly spread, therefore, that the problems of effective health care could not be solved solely by collectivized methods of financing. The system of health care delivery must also be improved, made more efficient. The prevailing patterns of health care, it was realized, clung to the horse-and-buggy model in an age of ever-more-complex technology. This had, indeed, been recognized by sophisticated leaders of the Committee on the Costs of Medical Care in 1932, but national complacence and the opposition of traditional interests had thwarted any significant changes. Unlike the patterns of producing other goods and services, health care remained a cottage industry.

With the widespread recognition of cultural lag in the health services—what, years before, Henry Sigerist had called the lag of medicine's sociology behind its technology—attention became increasingly focused everywhere on the contours of the health care delivery system. This required survey and analysis of the health manpower in the system; the patterns of providing ambulatory care (therapeutic and preventive); the organization and operation of hospitals; the role of government; the control and measurement of medical care quality; the process (if any) of planning to meet population needs, the promotion of research—all these aspects of health care *delivery*, as well as its financing. When these components of the health care system were examined, many problems were discovered: discrepancies between a rational scheme of organization and current realities.

A comprehensive, yet concise, presentation of these explorations of the American health care delivery system, in its many component parts, is the great contribution of this book, published first in 1977. The second edition brings to the reader the further developments of the 1980s. While improvements are recognized and reported, the viewpoint remains critical, as it must if progress toward effective meeting of health needs is to continue.

Many books have been written or compiled on the American health care system and its problems. Because of the system's complexities, most of these are understandably multi-authored; it is hardly feasible for a single scholar to understand in depth each of the many varied components of the field. The result of such compilations, however, is often a mosaic that does not make a picture. Dr. Jonas and his colleagues, on the other hand, have worked together in a remarkably integrated way. While each author has his or her own style and emphases, there is a unifying perspective. This is first to trace the major historical forces in back of each component of American health services that shape their current contours. Then, each element of the health care system is analyzed in a manner that highlights its essential character, along with unsolved problems, so that feasible pathways to improvements are clearly illuminated.

—MILTON I. ROEMER

Foreword to the First Edition

Since World War I our health care delivery system has evolved from one featuring the general physician and the community hospital to one having an incredibly complicated and bewildering array of providers and institutions. The change from a physician-dominated to a system-oriented model has brought into being a whole new language of health care and has made health care a focus of nationwide attention and sometimes indignation.

This evolution away from the "family doctor" began slowly in the 1920s, when the technological revolution in medicine was in its early stages. Technological change—which was stimulated by World War II and has grown in quantum leaps ever since—begat specialization, because the vast armamentarium of new drugs and technical procedures made care-giving much more complex than ever before. No longer could the general practitioner handle all health problems, including surgery, and keep up to date on all new knowledge. Thus the superspecialist has come to outstrip the nonspecialist in status and in access to academic and financial rewards. Attention to organ systems, or even one part of an organ, has become the acceptable M.D.–university model.

Not only has the physician become specialized; he has been subsumed into (while remaining dominant over) a complex health team, and the system he works in has become organized into a regionalized referral network of institutions providing varying levels of specialized patient care. The specialist imperative extends to other workers in the system, including those involved in the highly sophisticated technology of, for example, intensive-care units, renal dialysis, and organ transplant centers.

Inevitably this specialization has created an increasing gap in general continuing health care at the community level. There is a serious contradiction between the need to provide basic health services to the entire population and the specialist imperative resulting from the ever-increasing growth of scientific and technological knowledge.

As a result, a whole field of community medicine has emerged to redirect medical attention to general care. In July 1955, Cornell Medical College in New York City and the Navajo Tribal Council, which governs the 100,000 American Indian Navajo people, conducted an early experiment in this domain. The project was located in a remote area of the Navajo reservation in northern Arizona, 90 miles north of the general hospital at Fort Defiance, Arizona. The experiment was designed to find the most effective way to provide modern medicine to a culturally different, indigenous population; it was hoped that the lessons learned could help the U. S. Public Health Service improve the delivery of general rural health services to Indian people throughout the nation.

In that period of innocence, our language was informal; we had little of today's ubiquitous terminology. Thus, although our program involved "community participation," centered in a "neighborhood health center," and employed "primary care doctors," "nurse-clinicians," and "community health workers," we knew none of these terms. We did not speak of ourselves as "health teams" practicing "community medicine," although, in current parlance, that was what we were doing.

I use this example to show the rapid development of health care systems language and concepts during a 20-year period. In public health as well as in specialized technology, whole new principles have been formulated and a whole new vocabulary invented to describe them.

Because these enormous changes have occurred, both providers and consumers often have a confused picture of the current health care delivery system. It is essential that health care education keep pace with changes, but it has not always done so.

In this book Dr. Steven Jonas and his co-authors do much to remedy the lack of basic texts conveying the knowledge required by present and future decision-makers in the health care system. The book is basically descriptive in nature, examining the various elements in the delivery system and elucidating their interactions; it succeeds in describing this labyrinthine system lucidly and comprehensively. It does not neglect the economic ramifications of an industry that is now second only to defense in the Gross National Product, nor the political controversies raging over accountability and the right to health care. Importantly, the book is up to date in terminology, and thus will help meet the urgent need of health workers to communicate with one another and with the public at large.

KURT W. DEUSCHLE, M.D.
Mount Sinai School of Medicine

Preface

Health services, affecting as they do the lives of all of us, have become a major social issue. The rapidly rising costs of health services make them a major economic issue too. There are frequent political debates and innumerable statements of policy. Thus, the main topic of this book—how personal health services are organized and delivered—has come to interest a wide array of professionals, as well as many laypersons.

For these reasons, in describing the health care delivery system in the United States, we do not address ourselves to one specialized audience. The book is designed primarily as a text for introductory courses in health care delivery offered in medical schools, schools of public health, health services administration programs, nursing schools, schools of allied health professions and of social welfare; but it can also be used in such non-health-oriented academic programs as law, architecture, engineering, economics, political science, history, sociology, community planning, and the like.

Moreover, we have attempted to produce an integrated work that can be read by interested persons who are not students, but want to locate in one place the basic, essential information about health care delivery in the United States. We hope that health professionals, lay members of health-related boards, policy-makers, observers from abroad, and the concerned general public will find this book useful and enlightening.

We attempt to be reasonably objective in our description of the health care delivery system; this is not intended to be another "health care crisis" book. As we point out in the Introduction, over the years there has been a plethora of such books, many serving a useful purpose. However, we do not believe that there is actually a health care "crisis," as the word is customarily defined; rather, we think that our complex health care delivery system has a number of serious problems, most of which have a long history. In our analysis of the system, we recognize both its good points and its failings. Its outstanding strengths include a large and dedicated manpower pool, a strong institutional base, fine education and research establishments, and a supporting industry that has produced many significant technological advances over the years. Our society now faces the task of attempting to build creatively on the strengths in order to deal with the shortcomings.

The authors do, of course, hold individual opinions and, to a certain extent, a collective point of view. We represent a variety of health care professions, but in our work we are all involved in continuing analysis, evaluation, and program development in one or more parts of the system. In work of this type, one naturally tends more toward involvement with change and reform than toward defense of the status quo: we are aware of the system's strengths, but we are likely to be more directly concerned in our day-to-day work with its weaknesses. Thus, we have allowed ourselves the privilege of occasionally "editorializing," sometimes critically, without, however, succumbing to the natural temptation to offer our own sweeping prescriptions for change. Based on the facts as they are presented, we feel that readers who are so inclined should be able to develop their own proposals for reform.

We do feel that without some comments from us, however, this book would be very dry indeed. Some readers will undoubtedly feel that we have been too factual, whereas others will think that we have overeditorialized. Nevertheless, we hope that our descriptions are clear enough for the reader to be able to judge for him- or herself which of our subjective evaluations are closest to reality.

The reader should note several important technical features in the book. Most tables are from public sources, published on a regular, periodic basis. Part A of Appendix I ("Guide to Sources") briefly describes most of the important sources of health and health care data in the United States, and numbers each source. Each table in the text taken from a source listed in Appendix I is keyed to the Appendix. By using Appendix I, the interested reader can thus find the most recent versions of all tables from public, recurring sources. We hope that this feature will allow the book to remain up to date longer than most textbooks.

Part B of Appendix I lists the important categories of data (population, mortality, health manpower, and so on); the reader is told in which sources the data may be found. For example, in Appendix I, Part B, under "Institutions," there is a list of the principal recurring sources of data on health care institutions in the United States, keyed to the source descriptions in Part A.

Appendix II contains abbreviations.

Most of the chapters have fairly lengthy reference lists. This was done in order to document our material satisfactorily and to provide instructors with an ample selection of supplementary readings, if they wish to use the bibliographies for that purpose.

Please note that in general the male pronouns are used, only because that is the customary mode at this time and because the alternatives—using he/she or changing from male to female pronouns in alternate chapters—are artificial and linguistically cumbersome. We trust that readers will not invest this point of usage with political implications.

Acknowledgments

In part, the genesis of the first edition of our book is to be found in "The Delivery of Health Care," by Steven Jonas and Victor W. Sidel, Chapter 21 in *Practice of Medicine* (New York: Harper and Row, 1973). Portions of that work appear in this book, particularly in Chapters 2 and 6, and are used with the special permission of Harper and Row. Dr. Sidel's contributions to the earlier chapter are gratefully acknowledged, and the material is used with his permission as well.

The material in Chapter 7 attributed to *The American Health Care System*, by John Gordon Freymann, is used with the kind permission of Dr. Freymann and the publisher, Williams & Wilkins, Baltimore (© 1974).

Chapter 4, by Ruth Hanft, was not written in her official capacity. No official support or endorsement by the Department of Health and Human Services is intended or should be inferred.

Figure 2-1 is reprinted, with permission, from Kerr White's "Life and Death in Medicine," Copyright © September 1973 by Scientific American, Inc. All rights reserved.

Figure 2-2 is reprinted with permission from the *Medical Care Chart Book*, Sixth Edition, 1976, Department of Medical Care Organization, School of Public Health, University of Michigan.

In the first edition, Barbara Rimer contributed to Chapter 6, and Michael Enright and James Korjus contributed to what has become Chapter 11 in this edition. We acknowledge their contributions with thanks.

This book could not have been produced without the help of many people. For reading, commenting on, and helping with the preparation of various chapters of the first edition, we thank Patricia Bauman, Martha Blaxall, James Brindle, Helen Burnside, Robert Carroll, Tom Christoffel, Barbara Cohen, Kathleen Dolan, H. Jack Geiger, Bernard Glassman, Frederick Jerome, Howard Kelman, Marvin Leeds, Raymond Lerner, Thomas Mann, Joyce Page, Ian Porter, Wanda Robinson, Ruth Roemer, Joshua Sanes, Richard Seggel, Milton Terris, John Thompson, and Andre Varma. We received valuable help from student assistants. Among them are Charles Andrews, Daniel Ricciardi, Harold Rosenthal, and Zakhar Spektor.

For the second edition we thank Harold J. Jonas for his thorough review of the entire text of the first. His comments on both form and content were most helpful in the preparation of this edition. In addition, we are grateful to Professor Jonas for proofreading the typesetting of this edition. Andre Varma, Peter Rogatz, and John Last reviewed Chapters 3, 7, and 14, respectively, in detail. Their suggestions were very constructive. Robert Greifinger contributed to the preparation of Chapter 6, as noted in the authorship of that chapter. We thank him for his effort. The National Center for Health Statistics is thanked for making available valuable material from *Health United States, 1979*. We acknowledge the help of Richard W. Besdine, Peggy Gallup, and Lillian Merriam in the preparation of Chapter 8. We acknowledge the generosity of the Division of Biometry and Epidemiology, National Institute of Mental Health, in providing copies of NIMH publications used in the preparation of Chapter 9.

Many people participated in the typing and we are grateful to them all. For the first edition the dedication of Eleanor Lindwall and Eugenia DiGirolamo in the editor's office deserves special mention. They typed, and retyped, not only the editor's own chapters but also the entire manuscript. Their participation proved invaluable. For the second edition, Anne Marie McNally made an equally important contribution in manuscript typing.

Our editors at Springer Publishing Co., Ellen Tumposky for the first edition and Isabel Stein for both editions, were able, despite little direct knowledge of this rather technical field, to find that fine line between doing too much and too little. In their hands, on many occasions, ponderousness gave way to brevity and grace. Mrs. Stein added an exceptionally good job of technical editing for the second edition. Many thanks too are due to Carole Saltz and Nancy Schulz of Springer for their encouragement and help.

Our publisher, Ursula Springer, reviewed every chapter of the first edition in detail. Her suggestions were very helpful. More important, however, in accepting our book for publication in the first place, Dr. Springer demonstrated her faith that a group of generally young, generally unknown authors could produce something of value. We are grateful to our readers for their response to the first edition. It is that response which encouraged us to write this edition. It has also justified Dr. Springer's original faith in us. We gratefully acknowledge that the publication of the first edition was assisted by a grant from the Josiah Macy, Jr., Foundation.

Finally, the editor would like to thank his department chairman, Andre Varma, for graciously providing the environment of time and space which made the preparation of the second edition possible.

1

Introduction

Steven Jonas

The State of Health Care Delivery in the U. S.

About 50 years ago, a study of health care delivery in the United States summarized its findings in these terms (Committee on the Costs of Medical Care):

> The problem of providing satisfactory medical service to all the people of the United States at costs which they can meet is a pressing one. At the present time, many persons do not receive service which is adequate either in quantity or quality, and the costs of service are inequably distributed. The result is a tremendous amount of preventable physical pain and mental anguish, needless deaths, economic inefficiency, and social waste. Furthermore, these conditions are, as the following pages will show, largely unnecessary. The United States has the economic resources, the organizing ability, and the technical experience to solve this problem. (p. 2)

So commenced the final report of the Committee on the Costs of Medical Care, published in 1932. The committee, chaired by Ray Lyman Wilbur, a past president of the American Medical Association, had been created in 1927 to look into problems of health care delivery. Strikingly, the statement is entirely applicable to our current health care system.

In the 1960s and 1970s, observers of the U.S. health care system of differing political persuasions often spoke in terms of "crisis." For example, in 1968, an article called "Crisis in American Medicine" (Battistella and Southby) in the British journal *The Lancet* began:

> In terms of gross national product the U.S.A. spends more on health than does any other country. But costs are rising at such a rate that more and more people will find it difficult to get complete health care. This particularly applies to the poor, the old, the Negroes, and other disadvantaged groups. Doctors and hospital beds are distributed most unevenly both in broad

geographic regions and between States. There are indications, too, that the quality of care has been inferior, especially in terms of antenatal and infant mortality. The whole organization of medical care in the U.S.A. has failed to respond to changing disease patterns, the move from country to cities, industrialization, and the increasing proportion of old people in the population. (p. 581)

In 1970, the editors of *Fortune* said:

American medicine, the pride of the nation for many years, stands now on the brink of chaos. To be sure, our medical practitioners have their great moments of drama and triumph. But much of the U.S. medical care, particularly the everyday business of preventing and treating routine illnesses, is inferior in quality, wastefully dispensed, and inequitably financed. Medical manpower and facilities are so maldistributed that large segments of the population, especially the urban poor and those in rural areas, get virtually no care at all—even though their illnesses are most numerous and, in a medical sense, often easy to cure. (p. 9)

In a similar vein, Senator Edward M. Kennedy, speaking to an audience of doctors in New York City in 1971, said (Klaw):

America is beginning to realize that we have a health care crisis on our hands, and that the magnitude of the crisis is enormous. . . . I challenge even the most reactionary pillars of organized medicine, even the most affluent physicians in the most affluent suburbs of this rich city, to deny that a crisis exists, or that it exists for all Americans—not just the poor, not just the black, but each and every one of us. (p. xi)

Eliot Richardson, one of the Secretaries of the United States Department of Health, Education, and Welfare (USDHEW) in the Nixon administration, said in Senate testimony (1971):

In general our critical health problems today do not arise because the health of our people is worsening, or because expenditures on health care have been niggardly, or because we have been negligent as a nation in developing health care resources, or because we have been unconcerned about providing financial protection against ill-health. We must look elsewhere. I should like to suggest that our present concern is a function of two broad problems. The first is the inequality in health status and care, and in access to financing. The other is the pervasive problem of rising medical costs. . . . The impressive growth in the number of people covered by health insurance conceals the fact that only 29 percent of all personal health expenditures were paid by insurance in 1968. . . . The indices of general improvement in health pale in importance when we look behind them and see that the poor and non-whites are doing far worse than whites and those with decent income. . . . When we look beyond our borders and compare ourselves with other nations, any sense of accomplishment over our long-run gains in health status is mitigated by the fact that other advanced nations are doing better than we are. . . . These disparities point to a gap between what we have accomplished and what remains to be accomplished, between our achievements and our expectations, between what is and our impatience for what might be. . . . (pp. 72–74).

In 1973, the Research and Policy Committee of the Committee for Economic Development, the board of which is composed of representatives of many of the leading American corporations and banks, came to the following conclusions concerning the present system (Research and Policy Committee):

First, faulty allocation of resources is a major cause of inadequacies and inequalities in U.S. health services that result today in poor or substandard care for large segments of the population.

Second, the task of assuring all people the ability to cope financially with the costs of health care has been made realizable by the substantial base of coverage now provided by both private and public insurance plans.

Third, unless step-by-step alterations are made in the means of delivering services and paying providers, closing the gaps in financing would overburden an inadequate system and offer little prospect of materially improving the quality and quantity of medical services of the health of the American people. (p. 17)

Finally, in 1979, Congressman Ronald Dellums introduced a bill to create a National Health Service wih a statement that said in part:

We have in this country today a health delivery system where the quality of health care received is determined by race, language, national origin, or income level. Health is viewed as a commodity to be bought and sold in the marketplace, it is not viewed as a right of the people; a service to be provided by the Government. However, financing is not the only problem facing the people when it comes to the delivery of health care. Other, equally important, problems are the maldistribution of health manpower, the unequal access to services, the unreliable quality of care, and the lack of public control over health care. No matter how much we guarantee the payment of services to the people, it is of little comfort to them if there is no one around to provide the service.

There have indeed been many critical reports and studies (*Business Week;* Ehrenreich and Ehrenreich; *Harper's Magazine;* Jonas; Kennedy; Klaw; Knowles; Moskin: National Commission on Community Health Services; Citizens Board of Inquiry report; Health Task Force report; Ribicoff; Schorr; Sidel and Sidel; Silver; Somers and Somers). Milton Roemer has cited a series of them going back many years.*

On the other hand, some observers deny that a crisis exists. In 1972, in his book *The Case for American Medicine,* journalist Harry Schwartz wrote that cries of "crisis" were just so much hyperbole; United States medicine has been doing an outstanding job, and new research and sociological change is needed to improve the nation's health further (*American Medical News,* October 16, 1972).

In 1975, an AMA president extolled the merits of the present system: (*American Medical News,* November 17, 1975):

> The constantly improving American health system is the best in the world and must not be stifled by adopting a government-controlled national health insurance program, the American Medical Association told Congress.
>
> AMA President Max H. Parrott, testifying before Congress, said: "When considering a national plan for this country, it is necessary to take cognizance of the strengths of our own method of health care delivery. . . . This will assure that our excellent system will continue to improve and will not suffer the stifling effects experienced in other countries." He further stated, "American medical service and technology have developed at an unparalleled rate . . . presently there is more and better medical technology here than anywhere else in the world."

In 1978, the AMA Executive Vice-President, Dr. James Sammons, told a Senate Subcommittee that U.S. health care is "superior to any other in the world" ("Month in Washington," p. 2, 282). This view was confirmed by

---

*Roemer listed these studies as follows:
"Every few years, more recently in the last decade, there appears a book analyzing the serious defects of health care in America. In 1927, Harry H. Moore produced *American Medicine and the People's Health,* in the 1930's were the magnificent 27 volumes of the Committee on the Costs of Medical Care, in 1939 there was James Rorty's *American Medicine Mobilizes,* and in 1940 Hugh Cabot's *The Patient Dilemma.* After World War II Carl Malmberg wrote *140 Million Patients* in 1947, Michael Davis wrote *Medical Care for Tomorrow* in 1955, and Richard Carter wrote *The Doctor Business* in 1958. In 1965 there was Selig Greenberg's excellent *The Troubled Calling: Crisis in the Medical Establishment.* The year after Medicare, 1966, saw two critical outputs: *The American Health Scandal* by Raul Tunley and *The Doctors* by Martin L. Gross. In 1967 there was Fred J. Cook's *Plot Against the Patient* and in 1970 Ed Cray's *In Failing Health.*"

an editorial entitled "The Invisible Medical Crisis" in the *New York State Journal of Medicine,* which said: "The medical system in the United States is without question the best in the world" (Stolfi).

Finally, in 1979, shortly after Congressman Dellums made the indictment quoted above, Harry Schwartz, citing the existence of improving population death rates as proof that there is no crisis in the system for delivery of medical services, said:

Whatever happened to the national health care crisis?

You remember that crisis, don't you? Less than a decade ago, President Richard M. Nixon spoke of a "massive crisis" in the delivery of health care, while *Fortune* magazine wrote of American medicine standing "on the brink of chaos." The CBS television network devoted two hours of prime time and the reportorial talents of George Herman and Daniel Schorr to warn "don't get sick in America." NBC television joined in with Edwin Newman and "What Price Health?" And Senator Edward M. Kennedy chimed in to declare that "health care is the fastest growing failing business" . . .

[But] American medicine was never on the edge of chaos or in danger of collapsing. Many who raised such spectres were either uninformed or sought to use exaggerated descriptions of real problems to achieve socialized medicine here.

The debate, then, has centered on the soundness of the system, whether it is moribund or dynamic, whether it is "in crisis" or whether it is on the contrary smoothly functioning and effective. In our opinion, available statistical data, data from quantitative research, and descriptive analysis as presented in the chapters that follow confirm that major problems confront the health care system: rising costs; financial and other barriers to care; geographic maldistribution of manpower and facilities; overspecialization of providers; overutilization of hospitals; deficiencies in quality and quality control; a tendency, particularly among physicians, to stress the unusual at the expense of the commonplace; barriers to provider-patient communication; training and educational programs and research undertakings that are not always directly relevant to patient needs; an emphasis on treatment rather than prevention; and an orientation toward patients with acute, physical problems at the expense of patients who are chronically ill or have mental problems.

However, few if any of these problems are new; over time they have simply undergone gradual changes in magnitude. Indeed, many of the major problems considered by the Committee on the Costs of Medical Care and still pressing today originated in our country and those of our European forebears in the 17th, 18th, and 19th centuries (Freymann, Sections I, II). Thus it is not quite accurate to say we face a "crisis" in health care. Our health care delivery system has serious problems with deep historical roots embedded in the whole fabric of American society. This fact should not be a cause for complacency, however. As modern medical practice itself illustrates, it is often easier to deal with a crisis, even a major one, than with long-standing, chronic problems. Nevertheless, with its enormous resources, its dedicated health manpower pool, and its talent for problem-solving, the United States should be equal to the task.

In this book we undertake the difficult task of describing our health care delivery system. The United States presents a particular problem in this regard: in most industrialized countries there is a Ministry of Health that plays a central role in financing and operations and that often provides a framework for the various components of the system. The Ministry may not directly operate the system, but at least it creates the structure within which the system functions. In the United States, however, no such central organizational structure exists. There is of course a system; there are loci of power and control; but they are difficult to recognize and to describe.

In order to delineate the shape of this rather amorphous system, we will deal with the major components of any health care delivery system: the people for whom it provides care; the people who provide the care; the institutions and organizational structures within which they work; the financing mechanisms that allow the first three components to interact; and the government under which the system functions.

What Is Health Care and Who Is Served?*

The United States has one of the largest populations in the world, over 220,000,000 in 1980. The population is aging: the proportion of persons 65 and over is more than 10%. Many ethnic and national groups are represented. There is a broad range of social classes and large income differentials exist. Nonwhite persons are represented in the lower social class and income groups in a proportion greater than their representation in the total population. Unemployment, or the threat of it, substandard housing, and dysnutrition are major socioeconomic problems in rural as well as urban areas.

The crude death rate in 1980 was under 9 per 1,000 population and the infant mortality rate was about 13 per 1,000 live births. The major causes of death are heart disease, cancer, stroke, and accidents. The major causes of morbidity are upper respiratory infections, influenza, injuries, heart conditions, hypertension, arthritis, impairments of the lower limbs, impairments of the back and spine, asthma and hay fever, and mild emotional disorders.

*The bulk of the data presented in the balance of this chapter comes from the *Statistical Abstract of the United States,* 100th Edition, Washington, D.C.: U.S. Department of Commerce, USGPO, 1979, and *Health United States, 1979,* Washington, D.C.: USDHEW Pub. No. PHS (80)–1232, USGPO, 1979.

In Chapter 2, "What Is Health Care?," we discuss what constitutes health, disease, and illness, and consider the efficacy and utility of the several types of health services. In Chapter 3, "Population Data for Health and Health Care," we present the principal quantitative measures used to describe the population, its health and illness levels, how it uses the health care system, and how the health care system functions. Thus the reader is introduced to the first and most important component of any health care delivery system, the people whom it serves.

Inputs to the System

About 7,000,000 people work in the health care delivery system. They may be divided into three major groups: independent practitioners, dependent practitioners, and supporting staff, although the lines between the groups are at times unclear. The largest manpower categories are the nurses, clerical staff, hospital manual workers, physicians, dentists, pharmacists, and technicians. The physicians, of whom over 400,000 are active, are the dominant group. Indeed, as shall be seen in later chapters, this dominance is guaranteed by law.

The principal mode of physician organization is private practice. Excluding hospital house staff in training, about 80% of all physicians in active practice are in private practice. This means that they are self-employed private entrepreneurs, adminstratively responsible to no one but themselves. Since physicians are in a controlling position in the delivery of care, this mode of physician organization is one of the major features of the U.S. health care delivery system.

Chapter 4, "Health Manpower," provides basic information on supply, types, distribution, and education of health workers. There is not space in a book of this type to give due consideration to all of the categories of health worker. However, Chapter 5, "Nursing," is entirely devoted to the single largest health care provider group; it discusses nursing roles and functions, current issues in nursing, and key aspects of the relationships between nurses and other categories of providers. It is an example of the kind of analysis that can be carried out for each and every health manpower type.

Since physicians are the dominant manpower group, they receive the most attention throughout the book. Aspects of their work are discussed in chapters that deal primarily with the institutional and financing sectors. More detail on the distribution and functions of physicians can be found in Chapter 6, "Ambulatory Care," and Chapter 7 "Hospitals." Certain special aspects of the work of health care personnel are presented in Chapter 9, "Mental Health Services." In Chapter 14, "Measurement and Control of the Quality of Medical Care," the licensing system is discussed, along with the various modes of regulation and quality control that pertain to all health care personnel.

Various types of institutions provide health care services. The most frequently used type of care is ambulatory—care provided to patients other than in institutional beds. About 80% of ambulatory care is delivered in private doctors' offices; other sites include hospital ambulatory services, group practices, neighborhood health centers, and health department health centers. The most common loci for ambulatory care are described in Chapter 6.

Of the institutions housing and caring for patients in bed, hospitals are the most numerous. In the United States, there are more than 7,000, with more than 1.5 million beds. They are categorized in a variety of ways: by ownership, size, function, and average length of stay. There are three principal types of ownership: government (federal, state, and local); private not-for-profit (voluntary); and private for-profit (proprietary). There are four functional categories for hospitals in the United States: general, tuberculosis, mental, and other special. The American Hospital Association also defines the "community hospital": a nonfederal short-term general or other special hospital. It is the predominant type in the United States. The basic descriptive material on hospitals is presented in Chapter 7. Nursing homes and other nonmental-condition long-term care institutions, of which there are over 20,000, plus other long-term care services are described in Chapter 8, "Long-Term Care." Mental hospitals are discussed in Chapter 9, "Mental Health Services"; other government hospitals are touched upon in Chapter 11, while certain aspects of regulation of hospitals are considered in Chapter 13, "Planning for Health Care," and Chapter 14, on quality control.

Institutions for education and research in the health sciences are also important. Issues in health sciences education are considered in Chapter 4, "Health Manpower"; Chapter 5, "Nursing"; and Chapter 14.

American medical practice is organized primarily along the lines of the private enterpreneurial model, as pointed out above. Medical care is mainly provided on the basis of a private, direct contract, usually unwritten, between physician and patient, even when the source of payment is not the patient. Since medical care—that is, the treatment of sick persons by physicians—is the focus of the United States health care delivery system, and since medical care is provided primarily on a private basis, the organizational framework of the health care system is rudimentary compared to that found in other countries. The care provided by health care institutions themselves is discussed in Chapters 6, 7, 8, 9 and 11.

Financing

In the fiscal year 1980, the United States spent over $240 billion, 9% of its Gross National Product, on health care services. Expenditures on health care surpass the total GNP of most other countries in the world.

Most of the time, health care costs rise more rapidly than most other categories of consumer spending in the United States. Ultimately, of course, all money paid for health services comes from the people. However, there are three major means by which money is transferred from the people to the providers: government (about 39% of total expenditures); insurance companies (about 28% of the total); and direct payment (about 33% of the total). Government expenditures are both for services that it operates directly and for services obtained by patients from independent providers, in which case government is a third-party payor. The two major factors in the insurance mode of financing are Blue Cross/Blue Shield (not-for-profit) and the commercial (for-profit) companies, which share almost equally over 90% of the premium flow.

The major recipients of funds are the hospitals (39%), physicians (18%), dentists (7%), nursing homes (8%), and the drug companies (8%). The vast majority of health care personnel are paid on salary, although the independent practitioners are usually paid on a fee-for-service basis. Institutions for the most part operate on a global budget or on a cost-reimbursement basis.

Chapter 10, "Financing Health Care," considers these matters in depth, while Chapter 15, on national health insurance (NHI), looks at the implication of NHI for health care financing and of the present system of financing for NHI.

Government, Policy-Making, Quality, and the Future

Although the government operates no piece of the health care system in its entirety by itself, it is closely involved in one way or another in all of them: collecting and disseminating information, training personnel, operating institutions, providing services, participating in financing, supporting and carrying out research, planning, evaluating, and regulating. Some aspects of government activities in health care delivery are covered in the chapters on personnel, institutions, and financing. In Chapters 11 through 14, we look at some of the various functions of government not considered in earlier chapters.

In Chapter 11, we describe the major government activities in the delivery of personal health and medical services. Chapter 12 describes the process by which health and health care policies and legislation are developed in the United States Congress, as an example of the role of legislatures in the health care delivery system.

We then proceed to examine several important functions of the health care system in which government plays a critical, although not exclusive role: planning and quality control. Chapter 13 considers the health care planning process and major pieces of federal legislation that have appeared over time. Chapter 14 discusses the problems of quality assessment and regulation.

National health insurance by its very name means government participation at one or more jurisdictional levels throughout the country in the health care financing system. Chapter 15 first traces the history of proposals for NHI in the United States, then examines the major policy issues in and proposals for NHI in the early 1980s. Finally, it considers the relationship between NHI and health, and the prospects for passage of NHI legislation.

In the course of our book we describe some suggestions for change but do not propose a single plan for reform (or for revolution). We hope that after assimilating the facts as we see them and present them, the reader will be able to develop his or her own conclusions about what is to be done.

References

American Medical News. "AMA Hits Federal NHI Plans." November 17, 1975, p. 1.

American Medical News. "The Case for American Medicine. Chapter II: What Health Crisis? From the New Book by Harry Schwartz." October 16, 1972, Section 2, p. 1.

Battistella, R., and Southby, R. McK. "Crisis in American Medicine." *The Lancet*, March 16, 1968, p. 581.

Business Week. "The $60-Billion Crisis over Medical Care." January 17, 1970, Special Reprint.

Citizens Board of Inquiry into Health Services for Americans. Report. *Heal Yourself.* Washington, D.C., 1971.

Committee on the Costs of Medical Care. *Medical Care for the American People.* Chicago: University of Chicago Press, 1932. Reprinted, Washington, D.C.: USDHEW, 1970.

Dellums, R. "The Health Service Act: H.R.2969." *Congressional Record*, Vol. 125, No. 33, March 19, 1979.

Ehrenreich, B., and Ehrenreich, J. *The American Health Empire: Power, Profits, and Politics.* New York: Vintage Books, 1971.

Fortune (Eds). *Our Ailing Medical System: It's Time to Operate.* New York: Harper and Row Perennial Library, 1970.

Freymann, J. G. *The American Health Care System: Its Genesis and Trajectory.* New York: Medcom Press, 1974.

Harper's Magazine. "The Crisis in American Medicine." October 1960, p. 123.

Health Task Force of the Urban Coalition. Report. *Rx for Action.* Washington, D.C., 1969.

Jonas, S. *Medical Mystery: The Training of Doctors in the United States*. New York: W. W. Norton, 1979.

Kennedy, E. M. *In Critical Condition*. New York: Simon and Schuster, 1972.

Klaw, S. *The Great American Medicine Show*. New York: Viking, 1975.

Knowles, J. H., Ed. *Doing Better and Feeling Worse*. New York: W. W. Norton, 1977.

"Month in Washington," *New York State Journal of Medicine*, December 1978, p. 2277.

Moskin, J. R. "The Challenge to Our Doctors." *Look,* November 3, 1964, p. 26.

National Commission on Community Health Services. *Health Is a Community Affair*. Cambridge, Massachusetts: Harvard University Press, 1966.

Research and Policy Committee. *Building a National Health-Care System*. New York: Committee for Economic Development, 1973.

Ribicoff, A., with Danaceau, P. *The American Medical Machine*. New York: Saturday Review Press, 1972.

Richardson, E. L. "Health Care Crisis in America, 1971." Testimony before the Subcommittee on Health of the Committee on Labor and Public Welfare, U.S. Senate, February 22–23, 1971. Part 1, p. 72.

Roemer, M. Review Article. "The American Health Empire: Power, Profits, and Politics." *International Journal of Health Services*, 2, 119, 1972.

Schorr, D. *Don't Get Sick in America*. Nashville, Tenn.: Aurora Publishers, 1970.

Schwartz, H. *The Case for American Medicine: A Realistic Look at Our Health Care System*. New York: David McKay, 1972.

Schwartz, H. "Wherein Conventional Wisdom Is Asked, What Health-Care Crisis?" *The New York Times*, Sept. 11, 1979.

Sidel, V. W., and Sidel, R. *A Healthy State*. New York: Pantheon Books, 1977.

Silver, G. A. *A Spy in the House of Medicine*, Germantown, Maryland: Aspen Systems Corporation, 1976.

Somers, A. R., and Somers, H. M. *Health and Health Care*, Germantown, Maryland: Aspen Systems Corporation, 1977.

Stolfi, J. E. "The Invisible Medical Crisis." *New York State Journal of Medicine*, July 1978, p. 1216.

2

What Is Health Care?

David Banta

Introduction

It is a truism that the purpose of health care is to promote health. Yet most observers of the health care system would agree that it deals with disease, not with health. The education of health professionals, physicians in particular, focuses on pathology (Jonas; Millis), and medical practice is almost exclusively concerned with treatment of disease.

This chapter will present the case for a broader conception of health. It is doubtless easier to care for disease than to promote good health; moreover, such activities as health education lack the drama associated with the technology of university hospitals. One must also recognize the staggering limitations of knowledge in the psychological and social spheres. Yet the fact remains that if medical care providers do not begin to grapple with these uncertainties of their own accord, an ever more active consumer movement will surely demand action from them (Freymann, pp. 10, 328).

This chapter will also point out some of the limitations of contemporary medical knowledge. Since not all diseases can be prevented or cured, there is a clear implication that the caring function must be a vital part of medical practice. There is also some evidence that caring itself may be an effective method of therapy, both alone and in conjunction with effective curative medicine (Frank; Haggerty; Mechanic, pp. 129–130).

Finally, the chapter will attempt a modest look into the future. Medicine and health have always had a social definition: as society changes, its state of health and its view of what constitutes health change concomitantly. According to Dubos (1971), there is a "mirage of health" that constantly recedes into the future: the specific disease profile of a society may change, but disease itself remains.

What Are "Health" and "Disease"?

Health, disease, and illness are terms we use every day without thinking about precise definitions. It is easy to think of health as being the lack of disease, or of illness and disease as being interchangeable terms. In fact, health and disease are not simply opposites, and disease and illness do not mean precisely the same thing.

There is a philosophical distinction between the concepts of health and disease that goes back to antiquity. As Henry Sigerist (p. 57) points out: "The [ancient Greek] physicians had an explanation for health. Health, they believed, was a condition of perfect equilibrium. When the forces or humors or whatever constituted the human body were perfectly balanced, man was healthy. Disturbed balance resulted in disease. This is still the best general explanation we have." However, the cult of Asklepios concentrated on disease and miracle cures, and, with the rise of Christianity, the idea of disease was given a preferential place. The Greek ideal of health as a perfect balance had little meaning to the masses of that day, living as they did in poverty, sickness, and oppression. Later, scientific medicine began to develop, but the idea of miracle cures persisted, as it does in present-day medicine. It is a seductive dream: a cure that can compensate for the abuses the individual and society have perpetuated, correcting at a stroke the effects of smoking or of breathing polluted air or of eating saturated fats over a period of years.

Webster's Unabridged Dictionary reflects the conflict, defining health as "physical and mental well-being," but continuing, "freedom from defect, pain, or disease." Health statistics, of course, are actually disease statistics, and health care is often disease care. Jago (1975) lists 43 usages of "health" as an adjective, most of which add to the confusion. Examples include "health status," "health center," and "health worker."

The World Health Organization (p. 29) defines health as a "state of complete physical, mental, and social well-being, and not merely the absence of disease or infirmity." This definition has been criticized as being utopian (Dubos). To deal with this problem, Terris (1975) proposed a modification of the WHO definition: "Health is a state of physical, mental, and social well-being and ability to function, and not merely the absence of illness or infirmity." This definition, removing "complete," and adding "ability to function," has balance, positivism, and realism.

Disease is also frequently defined rather ambiguously. *Webster's* suggests "uneasiness or distress," and, more sweepingly, "any departure from health." Blakiston's *New Gould Medical Dictionary* terms disease "a failure of the adaptive mechanisms of an organism to counteract adequately the stimuli and stresses to which it is subject, resulting in a disturbance in function or structure of any part, organ, or system of the body."

Illness is another matter. While disease is a biomedical concept, illness is a state of being. As Cassell (p. 48) said: "Disease, then, is something an organ has; illness is something a man has." Illness has social and psychological as well as biomedical components. One can have a disease without feeling ill, as in asymptomatic hypertension. And one can surely be ill without being diseased.

More recent definitions of health have stressed life functioning, seeing health as the "state of optimum capacity for effective performance of valued tasks" (Parsons, 1958, p. 168) or as "personal fitness for survival and self-renewal, creative social adjustment, and self-fulfillment. The most exacting test of one's health is to stay alive and to retain the capacity for self-repair and self-renewal" (Hoyman, p. 189). This trend underlies the growing development of health status indices (Mushkin and Dunlop; Kaplan, Bush, and Berry). Although the early health status indices focused on mortality and morbidity, Bush and Fanshel have developed a promising functional index. Such an index becomes particularly important as government funding of health care increases. Cost-consciousness, along with an emphasis on evaluation, has developed because of the need to justify the expenditures of tax monies. If health is the ultimate goal of health services, then evaluation of health care activities is dependent on valid and reliable indicators of health.

Biological Factors in Health

Health is generally conceived of as a biological state. It is obviously dependent upon biological factors. Genetic endowment of the individual is the starting point, but health is to a large extent the result of the complex interaction of this soma with the environment (Burnett). The environment includes physical surroundings, social factors (largely beyond the control of the individual), and personal life-style.

The environment is a crucial determinant of health. In 1857 the tuberculosis death rate in Massachusetts was 450 per 100,000; by 1890, the figure had fallen to 250; by 1920 to 114; and by 1938 to 35.6 (Sigerist, p. 46) Yet the first specific antituberculosis therapy was not in general use until after 1938—convincing evidence that the prevalence of a disease can decline dramatically without effective medical care, probably owing to environmental factors.

An analysis of falling death rates and rising populations in England and Wales since 1841 has shown that changes considerably preceded any direct medical intervention. Death rates in England and Wales fell from about 22 per 1,000 in 1841 to around 6 per 1,000 in 1971. McKeown (1976, pp.

93–94) concludes that 92% of the fall between 1848 and 1901 and 73% from 1901 to 1971 is due to a reduction in the number of deaths from infectious diseases. Most of this reduction is due to a falling number of deaths from tuberculosis. Death rates due to respiratory tuberculosis fell steadily beginning in 1838, although chemotherapy for tuberculosis did not begin until 1948. However, after 1948, the rate of fall in the death rate did increase, indicating an effect of chemotherapy. McKeown also examined bronchitis, pneumonia, and influenza, after tuberculosis the greatest causes of mortality in the infectious disease era. The death rate for these conditions has been little affected by the introduction of antibiotics. McKeown concludes that improvement in nutrition was the most important influence in the fall in death rates. He estimates that hygienic measures, such as improvement in water supplies and sewage disposal, were responsible for about a fifth of the reduction. McKeown feels that: "With the exception of vaccination against smallpox, whose contribution was small, the influence of immunization and therapy on the death-rate was delayed until the twentieth century, and had little effect on national mortality trends before the introduction of sulphonamides in 1935. Since that time it has not been the only, or probably the most important influence" (McKeown, 1976, p. 94).

Diseases caused by microorganisms have been the scourge of man throughout recorded history and have been the largest biological determinant of death and disability. Now, although infectious diseases persist, they are of limited importance for most of the population of the United States. Figure 2.1 shows different categories of disease along with their impact on death, hospital admissions, and activity. Diseases of the circulatory system account for more than 50% of the deaths in the United States annually. But the most important cause of limitation of activity is apparently disease of the musculoskeletal system, including arthritis. Overall, chronic diseases have become the most prevalent and troublesome.

Chronic diseases are largely dependent on biological factors as well, although no specific etiology such as a microorganism can be identified for most such conditions (Burnett, pp. 2–3; Lalonde). The importance of genetic factors to the basic biological makeup of the individual is being recognized, and it is becoming increasingly apparent that congenital causes of sickness, disability, and death have been relatively unresponsive to changes in environment and in medical care. But the role of environmental factors is receiving the greatest attention. We now know beyond question that diet, air and water pollution, occupational hazards, and cigarette smoking are critical in the genesis of chronic disease. For example, epidemiological studies indicate that up to 90% of cancers may be related to environmental factors, including smoking and nutrition (Schneiderman; Higginson).

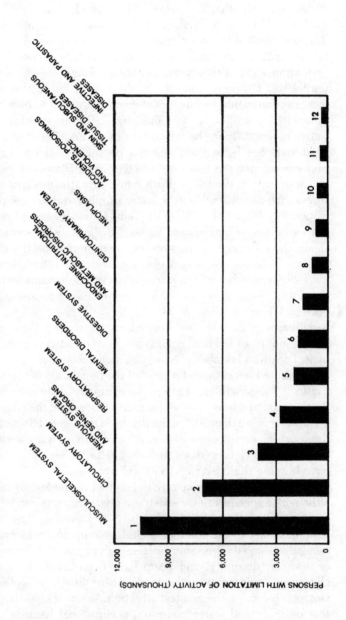

Figure 2.1 Disease categories: their impact on activity, hospital admissions, and death. (*Source:* K. White, "Life and Death in Medicine," *Scientific American, 229,* 23, 1973. Used with permission.)

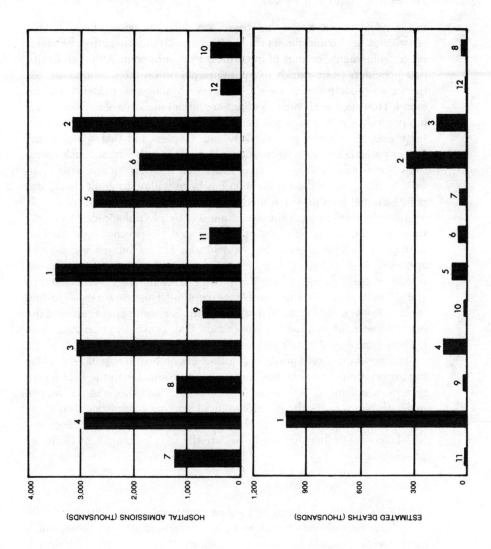

The essential point is that the interaction between genetic factors and the environment in producing individual disease is enormously complex (Cairns) and much research is needed to elucidate the relationship.

Perceptual Factors in Health

It is crucial to recognize that there are different perceptions of what constitutes health and illness (R. White). The stimuli that affect behavior range from vague feelings of uneasiness to severe pain. Although health care providers react quickly to a patient's pain, they often tend to dismiss the vague anxieties of careseekers unless physiological evidence can be found. However, such vague feelings are often indicative of real disease: it has been shown that such self-perceptions and symptoms predicted mortality over an 11-year period (Daly and Tyroler) and that symptomatic cancer patients do much worse than matched controls without such symptoms (Feinstein). This seems to indicate that self-perceptions have more validity than the medical profession has been willing to grant them, and points up one area in which medical practice is still ignorant.

An individual's perception is influenced by physiologic determinants such as chemical imbalances or hunger and by psychological factors. Perception is also affected by sociocultural factors influencing beliefs, attitudes, and values. Other cultures have conceptions of health and disease entirely different from those of the United States (Mechanic, pp. 129–130). And even in this country, perception of disease varies according to class (Koos; Kunitz et al.) and ethnic group. A classic paper examined the meaning of pain in Jews, Italians, and "Old Yankees" in an American hospital, and found rather remarkable differences (Zaborowski).

An important part of perceptual influences on health in today's world is the expectation the public has in coming into contact with the health care system. Medicine is overvalued by the public, and this is at the root of many problems facing the health care field, such as malpractice. It is likely that "right living" (Breslow, 1972, 1975; Belloc and Breslow; Belloc) and social changes, rather than medicine, are the keys to achieving a healthier population.

Social Factors in Health

Health has previously been defined in functional terms. Disease can be considered to be dysfunctional. Sickness can be seen as a social role, which carries with it certain rights and obligations (Parsons, 1951). Sick people are exempted from normal social obligations and are not considered responsible for their own state. Even when they have brought an illness upon themselves—as in a careless accident or lung cancer caused by cigarette smoking—they are not assumed to be responsible for the process of getting well. With increasing cost-consciousness in the health care sector, one hears more and more that people who have brought disease on themselves should somehow pay a higher price. A smoker might pay a higher health insurance premium, for example, or even be denied coverage under a national health insurance program. This proposal seems to be dangerous and inhumane. First, knowledge is not perfect enough to enable us to make such clear-cut causal determinations. And second, the logical extreme of this position is to deny care to those responsible for their own disease state unless they can pay for it; such a policy would lead to a class-bound system of health care perhaps even more pernicious than the one we have now.

The sick role also entails responsibilities. The sick person is expected to cooperate in his treatment and to return to normal functioning as soon as possible (Parsons, 1951). The physician shares society's disdain for hypochondriacs, who are felt to be using illness symptoms to gain special status.

The role of value systems and social structures is evident, as the example of other countries helps to make clear. People in developing countries may suffer from malaria or schistosomiasis without assuming the sick role or considering themselves sick (Susser). Every physician is familiar with patients who function well despite organic disease that should be incapacitating. A renowned physician described his long-standing competition with a famous faith-healer, some of whose patients go back to a functional status despite quite severe disease (Stead). The physician or other health care provider can also assume this healer's role of encouraging independence. In short, health is a relative, not an absolute, concept.

Society has increasingly viewed the medical profession as acting at the organic level in curing and preventing disease. But medicine must also function at the psychological level, giving reassurance to those who seek help, and at the social level, legitimizing the sick role. Further, society's categorization of health and disease changes over time. Within recent memory, social problems such as suicide and attempted suicide and drug addiction have been redefined, and are now considered to be illnesses (Mechanic, pp. 192–194). This broader conception of ill health carries dangers (Szasz; Illich) : for example, psychiatrists play an increasing role in the courts, where a person may be considered to be insane and locked up indefinitely. Psychiatry seems particularly prone to abuse in such ways (Mechanic, pp. 192–194).

Personal and Community Health Services

Given our broad definition of health, we may examine health services in a broad context as well. Health services have been defined as those services delivered by personnel engaged in medical occupations, such as physicians and nurses, plus other personnel working under their supervision; the physical capital involved, such as hospitals; and the other goods and services, such as drugs and bandages (Fuchs, 1966). Weinerman (1971) defines the health services system as "all of the activities of a society which are designed to protect or restore health, whether directed to the individual, the community, or the environment."

A critical distinction must be made between health care and medical care. Medical care is generally thought of as that care provided by a physician. It is generally restricted in scope, focusing on pathophysiological and social problems, and contains a strong element of "caring."

Health and health care services may generally be divided into two broad categories: personal and community (Jonas, p. 37). Personal health care services, familiar to everyone, deal directly with individuals for the maintenance of health or the control or cure of illness. Community health services are directed toward groups, not discrete individuals. The public today takes pure drinking water and sewage disposal for granted, but pure water has probably had a greater impact on health than any factor except nutrition. Other community health services include solid waste disposal; food, milk, and drug control and inspection; fluoridation of water; and control of air and noise pollution.

A number of health services—which we call "combined" services—have aspects of both community and personal health services. Mass immunization programs, by protecting each immunized indiviudal, protect the community as a whole. "Herd immunity" prevents epidemics. This is especially true of diseases caused by obligatory human parasites, like the now-eradicated smallpox virus. Other such combined community and individual services include tuberculosis and venereal disease case-finding and treatment programs, which gradually reduce the total number of sources of infection to healthy persons, and thus contribute to community health.

A definition of health care must take into account its boundaries and its providers. If health is to have a functional definition, stressing the positive, health care must in some way affect outcomes, by having an active role in improving or assisting in social functioning. Rudolph Virchow, the great German pathologist, fought on the barricades against Bismarck's government as a youth, and described his profession with these well-known words: "Medicine is a social science and politics is nothing else but medicine on a large scale" (Sigerist, p. 93). Should the physician be a revolutionary? Drs. Che Guevara and Salvador Allende thought so, but most physicians have seen their main task as helping people with their immediate ills. Yet in a day when cancer is the second greatest cause of death in the United States, and 40% of cancer could probably be controlled by changing the environment (Lilienfeld), can the physician stand by, merely providing personal care and ignoring a workplace exposing his patients to carcinogens, or a refinery whose fumes may be causing cancer? There is no easy answer to such a question.

There is also the danger, alluded to in the previous section, of defining health care too broadly, so as to encompass all areas of life. The patient generally initiates contact, seeking skilled assistance, and must be assumed to be in control of his overall life. But increasingly medicine is fostering a dependency role (Mechanic, pp. 15, 169), a situation made more acute in an era of chronic disease, where patients need care at frequent intervals for a period of years. Illich is particularly concerned about the social iatrogenesis that develops, with an individual losing control over his own life. The public has already lost sight of the fact that its own health behavior has far more impact on its health than medical care. There is also a risk in the tendency to broaden the definition of mental illness, thus taking away an individual's autonomy and personhood by calling him or her "sick" (Szasz). Health care could become a tyranny. For this reason, a somewhat limited definition seems more desirable.

The question of who provides health care is closely related to its definition. There are more than 12 health workers for every physician in the United States, yet when most people think of health care, they think of physicians. If health care is to live up to a dynamic definition, the contributions of such providers as social workers and medical administrators will need to be recognized by both the public and the health workers themselves. Physicians have perhaps been slowest to acknowledge these contributions; yet they too are beginning to be aware of the importance of teamwork in health care, and of the need for special efforts to foster such teamwork (Banta and Fox). At least one project is under way to train health care providers to be effective team members (Wise et al.).

Health Care as a Right

As early as 1787, Thomas Jefferson said: "Without health there is no happiness. And attention to health, then, should take the place of every other object. The time necessary to secure this by active exercises should be devoted to it in preference to every other pursuit. I know the difficulty with which a strenuous man tears himself from his studies at any given moment of the day; but his happiness, and that of his family depend on it. The most uninformed mind, with a healthy body is happier than the wisest valetudinarian" (Foley, p. 402). With the growing affluence of the United States, this seems to be an idea whose time has come. Although high-quality health care is certainly not available at present to the entire population, it is generally accepted that this country is in the process of different from "health as a right." Health is first and foremost the concern of the individual: he can strive for it, but the health care system cannot provide it. However, health *care* for all is a realizable goal.

The United States has been slow, however, to take the necessary steps. Up to the time of the enactment of Medicare in 1965, no unit of government had taken general responsibility for aiding nonindigent individuals when they were ill (R. White). The roots of this inattention can be found in the American ethic of freedom and equality. Harlow (R. White, p. 56) says it well: "There has been a stubborn insistence on protecting the individual's freedom by making him responsible for his own tragedy."

A significant percentage of people in the United States can be said to have a right to health care already. More than 150 million people have work-related health insurance, including more than 5 million enrolled in prepaid comprehensive group practices (Banta and Bosch). Of course, a time of high unemployment points out the fallacy of using this mechanism to assure access to health care. In addition, in 1976 about 20 million elderly people had a right to care under the Medicare program, and about 12 million poor people had such a right through Medicaid. However, the Congressional Budget Office estimated that in 1976 there were 21.5 million people with no health insurance of any kind (Bureau of the Census, Table No. 154). Even those who have chosen not to buy health insurance must be covered by a compulsory program. In a just and humane society, one does not turn a sick person away from a hospital for lack of health insurance.

Many who endorse the concept of health care for everyone are unsure how to put it into effect. Dr. Hanlin's prescription, "The best care—to everybody—now" (R. White, p. 66) is appealing, but "best care" is difficult to define. It is simply not feasible to make available everything any individual could want at all times. Likewise, health care providers cannot have everything they want to do a good job. Limits must be set to avoid falling into the "bottomless pit" of medical expenditure (Fuchs, 1974).

The Value We Place on Health

It is commonly felt among health professionals that all possible services should be provided by a health system. But are people willing to support health services to that extent? Health is certainly an important value, but it is not the only value. Achilles recognized this in the *Iliad*: "Either, if I stay here and fight beside the city of the Trojans, my return home is gone, but my glory shall be everlasting; but if I return home to the beloved land of my fathers, the excellence of my glory is gone, but there will be a long life left for me, and my end in death will not come to me quickly" (Homer, p. 209). Achilles chose to stay and die. The modern analogue might be the skydiver or skier who intentionally takes a risk for the sake of the thrill he derives from the sport. To the extent that the public is aware of risk factors, one could say that the person who smokes cigarettes, eats saturated fats, or refuses to wear seat belts is deciding that other values are more important than good health.

Society can invest more in justice, beauty, or knowledge, just as it invests in health (Fuchs, 1974). The yearly federal budget is to a large extent a reflection of the values and choices of society and its leaders. The aggregated requests of the health programs in the Department of Health and Human Services would far exceed the approximately $50 billion budget allocated for those health programs in 1979. Health economists deal with this problem of limited resources by speaking of marginal benefit and marginal cost. Is the added benefit—of a day in the hospital, for example— worth the added cost?

Every practicing physician confronts conflicting values every day in practice. A person may be fully knowledgeable about the risks of smoking but continue to smoke. Overeating, drinking alcohol, or not exercising are other examples of behavior with profound health implications which may be impossible to alter because the values of a person make that behavior more important than theoretical future health consequences. Such problems can only be dealt with by active intervention in matters which the society generally considers personal.

However, this society already intervenes rather aggressively in human behavior, particularly through the economic system. Navarro (1975) criticizes the recent emphasis on individual behavior as a way of avoiding the more important questions of the changes needed in society as a whole. As he says ". . . a far better strategy than self-care, and changes in life-style to improve the health of the individual would be to change the economic and social structure that . . . conditioned and determined that unhealthy individual behavior to start with." His example of an unhealthy diet is a convincing one. Specific corporate interests have economic needs to determine consumption and stimulate certain kinds of production. Navarro cites the well-known nutritionist, Dr. Jean Mayer, who maintains that the food conglomerates have a primary responsibility for the poor diet of United States citizens. One can readily recall seductive advertisements for snack food and fast-food restaurants, as well as the difficulty one sometimes faces in trying to find tasty fresh vegetables.

It may also not be necessary to intervene actively in affecting values and behavior in all cases. It has been pointed out that changing the definition of the "prime" designation for beef would have great potential benefits to health, because the marbling that allows the "prime" rating is made up of saturated fat. The National Institutes of Health is trying to produce a safe cigarette that preserves good taste—already the amount of tar and nicotine in the average cigarette has been reduced approximately 25% over the past 20 years. Air bags to replace seat belts is another example of engineering protection against risk factors. Some object that these regulations infringe on personal freedom, but society can no longer afford to be so passive in the face of mounting evidence of risk factors that could in many cases be controlled. Society has already determined that some interventions are necessary to protect the public, as when it made vaccination against smallpox compulsory, over the objections of a vocal minority.

Clearly, both personal and governmental action are needed. The society needs a health policy similar to that being developed in Canada, which will deal with four elements seen to affect health: human biology, environment, life-style, and health care organization (Lalonde). Sigerist said:

> . . . The people's health is the concern of the people themselves. They must be enlightened in matters of health. They must want it and take an active part in its administration. And since the protection of health is a task of great magnitude, the people will endeavor to fulfill it collectively through the state and its organs. That is why health is a primary concern of the people *and* of government. (p. 102)

The Efficacy of Health Care

There have been some remarkable improvements in health levels in the United States since 1900. The purpose of this section is to analyze the contribution of health and medical care to those improvements. Such measures as life expectancy and infant mortality rates are useful in understanding the reason for these improvements. Unfortunately, readily available statistics are all related to mortality, whereas data on morbidity are difficult to obtain and verify. Furthermore, there are not as yet any generally accepted direct measures of health itself. Thus, for long-term historical analysis of health levels, we are forced to rely upon mortality data.

Between 1900 and 1976 in the United States, the crude and infant mortality rates fell, while the life expectancy from birth rose (Table 2.1). However, while crude mortality declined almost 50% during that period, the infant mortality rate declined by about 86%. In fact, the major portion of the decline in the crude mortality rate is due to the remarkable drop in mortality that occurred generally in the younger age groups in the population. Table 2.2 shows the 1970 age-specific mortality rates as percentages of the 1900 age-specific mortality rates. The death rate for the 1 to 4-year-old age group in 1970 was only 4% of the rate in 1900, while for people over age 65 in 1970 it was still almost two-thirds of the 1900 rate. Note too the large gap in percentage improvement between the 15–35 age group and the 45–65 age group.

This evidence is corroborated if one looks at mortality data in yet another way. Table 2.3 shows the average number of years of life remaining at specific ages in 1900 and in 1970 and the percentage change in life expectancy at specified ages between those two years. The percentage

Table 2.1

Mortality Rate, Infant Mortality Rate, and Life Expectancy from Birth, U.S., 1900–1970

	Crude Mortality Rate (per 1,000 pop.)	Infant Mortality Rate per 1,000 Live Births[a]	Life Expectancy from Birth (in years)
1900	17.2	(99.9)	47.3
1920	13.0	85.9	54.1
1940	10.8	47.0	62.9
1960	9.5	26.0	69.7
1970	9.5	20.0	70.9
1977	8.8	14.1	73.2

Source: Data for 1900–1960 derived from R. D. Grove and A. M. Hetzel, *Vital Statistics Rates in the United States, 1940–1960* (National Center for Health Statistics, U.S. Dept. of Health, Education and Welfare, 1968), Tables 38, 51, and 53. Data for 1970 and 1977 are from *Health United States* (National Center for Health Statistics and National Center for Health Services Research), Tables 8, 9, and 10. (See Appendix I, A9.)
[a]Data available only from 1915.

Table 2.2

Age-Specific Mortality Rates, U.S., 1900 and 1970

Age Group (years)	Age-Specific Mortality Rate (per 1,000 pop.)		1970 Rate as % of 1900 Rate
	1900	1970	
1–4	19.8	0.8	4.0
5–14	3.9	0.4	10.3
15–24	5.9	1.3	22.0
25–34	8.2	1.6	19.5
35–44	10.2	3.1	30.4
45–54	15.0	7.3	48.7
55–64	27.2	16.6	61.0
65–74	56.4	35.8	63.5
75–84	123.3	80.0	64.9
85 and over	260.9	163.4	62.6

Source: Statistical Abstract of the United States, 1974 (Bureau of the Census, U.S. Dept. of Commerce, 1974), Table 83. (See Appendix I, A1.)

increase in life expectancy is a large one. Further, in 1976, one could
expect to live 23.6 years longer from birth than one could in 1900. However, upon reaching age 65, one could expect to live only 4.1 years longer
than one could have in 1900. Tables 2.2 and 2.3 thus indicate that the most
important factor in the fall in the crude mortality rate and the rise in life
expectancy from birth is the decrease in the infant mortality rate. If many
more individuals survive the first year of life to then live into their sixties or
seventies, the overall life expectancy of any one group of such fortunate
infants is going to rise.

Figure 2.2 indicates how the important causes of death changed between 1900 and 1974. In 1900, the ten leading causes of death included
influenza and pneumonia, tuberculosis, and gastritis. Although some of
these are still in the top ten causes of death, their relative importance has
changed. Diseases of the heart and blood vessels now account for more
than half of all deaths, whereas they accounted for less than 20% in 1900.
Diseases of early infancy remain in the top ten, but are much less important
as a contributor to the overall death rate.

Since the improved life expectancy in 1976 results primarily from the
change in infant and child mortality, it is worthwhile to look specifically at
that group of illnesses. The major killers of infants and young children early
in the century were the major infectious diseases, including infantile
diarrhea, tuberculosis, typhoid fever, measles, diphtheria, and influenza
and pneumonia. Most of the decline in infant mortality has resulted from
the decline in infectious diseases. Some diseases were probably affected
most by nutrition, as in the case of tuberculosis. Others, such as infantile

Table 2.3

**Average Remaining Lifetime in Years at Specified Ages, U.S., 1900 and
1976, and Percent Change between 1900 and 1976**

Age in Years	Life Expectancy		Years	
	1900	1976	Difference	% Change
0	49.2	72.8	23.6	48.0
5	55.0	69.1	14.1	25.6
15	46.8	59.3	12.5	26.7
25	39.1	50.0	10.9	27.9
35	31.9	40.6	8.7	27.3
45	24.8	31.5	6.7	27.0
55	17.9	23.2	5.3	29.6
65	11.9	16.0	4.1	34.5
75	7.1	10.1	3.0	42.3
85	4.0	6.1	2.1	52.5

Source: Statistical Abstract of the United States, 1971, 1974, and 1978 (Bureau of the
Census, U.S. Dept. of Commerce, 1971 and 1974, and 1978).
(See Appendix I, A1.; see p. 70 in 1978 edition.)

Figure 2.2   Percent of all deaths, by specific causes of death,* U. S. 1900 and 1974. *Sources:* For 1900: U. S. National Office of Vital Statistics. *Vital Statistics of the United States, 1950, Vol. 1,* Washington, D.C., 1950, Table 2.26, p. 170; the 1900 data are from death registration states only. For 1974: U.S. Dept. of HEW. Public Health Service, National Center for Health Statistics. *Monthly Vital Statistics Report,* Vol. 23, No. 13, May 1975, Table C. p. 3. (See Appendix I, A4)

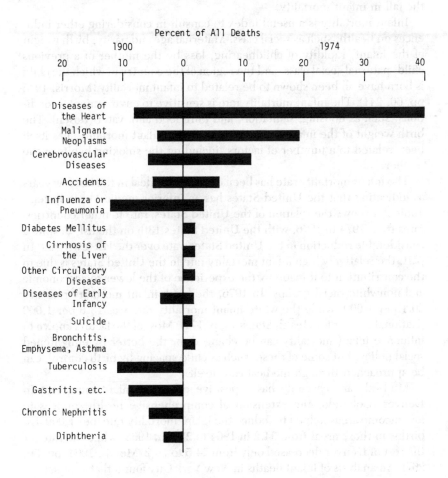

diarrhea and typhoid fever, were probably more affected by environmental sanitation. Diphtheria was on the decline prior to the development of a vaccine, but the vaccine probably contributed greatly to the near disappearence of the disease. Finally, pneumonia was probably affected by improved environment. As mentioned earlier, McKeown was unable to demonstrate an effect of the introduction of antibiotics. Thus, personal health services do not appear to have made an important contribution to the fall in infant mortality.

Infant mortality is a useful index to consult in considering other influences on health, such as social class. Maternal age and parity, birth weight of the infant, rapidity of childbearing, loss by the mother of a previous child, paternal social class, and the region of the country in which the child is born have all been shown to be related to infant mortality (Morris, 1975 pp. 60, 241). The infant mortality rate is sensitive to environmental conditions, such as housing, sanitation, and pure food and water (Rosen). The birth weight of the infant, one of the factors in infant mortality, has itself been related to a number of factors, including the smoking habits of the mother.

The infant mortality rate has been cited a great deal in the last few years as indicating that the United States has an inferior medical care system. Table 2.4 shows the relation of the United States' rate to other countries' rates from 1974 to 1976, with the United States 13th on the list, despite a considerable reduction in the United States' rate over the last few years. In part, the relatively high infant mortality rate in the United States is due to the contribution to it made by the experience of the lower socioeconomic and nonwhite racial groups. In 1976, the black infant mortality rate was 30.1 per 1,000, while the white infant mortality rate was 13.6 per 1,000 (National Center for Health Statistics, p. 171). Most of the factors known to influence infant mortality can be changed for the better by enlightened social policy, but some of these, such as child spacing by birth control, can be approached through medical care itself.

Medical care certainly has a positive effect on infant mortality. In Denver, Colorado, the extension of comprehensive health services to low-income areas helped to reduce the infant mortality rate (per 1,000 live births) in those areas from 34.2 in 1964 to 23.5 in 1968, while the rate for the rest of Denver decreased only from 24.5 to 19.2 (Morris, 1964, pp. 56, 267). An analysis of infant deaths in New York City found that adequacy of care was strongly associated with infant birth weight and survival, and estimated that adequate health services could reduce the overall 1968 rate of 21.9 per 1,000 live births as much as 33% to 14.7 per 1,000 (Kessner et al.).

However, the value or efficacy of health care in general has come under increasing scrutiny (Office of Technology Assessment). The rapidly rising costs of medical care have fostered a climate of questioning the value of the care provided, and such critics as McKeown and Illich have been widely quoted. It has been estimated that only 10% to 20% of procedures employed by health professionals have objective, controlled clinical trials to support the view that they will be helpful (K. White). Clinical physicians will counter the evidence with "clinical experience," but in a scientific age that is not sufficient. Physicians have unconscious reasons for wishing therapy to succeed, and each sees a limited spectrum of the population and its problems (Mechanic, p. 11). The practitioner is unable to avoid bias or to compare therapies to a control, and these are essential aspects of a controlled clinical trial. Perhaps the greatest problem overall is the dearth of scientific evidence on efficacy and safety (Office of Technology Assessment).

The technology most questioned is what Thomas (1975) has called "half-way technology"—technologies that deal with the symptoms of a condition without affecting the underlying disease process. These technologies, such as renal dialysis, respirators, and cardiac monitors and pacemakers, have come to dominate modern medicine. A mechanical orientation, traced by McKeown to Descartes, has developed. As

Table 2.4

Infant Mortality Rates,* Selected Countries, 1974–1976

Rank	Country	Rate
1	Sweden (1976)	8.3
2	Japan (1976)	9.3
3	Denmark (1976)	10.3
4	Netherlands (1975)	10.6
5	Switzerland (1976)	10.7
6	Finland (1974)	11.0
7	Norway (1975)	11.1
8	England and Wales (1976)	14.2
9	France (1974)	14.7
10	Scotland (1976)	14.8
11	Hong Kong (1975)	14.9
12	Canada (1974)	15.0
13	United States (1976)	15.2
14	German Democratic Republic (1975)	15.9
15	Belgium (1975)	16.2
16	Ireland (1974)	17.8
17	Austria (1976)	18.2
18	Spain (1975)	18.9
19	German Federal Republic (1975)	19.7
20	Czechoslovakia (1975)	20.9

Source: National Center for Health Statistics, Department of Health, Education and Welfare, 1979. (See also *Statistical Abstract,* section on "Comparative International Statistics," Appendix I, A1.)
*Rate represents deaths under one year of age per 1,000 live births.

Freymann (p. 172) says: "Cartesian mechanism and dualism encourage the naive faith that because the universe is composed of elemental particles, the total explanation of its complex systems can be found in information derived from these particles. There are many examples of this faith in medical literature." The resources of the physical and chemical sciences have intensified this "engineering" approach during this century. Although perhaps 40% of cancers could be prevented based on what is now known about them (Lilienfeld), our society will spend literally billions of dollars attempting to cure these cancers every year.

In a much-quoted analysis, Cochrane questions the efficacy of many of these interventions. An interesting example is the coronary care unit. A study carried out in Britain (Mather et al.) compared treatment of patients with acute myocardial infarction randomly allocated to treatment at home or to specially equipped and staffed coronary-care units in hospitals. The patients treated at home did slightly better overall. Similarly, questions have been raise about the value of electronic fetal monitoring (Banta and Thacker); therapy for adult-onset diabetes (Cochrane); coronary bypass surgery (Office of Technology Assessment); and tonsillectomy (Office of Technology Assessment).

However, even though it is not possible to show that personal health services substantially influenced the health of the population (as it can currently be measured), such services are certainly important to the health of individuals with various disease processes (Haggerty). McDermott categorizes the services of the personal physician into four functions: technologic use, Samaritanism, physiologic supportive management, and the capability to report negatives authoritatively and thus help maintain peace of mind. As he notes, we lack indicators to measure the effectiveness of these categories of care, unless we are content with the crudeness of the mortality measures. We have begun to develop mechanisms for addressing the lack of evidence on medical technology, notably through 1978 legislation to establish a new National Center for Health Care Technology in the Department of Health and Human Services. A major challenge for the future is to greatly expand the scientific basis of medical treatment.

The Caring Function

Health professionals sometimes become so involved in delivering services that they neglect medicine's traditional role, caring for people. As Sigerist says:

> Disease, then, is a biological process. . . . But this process takes place in man, and thus always involves the mind. . . . Disease, a destructive process that threatens life, may destroy only a few cells that can easily be replaced, but it may destroy the entire organism and with it the individual. For this reason, man suffers and is afraid: disease reminds him that he is mortal, that he must

die sooner or later, and if the illness is serious, it may be very soon. . . . Elementary fears, age-old views, come from the depth of the unconscious, breaking through the thin crust of education. (p. 93)

Although care has a long history, it is little talked about in today's technological world of medicine. But the public is beginning to demand more than machines.

Studies have supported the importance of care (Haggerty). It has been shown that patients with acceptance—measured by a scale including trust in the surgeon, optimism about the outcome, and confidence in their ability to cope—healed faster in a trial involving eye surgery (Frank). Another study showed that when mothers were reassured and given an opportunity to ask questions, their children undergoing tonsillectomy adapted more easily to the hospital and recovered faster after surgery (Skipper and Leonard). Perhaps more important, it is known that disability from chronic disease is probably more dependent on the patient's attitudes than on his actual physical state (Mechanic, pp. 117–119, 133–134).

Studies of primary-care settings have indicated that a large majority of patients present either with psychological problems or with physical complaints that a physician is trained to regard as trivial (Mechanic, p. 119). Yet caring is really the essence of health care. The conclusions of the 1972 Sun Valley Forum on "Medical Cure and Medical Care" are germane: "Traditionally, medical care has served as much to relieve pain and anxiety and system function as it has to effect cures. Medical care is a highly personalized service with both physical and psychologic elements; these are highly related in the consumer's motivation to seek service and in the physician's ability to achieve cooperation by his advice and to change behavior to be conducive to health. There was widespread agreement that both the 'curing' and 'caring' functions are central to high-quality care, and that models for delivering health services must allow for the effective integration of both concerns" (Sun Valley Forum on National Health).

It seems clear that if the traditional system is unable or unwilling to provide practitioners to deal with problems in a warm and caring way, the public will either force it to change or will find other types of providers who can meet those needs. As McKeown (1971) notes, "Since most serious diseases and disabilities are likely to prove relatively intractable if they cannot be prevented, the role of therapeutic medicine should be modified to include as the major commitment the concept of care. Such a change would carry important implications for medical science and service and should affect the content and orientation of medical education."

The Future of Health Care

Too often, health care is thought of as modern biomedicine. But, traditionally, health care has included both a "curing" and a "caring" function.

We are also again realizing the importance of our physical and social environments for health. The recent critiques of medical care should not obscure the value of much of modern medical technology. Hopefully, we are developing a more rational perspective that pays more attention to the environment while at the same time assuring caring providers (Sobel, pp. 3–6).

The engineering approach to disease is not going to be abandoned, nor should it be. The major criticism of this approach is that it has limited applicability; but research will surely produce new and valuable advances. Advances that have been predicted include genetic transfer, understanding the genetic origin of many diseases, regeneration of tissues, slowing of aging, and increased epidemiological knowledge resulting from data banks. But even here, a perspective is important. Perhaps the most important genetic research concerns the effect of the environment on a given genetic heritage.

One can also predict that the importance of care will not decline. The future in technologically advanced countries probably includes caring for a group of intractable problems made up of congenital, psychological, and geriatric conditions (McKeown, 1971; Weinerman, 1965). At best, the many mild emotional, sexual, and social problems of adjustment for which people seek care will surely not disappear. And diseases of aging, with death coming after a prolonged course of chronic disease, will remain.

In 1972, a panel of 102 "experts" were asked to predict future events in health care. The results are interesting because they go beyond the technical advances mentioned above. Predicted changes included the disappearence of solo practice (the entire population being served by strategically located neighborhood health centers); the extension of national health insurance to cover more than 95% of the population; and effective coordination of medical care disbursement and planning on a regional basis throughout the country. Most of the changes were predicted to occur before the end of ten years from the date of the survey (McLaughlin and Sheldon).

The Future of Man

Earlier sections of this chapter have argued that the concept of health depends greatly on psychological, social, and cultural factors. Thus, the future of health and health care is intertwined with our view of ourselves and how we act on that view. Enduring traits of the American character include self-reliance and independence, propensity to participate in local affairs, innovativeness, and a sense of efficacy and optimism (Inkeles). Recent changes include growing social tolerance, a decline of the "Protestant ethic," and decreasing political confidence. The change in such ideals as frugality, industry, and initiative have profound implications for the health system.

These questions have also been considered by the Stanford Research Institute, which cites survey and poll data indicating changing attitudes toward spiritual and transcendental experience, questions as to the continuation of the growth-and-consumption ethic of business, and a changing attitude within science itself toward subjective experience, varied states of consciousness, psychic phenomena, and so forth (Harman). A recent book examines the value of such interventions as religious and secular healing, healing by the laying on of hands, yoga, and biofeedback (Sobel).

Some of the implications for health care are described in a report from the Stanford Research Institute (Harman). They include a broadened definition of health, reduced status for professionals, recognition that the whole society is the environment that affects health, blurring of the distinction between mental and physical illness, changing attitudes toward death, and control over medical technology.

Summary and Conclusions

This chapter has argued for a broadened conception of health and health care, and has supported the idea of health care as a right. Evidence has been cited that curative medicine is less efficacious than the public, or even the professions, believes. This and other considerations lead to the conclusion that "caring" in medicine and health care must and will increase. However, it is recognized that within limits the individual can still determine his or her own destiny, although many factors in society act to produce unhealthy behavior. Unquestionably, great possible health benefits could result from controlling the physical and social environment.

However, it is important to emphasize that treating disease is not the same as creating health. Dubos sees health as a mirage that will continue to recede just beyond reach; he believes that this is all to the good. "Human life implies adventure, and there is no adventure without struggles and dangers. . . . Attempts at adaptation will demand efforts, and these efforts will often result in failure. . . . Disease will remain an inescapable manifestation of his struggles. While it may be comforting to imagine a life free of stresses and strains in a carefree world, this will remain an idle dream. Man cannot hope to find another Paradise on earth, because Paradise is a static concept while human life is a dynamic process" (p. 278).

References

Banta, D., and Bosch, S. "Organized Labor and the Prepaid Group Practice Movement." *Archives of Environmental Health, 29,* 43, 1974.

Banta, D., and Fox, R. "Role Strains of a Health Care Team in a Poverty Community." *Social Science and Medicine, 6,* 697, 1972.

Banta, D., and Thacker, S. "Assessing the Costs and Benefits of Electronic Fetal Monitoring." *Obstetrical and Gynecological Survey, 34,* 627, 1979.

Belloc, N. B. "Relationship of Health Practices and Mortality." *Preventive Medicine, 2,* 67, 1973.

Belloc, N. B., and Breslow, L. "Relationship of Physical Health Status and Health Practices." *Preventive Medicine, 1,* 409, 1972.

Blakiston's *New Gould Medical Dictionary,* 2nd Ed. New York: Blakiston Division, McGraw-Hill, 1956.

Breslow, L. "A Quantitative Approach to the World Health Organization Definition of Health: Physical, Mental and Social Well-Being." *International Journal of Epidemiology, 1,* 347, 1972.

Breslow, L. Chairman. "Theory, Practice and Application of Preventive Medicine in Personal Health Services." Task Force III Report, The National Conference on Preventive Medicine, *Summaries and Recommendations.* Fogarty International Center, Bethesda, Maryland, November 1975.

Bureau of the Census. *Statistical Abstract of the United States, 1979.* Washington, D.C.: U.S. Department of Commerce, USGPO, 1979.

Burnett, M. *Genes, Dreams, and Realities.* New York: Basic Books, 1971.

Bush, J., and Fanshel, S. "A Health Status Index and Its Application to Health Services Outcomes." *Operations Research, 18,* 1021, 1970.

Cairns, J. "The Cancer Problem." *Scientific American, 64,* 1975.

Cassell, E. *The Healer's Art.* Philadelphia: Lippincott, 1976.

Cochrane, A. *Effectiveness and Efficiency.* London: Nuffield Provincial Hospitals Trust, 1971.

Daly, M., and Tyroler, H. "Cornell Medical Index Response as Predictor of Mortality." *British Journal of Preventive & Social Medicine, 26,* 159, 1972.

Dubos, R. *Mirage of Health.* New York: Harper and Row, Perennial Library, 1971.

Feinstein, A. "Symptoms as an Index of Biological Behaviour and Prognosis in Human Cancer." *Nature, 209,* 241, 1966.

Foley, J.P., Ed. *Jeffersonian Cyclopedia: A Comprehensive Collection of the Views of Thomas Jefferson.* Vol. I. New York: Russell and Russell, 1967.

Frank, J. "Mind-Body Interactions in Illness and Healing." Presented at the May Lectures, "Alternative Futures for Medicine," April 4, 1975, Airlie House, Airlie, Virginia.

Freymann, J. *The American Health Care System: Its Genesis and Trajectory.* New York: Medcom Press, 1974.

Fuchs, V. "The Contribution of Health Services to the American Economy." *The Milbank Memorial Fund Quarterly, 44,* 65, 1966.

Fuchs, V. *Who Shall Live?* New York: Basic Books, 1974.

Haggerty, R. J. "The Boundaries of Health Care." In Sobel, D. S., Ed., *Ways of Health.* New York: Harcourt Brace Jovanovich, 1979, pp. 45–60.

Harman, W. "New Images of Man: What to Do until the New Paradigm Arrives." Presented at the May Lectures, "Alternative Futures for Medicine," April 4, 1975, Airlie House, Airlie, Virginia.

Higginson, J. "A Hazardous Society? The Role of Epidemiology in Determining the Individual versus Group Risk in Modern Societies." Rosenhaus Lecture.

American Public Health Association Annual Meeting, November 17, 1975, Chicago, Illinois.

Homer. *The Iliad*. Translated by R. Lattimore. Chicago: The University of Chicago Press, 1951.

Hoyman, H. "The Spiritual Dimensions of Man's Health in Today's World." In Belgum, D., Ed., *Religion and Medicine*. Ames, Iowa: Iowa State University Press, 1967.

Illich, I. *Medical Nemesis*. New York: Pantheon Books, 1976.

Inkeles, A. "Continuity and Change in the American Character." In Lipset, S. M., Ed., *The Third Century*. Stanford, California: Hoover Institution Press, 1979, pp. 389–416.

Jago, J. " 'Hal'—Old Word, New Task—Reflections on the Words 'Health' and 'Medical.' " *Social Science and Medicine*, 9, 1, 1975.

Jonas, S. *Medical Mystery: The Training of Doctors in the United States*. New York: W. W. Norton & Company, 1979.

Kaplan, R. M., Bush, J. W., and Berry, C. C. "Health Status: Types of Validity and Index of Well-Being." *Health Services Research*, 11, 478, 1976.

Kessner, D., et al. *Infant Death: An Analysis by Maternal Risk and Health Care*. Washington, D.C.: Institute of Medicine, National Academy of Sciences, 1973.

Koos, E. *The Health of Regionville*. New York: Hafner Publishing Co., 1954.

Kunitz, S., et al. "Changing Health Care Opinions in Regionville, 1946–1973." *Medical Care*, 13, 549, 1975.

Lalonde, M. *A New Perspective on the Health of Canadians*. Ottawa, Canada: Government of Canada, 1974.

Lilienfeld, A. Personal communication. June 24, 1975.

McDermott, W. "Medicine: The Public Good and One's Own." *Perspectives in Biology and Medicine*, 21, 167, 1978.

McKeown, T. "A Historical Appraisal of the Medical Task." In McLaughlin, G., and McKeown, T., Eds., *Medical History and Medical Care*. New York: Oxford University Press, 1971, pp. 27–50.

McKeown, T. *The Role of Medicine, Dream, Mirage, or Nemesis?* London: The Nuffield Provincial Hospitals Trust, 1976.

McLaughlin, C., and Sheldon, A. *The Future and Medical Care*. Cambridge, Massachusettes: Ballinger Publishing Company, 1974.

Mather, H., et al. "Acute Myocardial Infarction: Home and Hospital Treatment." *British Medical Journal*, 3, 334, 1971.

Mechanic, D. *Politics, Medicine, and Social Science*. New York: Wiley, 1974.

Millis, J. "A Rational Policy for Medical Education and Its Financing." New York: The National Fund for Medical Education, 1971, pp. 53–58.

Morris, J. *Uses of Epidemiology*. Baltimore: Williams & Wilkins, 1964.

Morris, J. *Uses of Epidemiology*. Edinburgh, Scotland: Churchill Livingstone, 1975.

Mushkin, S. J., and Dunlop, D. W. *Health: What Is It Worth?* New York: Pergamon Press, 1979.

National Center for Health Statistics, National Center for Health Services Research. *Health United States: 1979*. Hyattsville, Maryland: USDHEW Publication No. (PHS) 80–1232, USGPO, 1980.

Navarro, V. "The Industrialization of Fetishism or the Fetishism of Industrialization, A Critique of Ivan Illich." *International Journal of Health Services*, 5, 347, 1975.

Office of Technology Assessment, Congress of the United States. *Assessing the Efficacy and Safety of Medical Technologies*. Washington, D.C.: USGPO, 1978.

Parsons, T. *The Social System*. Glencoe, Illinois: The Free Press, 1951.

Parsons, T. "Definitions of Health and Illness in the Light of American Values and Social Structure." In Jaco, E., Ed., *Patients, Physicians, and Illness*. Glencoe, Illinois: The Free Press, 1958.

Rosen, G. *A History of Public Health*. New York: MD Publications, 1958.

Schneiderman, M. "Cancer—A Social Disease?" Presented at the Interagency Collaborative Group on Environmental Carcinogenesis, June 11, 1975, National Institutes of Health, Bethesda, Maryland.

Sigerist, H. *Medicine and Human Welfare*. College Park, Maryland: McGrath Publishing Co., 1970.

Skipper, J., and Leonard, R. "Children, Stress, and Hospitalization." *Journal of Health and Social Behavior*, 9, 275, 1968.

Sobel, D. S., Ed. *Ways of Health*. New York: Harcourt Brace Jovanovich, 1979.

Stead, E. "Excellent Care: The Clinician's View." In Walker, E.C., et al., Eds., *Evaluation of Care in the University and Community Hospital*. Hartford, Connecticut: Connecticut Health Services Research Series, 1971.

Sun Valley Forum on National Health. "Medical Cure and Medical Care." *Milbank Memorial Fund Quarterly*, 50, 231, 1972. (Summary)

Susser, M. "Ethical Components in the Definition of Health." *International Journal of Health Services*, 4, 539, 1974.

Szasz, T. *The Manufacture of Madness*. New York: Harper & Row, 1970.

Terris, M. "Approaches to an Epidemiology of Health." *American Journal of Public Health*, 65, 1037, 1975.

Thomas, L. *Lives of a Cell*. New York: Viking Press, 1975.

Weinerman, E. R. "Anchor Points Underlying the Planning for Tomorrow's Health Care." *Bulletin of the New York Academy of Medicine*, 41, 1203, 1965.

Weinerman, E. "Research on Comparative Health Service Systems." *Medical Care*, 9, 272, 1971.

White, K. "International Comparisons of Health Services Systems." *Milbank Memorial Fund Quarterly*, 46, 117, 1968. (Personal communication: Dr. White stated in 1975 that he considered this estimate to be still generally accurate.)

White, R. *Right to Health: The Evolution of an Idea*. Ames, Iowa: The University of Iowa Press, 1971.

Wise, H., et al. *Making Health Teams Work*. Cambridge, Massachusettes: Ballinger Publishing Co., 1974.

World Health Organization. "The Constitution of the World Health Organization." *WHO Chronicle*, 1, 29, 1944.

Zaborowski, M. "Cultural Components in Responses to Pain." *Journal of Social Issues*, 8, 16, 1952.

3

Population Data for Health and Health Care

Steven Jonas

Introduction

Quantitative analysis provides a basic means of describing, and thus understanding, the population served by our health care delivery system. Quantitative analysis of populations—especially in terms of number, health
status, and health care services utilization—serves to elucidate the populations' place in and relation to the delivery system.

Because of the nature of most data-gathering and reporting on the one
hand, and book-writing and publishing on the other, most of the data in this
chapter will be two to four years out of date by the time this book first
appears. Some data will be presented, of course, particularly in relation to
change and rates of change, major issues in any health care delivery
system. However, it is intended that the reader should use this chapter
(and indeed all sections of the book in which data appear) in conjunction
with Appendix I, "Guide to Sources." Thus, when we discuss population,
for example, the reader will not be dependent on estimated census data for
1978 or 1979; Appendix I tells him where the most current data may be
found. We are concerned, then, not with numbers per se, but with the
principles and purposes of using numbers in describing a population.

Quantitative Perspectives

There are three major quantitative perspectives from which a population
can be viewed in relation to health and health care services. First is the
number of people, and what are called "demographic" characteristics, from
the Greek "describing the people." Among the important demographic
characteristics are geographic distribution, age, sex and marital status, and
such social characteristics as ethnicity, income, education, employment,
and measures of social class. Second is the actual *health status* of the
population, or conversely, the *sickness status;* these can be characterized
in terms of mortality (death) and morbidity (sickness). Mortality

and morbidity may be counted for the population as a whole, in which case the resultant numbers or rates are described as "crude," or may be counted by cause, or by demographic characteristics used in describing segments of the population. The third perspective is utilization of health services: who uses how many of what kinds of services. Utilization can be measured from the point of view of the consumers, e.g., what is the per-person physician visit rate, or from the point of view of the provider, e.g., how many visits does a particular physician give. When one knows how many people there are, what their health status is, and the levels at which they utilize services, one has quantitatively characterized a population in relation to health and health care fairly well.

Numbers and Rates

Population, health status, and utilization data all can be presented in two forms: as numbers and as rates. A *number* represents simply a count of conditions, individuals, events. A *rate* has two parts, a numerator and a denominator; the numerator is a number of conditions, individuals, events counted, while the denominator is a larger group (usually) of conditions, individuals, events from among which the numerator is drawn. It is customary to give the rate as applying during a particular time period. For example, one could count 1,000 deaths occurring in a particular population during a year. This *number* of deaths becomes a *rate* if one counts the population, finds that number to be 100,000 and then says that the mortality *rate* is 1,000/100,000, per year. The rate can be expressed as a percentage (in this case, 1%), or as a rate per thousand (in this case, 10), or any other expression that is useful. The multipliers are usually in powers of 10 and the magnitude is usually chosen so as to make the rate a number of reasonable size. Thus, the more infrequent the event being counted by the numerator, the greater the magnitude of the denominator. For example, crude death rates for a whole population, all causes, are usually given as per thousand population, whereas rarer cause-specific mortality rates are given as per 100,000 or even as per 1,000,000. This is done so that the rate itself will not appear as a fractional number.

Denominators, as well as numerators, can be fairly specific. In discussing deaths from lung cancer related to cigarette smoking, for example, a rate can be determined for the number of deaths per year from lung cancer in males over page 45 who have smoked 2 or more packs of cigarettes per day for 20 years or more (the numerator), per all males over 45 who have smoked 2 or more packs of cigarettes per day for 20 years or more (the denominator). The units of the numerator and the denominator in health indices, however, are usually different. For example, in cause-specific mortality rates, the unit for the numerator is deaths by cause, while the unit for the denominator is persons.

Although rates are usually fractions, they will occasionally be whole numbers. For example, in measuring total morbidity in a population, one may find that the number of diagnosed disease conditions is greater than the number of people. The rate then is usually given with a denominator of 1, e.g., in the population of a central African city there are 2.5 disease conditions per persons. This usage also occurs in utilization rates, e.g., the physician-visit rate in the United States is approximately 5.0 per person. A very important use of rates is to measure changes over time, e.g., the death rate for condition X went down from one year to the next. Health care service utilization rates are not usually given in terms of numerators and denominators. Hospital admission rates that are specific for a particular hospital, for example, are not usually given as per person, but simply as per unit of time, as follows: in 1975, the admission rate for hospital Y was 1,000 per month. This practice prevails because the sizes of the populations served by most providers are not known.

The Purposes of Quantification

Description. Quantification has two major purposes in relation to understanding a health care delivery system. First, quantification is descriptive. It describes the size of the population under consideration. Demographic characteristics such as location (Do many people live near marshes in which malaria-carrying mosquitoes live?) and age distribution (Are there many infants and/or old people?) give some indication of the population's relative disease risk. Disease-specific mortality and morbidity rates point out the major health and illness problems in the population. The infant mortality rate gives some indication both of general health levels and the availability of medical care.

Crude and disease-specific mortality and morbidity rates can be distributed by place, age, sex, ethnic group, and social class to show which population subgroups are being affected by which diseases. An analyis of such data reveals what diseases and conditions of ill health the population has, and which subgroups of the population are affected by what problems.

Utilization data also show how the population uses the health care system. As we noted above, utilization of health services can be viewed from the consumer's perspective—how many times the average person sees a physician per year, and what the sources of care are—or from the point of view of the provider—how many patient visits the average physician gives in a year. Again, these kinds of data can be subdivided according to the various demographic characteristics of the population—i.e., what is the average annual per-person physician visit rate by age, sex, geographic location, social class, and the like. From the provider side, the demographic makeup of the group of patients admitted to a particular hospital in the course of a year can be examined. In addition, there can be demographic analyses of the providers themselves, both individual and institutional; that is, one can determine the average number of visits provided annually by physicians according to their age, practice location, and specialty. Thus, descriptively, quantification tells us how many of what kind of people are at risk, what kinds of diseases and conditions of ill health they have, how those problems are distributed in the population, and, finally, who goes where for how many of what kinds of health services, delivered by which types of providers.

Program-planning. The second purpose of quantification in health care delivery is prospective. Description can reveal the existence of problems; if there is a desire to do something about the problems, data can be used for prospective program-planning. Once new programs are under way, data can be used to evaluate their effects and effectiveness. Thus data are necessary for logical program planning, as they are in most fields of human endeavor. However, it must be remembered that they are not sufficient: the agencies and institutions that control the health care delivery system must first make a policy decision to undertake program-planning and to implement a suitable plan before the prospective use of data has any real meaning. We discuss the problems of health care program-planning in the United States in some detail in Chapter 13.

To illustrate the use of data prospectively, let us take the hypothetical case of planning a hospital for a medical school in a suburban/semirural area. A program is to be designed for this hospital that will help meet the health care needs of the community as well as the educational and research needs of the medical school, since the three functions of any medical school, in theory at least, are patient care (service), teaching, and research. It is to be hoped, of course, that these three activities can be made congruent.

Let us look at some of the questions we would need to answer in undertaking intelligent, rational program-planning for a new medical school hospital. First, a proposed service area would be delineated by counting population, determining population density, examining modes of transportation, and evaluating existing health care resources, particularly the more complex and sophisticated ones already in use. Thus, the questions are defined. Among them are:

- How many people are there and where are they located?
- What are the rates of population change?

- What are the age, sex, and marital status distributions?
- What are the social class and ethnic makeups of the population?
- What diseases do they get?
- What diseases do they die of?
- What are the existing health care resources?
- How are they used?
- What do existing providers see as their needs?
- How do they view the new facility and how will they relate to it?

The answers to these and many other similar questions indicate the health and health care needs of the population to be served. Going a step further, taking into account existing health care services and what they do, the data identify the *unmet* health and health care needs of the population. An analysis of the provider utilization patterns shows what the providers are doing, and what they are not doing, and indicates what *their* needs are. In planning any new health care facility, it is essential to know how it is going to relate functionally to existing providers, both individual and institutional. Finally, as we noted above, educational and research needs must be taken into account.

Amalgamating, classifying, and analyzing all these data is the basis for rational program-planning. The data enable us to make intelligent decisions on facility design, location, services, space allocation, administrative structure, community relations, staffing and personnel policies, teaching and research programs, capital cost, expense budget, and so on. In general one can say that intelligent decisions depend on intelligent use of data; unfortunately, such use does not always obtain in the United States.

Population

Number. A census enumerating the population of the nation is required at least once every 10 years by the Constitution of the United States (Bureau of the Census, p. 1). Its orginal purpose was to provide the basis for the apportionment of seats in the House of Representatives of the United States Congress. A census has been carried out every 10 years since 1790. Although every effort is made for completeness, the Bureau has estimated that it undercounted in 1970 by 2.5% (Bureau of the Census, p. 1). In addition to the decennial censuses, the Bureau makes interim estimates on various parameters based on information gathered from population samples and a variety of other sources. The resident population as of April 1, 1970 was officially reported as 203,211,926 (Bureau of the Census, Table 1). In addition, there were about 1 million armed services persons resident abroad. (By January 1, 1974, with the virtual end of American involvement in Vietnam, the number of armed service persons abroad dropped to just over one-half million.)

Births, deaths, immigration, and emigration produce changes in population size. During the 1970s, the population growth rate averaged about 0.8% per year, whereas during the 1960s the population had grown at the rate of about 1.3% per year. This decline stems primarily from a decline in the birth rate, which we shall consider in more detail below. The bearing on health services of such matters as population size, growth rate, and birth rate should be obvious. By April 1, 1979, one year before the next decennial census was taken (with results being published too late to be included in this chapter), the Bureau of the Census estimated the U. S. population to be 219.9 million.

Demographic characteristics. In 1970, 68.6% of the population lived in what are called Standard Metropolitan Statistical Areas (SMSAs) (Bureau of the Census, Table 16). The definition of a SMSA is determined by the federal Office of Management and Budget, an agency of the Executive Branch (Bureau of the Census, p. 935). As of March 1976, an SMSA had to include at least: (a) one city with a population of 50,000 or more (75,000 in New England), or (b) a city with a population of 25,000, plus surrounding areas with a population of at least 1,000 per square mile to produce, "for general, economic and social purposes, a single community" with a "combined population of 50,000," and a total population in the city and contiguous areas of at least 75,000. In addition, an SMSA must include the county in which the central city is located, and adjacent counties that are "determined to be metropolitan in character" (Bureau of the Census, p. 935).

In 1977, approximately 73% of the U. S. population lived in SMSAs (Bureau of the Census, Table 14). The comparable figures for 1940 and 1960 are 53% and 63% (Bureau of the Census, Table 16). As of 1978, it was estimated that the U. S. population was 49% male, 87% white, and had a median age of 29.7—30.6 for whites, 24.3 for blacks (Bureau of the Census, Table 27). In terms of age distribution, in 1978, 38% of the population was under 21, 52% between 21 and 65, and 10% were age 65 and over (Bureau of the Census, Table 29). In 1978, about 70% of males and 64% of females over 18 were married (Bureau of the Census, Table 48). In 1970, more than 2 million Americans were inmates of institutions, nearly 1 million in homes for the aged, about 435,000 in mental hospitals, more than 325,000 in prison, more and 200,000 in homes for the mentally retarded, and approximately 85,000 in tuberculosis and other chronic-disease hospitals (Bureau of the Census, Table 75).

Social class status is often thought to be a valuable parameter by which to cross-tabulate population, health and illness, and utilization data.* Unlike the government of England, the U. S. government has not developed a "social class" index by which it cross-tabulates its demographic data. Thus, one is forced to use ethnicity and income as rough indicators of, at least, relative social class. This is unfortunate, because social class is really determined by the combination of a number of factors: income, education, employment, and dwelling-place. A great deal of such information is in fact collected by the government, but an index has not been created.

The information we have been presenting so far comes from Section 1 of *Statistical Abstracts*, "Population." Additional information necessary to develop a comprehensive profile is contained in the following other sections of *Statistical Abstracts:* Education; Social Insurance and Welfare Services; Labor Force, Employment, and Earnings; and Income, Expenditures, and Wealth.

How the Vital Statistics Data Are Collected

Traditional in public health, "vital statistics" consist of births, deaths, marriages, and divorces. In the United States, primary responsibility for collecting these data lies with the states. Not all states collect all categories of data. In most states that do collect these data, the Department of Health is responsible; where possible, state health departments rely on county and other local health departments to do the actual counting. The locally accumulated data are then organized at the state level and transmitted to the federal level. The District Government for Washington, D.C., carries out the above responsibilities in that city.

A National Death Index is being established by the National Center for Health Statistics (NCHS), beginning with deaths occurring in 1979. † NCHS will develop and maintain a national computer file for indexing and searching purposes, updating it in each subsequent year with data from computer tapes obtained from the state Vital Statistics offices under a contractual arrangement. These tapes will provide a standard minimum data set for each death and will make it possible for NCHS to compare

---

*A detailed discussion of this very important subject area, with an extensive bibliography, is presented in *The Health Gap*, edited by Robert Kane, M.D. (New York: Springer, 1975). See also: *Health Status of Minorities and Low Income Groups*. Washington, D.C.: Office of Health Resources Opportunity, DHEW, Pub. No. (HRA) 79–627, USGPO, 1979.

† This paragraph was supplied by the office of Ruth Hanft, Deputy Assistant Secretary of the USDHHS for Health Research, Statistics and Technology, 1980.

listings of individuals provided by users of the index with the national file and then indicate to the user any probable matches along with the appropriate state death certificate numbers and the name and address of the vital registration areas in the states where the deaths occurred. The user will then make the necessary arrangements with the state offices for the procurement of death records or any specific information, such as cause of death. Use of the National Death Index will be limited to statistical purposes in accordance with NCHS's contracts with the states. The index is designed primarily to facilitate prospective studies to determine the relationships between chronic degenerative diseases, such as cancer, and environmental, occupational, medical, and life-style factors. Because no national index or registry currently exists and because death registration is a responsibility of the states, investigators conducting many types of prospective mortality studies must now contact many or all individual state Vital Statistics offices in order to ascertain even the fact of death for persons in their studies.

The collection of mortality data in the United States did not begin on an annual basis until 1900. At that time, 10 states and the District of Columbia became "death registration states" to carry out that task and forward the results to the federal government (Bureau of the Census, p. 57). Until 1946, the Bureau of the Census assembled the vital statistics at the national level. From 1946 to 1960, the work was performed by the Bureau of State Services of the United States Public Health Service, Since 1960, the National Center for Health Statistics, USDHHS, has carried out the function. Beginning in 1915, 10 states and the District of Columbia formed a "birth registration area," collecting birth data on an annual basis. By 1933, all states were in both the birth and death registration areas. Fetal deaths have been counted annually since 1922. The corresponding "marriage registration area," first formed in 1957, included 41 states, the Virgin Islands, Puerto Rico, and the District of Columbia by 1978. The "divorce registration" area was established in 1958, and by 1978 covered 28 states and the Virgin Islands (Bureau of the Census, p. 58).

Vital statistics rates are calculated by the National Center for Health Statistics and are based upon the actual number of persons counted by the Bureau of the Census on April 1 of each decennial year, as well as the midyear estimates made by the Bureau of the Census for other years. Death statistics are based on a 10% sample of all reported deaths. Fetal deaths and stillbirths are not included, nor are deaths among Armed Service persons abroad. Cause-specific mortality data are classified according to the *Ninth Revision International Classification of Diseases, Adapted for Use in The United States (1979)*, the so-called ICDA. The use of a system at least parallel to the "International Statistical Classification of

Diseases, Injuries, and Causes of Death," produced by the World Health Organization, is required for WHO membership (Bureau of the Census, p. 57), and the ICDA is such a system. The ICDA–9–Clinical Modification (ICDA–9–CM) is an extension of the ICDA–9, which all hospitals in the U. S. receiving federal funds are required to use.

Natality

In 1978, about 3.3 million babies were born in the United States (National Center for Health Statistics, 1980d). The annual rate was 15.3 live births per 1,000 population rate, up from the lowest rate recorded in recent years, 14.8 in 1975–1976. That rate represented a low point in a birth rate that had been steadily dropping from a post-World-War-II high of 25, achieved in 1955 (Bureau of the Census, Table 80). The fertility rate (annual births per 1,000 resident females 15 to 44 years of age) for 1978 was 66.6, down from the post-World-War-II high of 118.5, but up slightly from the low of 65.8 recorded in 1976 (Bureau of the Census, Table 83). This declining birth rate still produces net population growth each year (Bureau of the Census, Table 2).

Mortality

The crude death rate (total deaths per 1,000 population) in the United States for 1979 was 8.8 (National Center for Health Statistics, 1980b). This was a decline from a rate that had generally hovered between 9.4 and 9.5 from 1955 through 1974, going no higher than 9.7 (once, in 1968), and no lower than 9.3 (twice, in 1955 and 1971) (Bureau of the Census, Table 104).

Mortality data are rather neatly reported. There is one primary reporting authority, the local health department, or, where none exists, the state health department acting in its place. Death is a well-defined event in the vast majority of cases, although with recent advances in medical technology, the possibility of dispute has arisen. Determination of cause of death has presented some problems from time to time, since it is left up to the physician certifying that the patient is dead, in most cases, and physicians do have varying diagnostic styles, opinions, and abilities. Furthermore, there have been changes in the technical definitions of causes of death over time.* For example, is diabetes or coronary artery disease the cause of death in a patient who dies from a heart attack that resulted from complica-

---

*For a detailed discussion of this problem, see "Estimates of Selected Comparability Ratios Based on Dual Coding of 1976 Death Certificates by the Eighth and Ninth Revisions of the International Classification of Diseases." *Monthly Vital Statistics Report, 28,* No. 11, Supplement, February 29, 1980.

tions secondary to diabetes? The reporting authorities have rules to cover these instances, however, and most physicians follow them, so that this last problem is not too serious. Finally, since both hospitals and funeral directors are legally required to report all deaths, with rather serious penalties for failure to comply, we can assume that most deaths are reported.

A great deal of data concerning differential death rates by the basic demographic variables of age, color, and sex can be found in *Monthly Vital Statistics Report, Vital Statistics of the United States*, the *Statistical Abstract*, and special studies published in *Vital and Health Statistics*, Series 20.* Mortality is relatively high during the first year of life, drops to a relatively low level until the mid-40s, and then begins to climb again (Bureau of the Census, Tables 104, 105). For the total population, males have a higher mortality rate than do females, at all ages. As the population grows older *in toto*, the preponderance of females over males in the older age group increases. Although the crude death rate for nonwhites is lower than for whites, the age-specific death rates for nonwhites are higher than for whites at all ages until 80. The crude death rate is lower for nonwhites because the nonwhite population is younger.

Cause-specific mortality rates. Turning to cause-specific mortality rates, the 10 leading causes of death in 1979 (excluding the diagnostic categories of "symptoms and ill-defined conditions" and "all other diseases") were, in order: heart disease; cancer; stroke; accidents; chronic obstructive pulmonary disease; influenza and pneumonia (primarily pneumonia); diabetes mellitus; cirrhosis of the liver; suicide; and "certain conditions originating in the perinatal period." Homicide was eleventh (National Center for Health Statistics, 1980b). In 1960, the 10 leading causes of death were heart disease; cancer; stroke; accidents; certain diseases of early infancy; influenza and pneumonia; diabetes mellitus; congenital anomalies; cirrhosis of the liver; and suicide. Homicide was well down on the list (Bureau of the Census, Table 110).

Infant mortality. The *infant* mortality rate is the number of deaths under the age of one year among children born alive, divided by the number of live births. Since infant mortality appears to be related to a variety of socioeconomic, environmental, and health care factors, as was pointed out in Chapter 2, some authorities (Morris, pp. 56 ff., 267; Rosen, p. 342) consider it to be a fairly sensitive indicator of general health levels in a population. In 1979, the infant mortality rate in the United States was 13 per 1,000 live births (National Center for Health Statistics, 1980b). The rate has been declining steadily since 1940, when it was 47 (Bureau of the

*For a description of these publications, see Appendix I.

Census, Table 108). In fact, the infant mortality rate has been falling since it was first recorded in this country at 99.9 in 1915 (Grove and Hetzel, Table 38).

The most striking feature of the U. S. infant mortality rate is that although it has consistently fallen over the years, the nonwhite rate has just as consistently remained almost double the white rate. Detailed examinations of the relationship between ethnicity, other factors, and infant mortality are contained in *Vital and Health Statistics*, Series 22, Number 14, "Infant Mortality Rates: Socioeconomic Factors," and a publication of the office of Health Resources Opportunity (1979, pp. 35–39).

A study in New York City of factors related to infant mortality in 140,000 births is to be found in a comprehensive work sponsored by the National Academy of Sciences (Kessner et al.), mentioned in Chapter 2. It finds that in this time of relatively low overall infant mortality rates, with the infectious diseases that formerly took the lives of many infants in the main under control, "generally, adequacy of [health] care . . . is strongly and consistently associated with infant birth weight . . . and survival" (Kessner et al., p. 1). Kessner and his co-authors also concluded from their study that "the survival of infants of different ethnic groups varies widely; . . . there is consistent association between social classes as measured by the educational attainment of the mothers and infant birth weight and survival; . . . within categories of mother's educational attainment, there are consistent trends relating the adequacy of care . . . to infant survival; . . . there is a gross misallocation of services by ethnic group and care when the risks of the women are taken into account. . . ." (pp. 2–3).

Marriage and Divorce

Turning to the remaining vital statistics, by 1979, the marriage rate stood at 10.3 per 1,000 population (National Center for Health Statistics, 1980b), down from a post-World-War-II high of 11.1 in 1950 (Bureau of the Census, Table 117). The divorce rate, which had stood at 2.6 per 1,000 population in 1950 (Bureau of the Census, Table No. 117), had reached 5.3 in 1979 (National Center for Health Statistics, 1980b), 50% of the marriage rate! Detailed analysis of marriage and divorce statistics can be found in *Vital and Health Statistics*, Series 21, "Data on Natality, Marriage and Divorce."

Morbidity

Morbidity refers to sickness, illness, disease. Like mortality, morbidity data can be expressed as rates and can be cross-tabulated with the broad range of demographic characteristics. Morbidity data are extremely important in characterizing the health status of a population. Mortality data alone are not adequate for that purpose, for several reasons. Many diseases and conditions of ill health that are widely prevalent in the population—particularly in a country like the United States, in which communicable disease, with a few exceptions, is not a major problem—do not appear in mortality figures. Such conditions include arthritis, low-back pain, the common cold, mild emotional and sexual problems, and the like. Other diseases that do kill do so rarely in relation to their appearance in the population. Included in this category are duodenal ulcer and gall bladder disease. When looking at morbidity, one learns not only which are the important diseases and the patterns of their distribution in the population, but also how they affect people in terms of limitation of activity.

To understand morbidity data, we must understand the terms incidence and prevalence. *Incidence* is the number of new cases of the disease in question occurring during a particular time period, usually a year. *Prevalence* is the total number of cases existing in a population during a time period or at one point in time ("point-prevalence").

Reporting and sources of data. Reporting mobidity is not nearly so simple as reporting mortality. When is a person sick? Who decides? The physician? The patient? The problems of perception of illness, and of the sick role, were referred to in the previous chapter. Furthermore, although it is thought that the determination of cause of death by physicians is reasonably reliable, the accuracy of physician diagnosis in illness is more questionable (Koran).

Although the law requires that all deaths be reported, only certain categories of sickness, the infectious diseases, must be reported. The list appears in *Morbidity and Mortality Weekly Report*. Among the 44 such diseases only 10 can be considered significant in the United States: chickenpox; gonorrhea; hepatitis A, B, and unspecified; measles; mumps; German measles; Salmonellosis; shigellosis; tuberculosis; and syphilis (Center for Disease Control). Of these, four are common childhood viral diseases, while two are venereal diseases. Clearly there are no reporting requirements for many categories of disease important in the United States.

It is known that physicians fail to report certain diseases, even when legally required to do so. Some private physicians will not report venereal disease in private patients, on the grounds of avoiding "embarrassment." Tuberculosis reporting, other than from institutions, is inhibited by the possible economic consequences: some employers automatically fire persons with tuberculosis. (Although the disease is one of low infectivity, it is commonly thought to be highly contagious, even by some health professionals.) Many physicians fail to report cases of the common childhood viral infections because they consider them to be "inconsequential."*

In mortality, there is only one possible source of data, and it isn't the patient. In morbidity, however, both providers and patients can obviously be data sources; as a result, quite different pictures can be obtained. Providers can report morbidity in terms of diagnostic categories and also in terms of patient chief complaints; that is, what the patient reports to the physician as being the problem. (Patients don't usually come to a physician saying "I've got diabetes mellitus, Doc," but rather something like, "I've been feeling kind of weak, and I'm drinking a great deal of water and urinating a lot.") Patients can also report chief complaints directly in a survey. From a chief complaint profile for a population, obtained from either source, some estimates of the morbidity patterns can be obtained. One advantage of deriving information directly from patients is that certain patients with certain types of illnesses will never come to medical attention. Thus morbidity surveys that only gather information from providers will not give a complete picture.

Other than reportable communicable disease data published by the Center for Disease Control in *Morbidity and Mortality Weekly Report*, the regular sources of morbidity data in the United States are from the National Center for Health Statistics. They include the Health Examination Survey, since 1970 the Health and Nutrition Examination Survey (HANES), and the Health Records Survey, the results of which are published periodically in *Vital and Health Statistics*, and the Health Interview Survey, the Hospital Discharge Survey, and the National Ambulatory Medical Care Survey, the result of which are published in both *Vital and Health Statistics* and *Monthly Vital Statistics Report*. Together these activities constitute the National Health Survey (National Center for Health Statistics, 1963). Series 1 of *Vital and Health Statistics* contains the general methodological and historical accounts.

The first HANES was initiated in 1970 and data collection began in 1971; HANES II data collection began in January 1976 and ended February

---

*For example, we can estimate that just before the introduction of the measles vaccine in the mid-1960s, the measles reporting was around 10%. Almost all children get measles before their fifth birthday. There were about 4,000,000 births annually in the U. S. at that time, but only 400,000 cases of measles were reported annually. Since, on the average, 4,000,000 children were getting the disease each year, the reporting rate was about 10%.

1980.* This survey is a modification of the Health Examination Survey begun in 1960. Its purposes are to measure the prevalence of certain health and nutritional conditions, to monitor nutritional indicators and changes in them over time, and to provide normative data with respect to health characteristics for the civilian noninstitutionalized population of the United States, aged one month to 74 years. Upon completion of brief household interviews, a subsample of persons is selected for the collection of more detailed medical history and nutritional information and clinical examination at a mobile examination center. The specific information collected in each cycle of HANES varies, but in general it includes dietary intake, physical measurements, biochemical characteristics, and demographic and socioeconomic characteristics, along with an appropriate medical history. The principal mechanism for release of data is Series 11 of the *Vital and Health Statistics* series.

The Health Interview Survey is another one of the ongoing activities of the National Center for Health Statistics. The results are published continuously in Series 10 of *Vital and Health Statistics*. Appendix I of most numbers in the series, "Technical Notes on Methods," describes the methodology in some detail. Using a sampling method, questionnaires are administered to members of selected households concerning "personal and demographic characteristics, illnesses, injuries, impairments, chronic conditions, and other health topics" (National Center for Health Statistics, 1979c, p. 36). This produces data on "incident of acute conditions, limitation of activity, persons injured, hospitalizations, disability days, dental visits, and physician visits" (National Center for Health Statistics, 1979c, p. 6). Thus both morbidity and utilization data are collected from the population perspective. Special studies produced details of conditions affecting the digestive system in 1968, skin and musculoskeletal systems in 1969, the respiratory system in 1970, and the circulatory system in 1972. "Impairments" was the special topic in 1971 and "miscellaneous conditions" in 1973 (National Center for Health Statistics, Oct. 1974c, p. 5). The cycle was recommenced in 1975, with studies on chronic digestive conditions for 1975 and use habits among adults of cigarettes, coffee, aspirin, and sleeping pills for 1976.

Incidence of morbid conditions. In 1978, the incidence of acute conditions was 218 per 1,000 persons per year, which was similar to the rate in the two previous years (National Center for Health Statistics, 1979c, p. 1). Most common were upper respiratory conditions (27%), followed by influenza (23%) and injuries (15%). Acute conditions were associated with

*This paragraph was supplied by the office of Ruth Hanft, Deputy Assistant Secretary of the USDHHS for Health Research, Statistics and Technology, 1980.

almost 1,000 days of restricted activity per 100 persons per year (National Center for Health Statistics, 1979c, Table A). Details of the data on acute conditions are contained in periodic publications in Series 10 entitled "Acute Conditions: Incidence and Associated Disability." It was found that 14.2% of the population experienced limitation in all activity owing to chronic conditions (National Center for Health Statistics, 1979c, Table C). The major chronic conditions causing limitations in activity in 1974, the most recent year for which such data are available, were heart conditions, arthritis and rheumatism, impairments of back or spine, hypertension, and impairments of lower extremities and hips (National Center for Health Statistics, 1977, Table 4).

Turning to data collected from the provider perspective, the Health Records Survey conducted three reviews of nursing homes and their patients in the United States, in 1963, 1964, and 1969, but there have been no recent studies. Sampling methods were used and information was collected about the institutions, the patients or residents, and personnel. The results of these surveys were published in Series 12 of *Vital and Health Statistics*. The Health Examination Survey, succeeded in 1971 by HANES, involved a series of direct examinations of population samples, which were carried out over the years by NCHS staff from specially designed mobile units. Until the early 1970s, there were three "cycles" of examinations: Cycle 1 on persons 18–79 years of age, conducted between 1959 and 1962; Cycle II on persons 6–11 years of age, conducted between 1963 and 1965; and Cycle III on persons 12–17 years of age, conducted between 1966 and 1970 (National Center for Health Statistics, 1975, p. 1). The voluminous data produced by the Health Examination Survey and the HANES is published in Series 11 of *Vital and Health Statistics*. Some data from the HANES also appears periodically in *Advance Data from Vital and Health Statistics* (see Appendix 1, A6).

The Hospital Discharge Survey (HDS) reports on morbidity and mortality as it occurs in hospitals. These data do provide a rather accurate picture of the illness profile of those in hospitals. It must be remembered, however, that the overwhelming majority of ill persons do not require hospitalization; thus, the morbidity profile of the population as a whole does not match that seen in hospitals. The results of the HDS appear in *Vital and Health Statistics*, Series 13. In the mid-1970s, some data were published in *Monthly Vital Statistics Report*. The HDS is carried out on a sampling basis in nonfederal, short-stay hospitals (hospitals with 6 or more beds and an average length of stay of 30 days of less). Almost 70% of hospital discharges from those hospitals are accounted for by 6 diagnostic groups: diseases of the circulatory system, 13%; diseases of the digestive system, 12%; complications of pregnancy, childbirth, and the puerperium, 12%; accidents, poisonings, and violence, 10%; diseases of the genitourinary system, 10%; and diseases of the respiratory system, 10% (National Center for Health Statistics, 1980a, Table 14). The five most common specific diagnoses are: malignant neoplasms; mental disorders; chronic ischemic heart disease; fractures, all sites; and diseases of the urinary system.

Finally, the most recent component of the National Health Survey is the NAMCS, National Ambulatory Medical Care Survey (National Center for Health Statistics, 1974a, 1974b). Although the NAMCS will eventually cover all loci of ambulatory care, it began by concentrating on private physicians' offices, which in the mid-1970s accounted for about 80% of all physician office visits (National Center for Health Statistics, 1979b). The data are collected on a sampling basis from a stratified random sample of all office-based allopathic and osteopathic physicians in the contiguous United States, excluding anesthesiologists, pathologists, and radiologists. Simple questionnaires on each patient seen during a given time period are filled out. Morbidity, patient demographic data, and utilization data are collected, as well as data on practice characteristics.

Morbidity data are collected from two perspectives: patient's reason for coming to the office and physician's diagnosis. In 1977, the ten leading patient's reasons for coming to the office were: general medical exam; routine prenatal exam; symptoms referable to the throat; blood pressure test; postoperative visit; cough; head cold, upper respiratory infection; back symptoms; skin rash; and gynecological exam (National Center for Health Statistics, 1980c, Table 14). These account for about 27% of all visits. The ten leading physicians' diagnoses were: special conditions and examinations without sickness; diseases of respiratory system; diseases of circulatory system; diseases of nervous system; accidents, poisonings, and violence; diseases of the genitourinary system; diseases of the musculo-skeletal system; diseases of the skin; symptoms and ill-defined conditions; and mental disorders (National Center for Health Statistics, 1980c, Table 13). These categories accounted for over 80% of diagnoses. In addition to general survey data such as these, NAMCS also publishes a variety of special studies by physician specialty, patient demographic characteristics, and diagnostic category in *Advance Data* and *Vital and Health Statistics* (National Center for Health Statistics, 1980c, pp. 12–13).

It should be clear that although we do know a great deal about how to characterize the health and illness status of our population, many aspects of this process are still not well understood. For example, we have yet to solve the problem of constructing a health status index for individuals (see Chapters 2 and 13) that would be broadly useful and easily determined (Anderson; Balinsky and Berger; Bergner, et al.; Bush et al.; Kaplan, et al.; Sackett, et al.). There is still a great deal to be done.

Utilization of Health Care Services

Introduction

We come finally to the third data perspective concerning health—that is, how the population utilizes the health care delivery system. We have pointed out that in quantifying utilization of health services, the same series of events can be counted either from the patients' or from the provider's perspective. As we shall see below, the results of the two types of counts are not always the same; thus, when discussing utilization, one has to be very careful to distinguish the two approaches.

To understand this problem compare the data on hospital ambulatory services utilization as reported by the Health Interview Survey, or HIS (patient perspective), with that reported by the American Hospital Association (provider perspective). For 1975, the Health Interview Survey reported that patients said that they made about 137 million visits to hospital clinics and emergency units (National Center for Health Statistics, 1979b, Table C). For the same year, the American Hospital Association's "Hospital Statistics" reported that patients made about 255 million visits to hospital outpatient services (American Hospital Association, 1976, Table 1).

The causes of the discrepancy are open to conjecture (Jonas). It is probably fair to say that neither figure is valid. (About 10% of the difference is accounted for by the fact that the HIS does not count visits by members of the Armed Forces to Defense Department Hospitals, while the AHA does.) If this is so, the discrepancy is the result of underreporting by patients to the HIS on the one hand, and overreporting (double-counting) by the AHA on the other. One of course does not know the degrees of underreporting and overreporting.

It must be borne in mind, however, that if the Health Interview Survey figures for hospital ambulatory visits are low, the comparable figures for private physician office visits may well be low, too. This could have a serious effect on health care planning, since it is customary to use the HIS figure for the average annual per-person physician rate (in the mid-1970s, around 4.5) as a base-line datum. Interestingly, in a paper on factors in the rise in health care costs, Nancy Worthington of the Social Security Administration estimated (without giving her sources) the average annual per-person physician rate for 1973 at over 8 (Worthington, 1975, Table 4).

Adding to the confusion is a discrepancy on physician office-visit rates between those reported by the HIS and the NAMCS. For 1975, in the HIS patients reported making 718 million office visits (National Center for Health Statistics, 1979b, Table C), while for the same year physicians reported to the NAMCS that they recorded 568 million office visits (National Center for Health Statistics, 1980c, Table A). The discrepancy is not nearly as large as it is for hospital outpatient visits, but it is in the other direction; that is, patients report *more* visits than providers do. It is possible that the new National Medical Care Utilization and Expenditure Survey (NMCUES) may help to resolve the problem since it, in part, will look at the same encounter from both the provider and patient perspectives, at least for Medicaid patients.

The NMCUES,* co-sponsored by the National Center for Health Statistics and the Health Care Financing Administration, is composed of four separate but interrelated surveys designed to: (1) provide a statistical base for the USDHHS's health care cost-containment effort; (2) provide updated, comparable measures of utilization and expenditures for monitoring national health insurance programs; and (3) provide data on trends and costs over time of health care services for different population subgroups (e.g. the poor, the elderly, and the uninsured). This survey began in the calendar year 1980 and is planned to be repeated on a biennial basis. The activities of the NMCUES are divided into four parts: (1) the Household Survey (HS), a national probability sample of 8,000 households in the civilian noninstitutionalized population; (2) the State Medicaid Household Survey (SMHS), in which 4 samples of 1,000 households in the civilian noninstitutionalized population with one or more Medicaid beneficiaries in the states of California, New York, Michigan, and Texas are utilized to provide estimates of the utilization experiences of the Medicaid populations; (3) the Medical Provider Survey, a survey of the doctors and hospitals providing care to a 25% sample of the Medicaid enrollees in the SMHS who have given written permission to release data from their providers; and (4) the Administrative Records Survey, a records survey that will obtain information from the administrative records of the Medicare and Medicaid programs for comparison with that reported in the HS and SMHS samples.

Utilization of Ambulatory Services

As we have noted, the Health Interview Survey (HIS) provides patient-perspective data for the utilization of ambulatory services. According to the HIS, in 1978, there were approximately 4.8 physician visits per person. † and about 75% of the population made at least one visit (National Center for Health Statistics, 1979c, p. 4). These figures have been fairly steady in recent years. In general, females made more visits than males, and, as might be expected, the visit rate increased with age. In the same year, the

---

*This paragraph was supplied by the office of Ruth Hanft, Deputy Assistant Secretary of the USDHHS for Health Research, Statistics and Technology, 1980.

† This figure includes telephone contacts, which account for about 12.5% of all "visits" reported by patients. Subtracting the telephone contacts, there were about 4.3 office visits per person, according to the HIS.

average number of dental visits per person was 1.6, with slightly less than one-half of the population making a dental visit in the year.

For place of visit, 1975 data, reported in a more detailed analysis of patient visits entitled "Physician Visits" (National Center for Health Statistics, 1979b), indicated that, excluding telephone contacts, about 78% of the total visits took place in the physician's office, less than 1% in the home, 15% in a hospital clinic or emergency room, 1% in an industrial health service, and 6% "other." "Physician Visits" also provides some useful information on the relationship between various sociodemographic variables and utilization variables.

There are several sources for provider data on the utilization of ambulatory services. The most comprehensive is the National Ambulatory Medical Care Survey, explained above. For 1977, the NAMCS reported 570 million visits to what it called "nonfederally employed office-based physicians" (National Center for Health Statistics, 1980c, p. 1). The NAMCS provides data on visits by age, color group, sex, geographic region, metropolitan/nonmetropolitan living area, type of physician and duration of visit, as well as morbidity, as we saw above.

The other major source of provider-perspective ambulatory service utilization data is the American Hospital Association's annual publication *Hospital Statistics*, published each summer. Until 1970, it appeared as part of the AHA's "Guide Issue" to hospitals in the United States, but since 1971, it has been issued separately. For 1978, the AHA reported 264 million outpatient visits including 83 million visits to hospital emergency units, and the balance to clinics and other units, such as outpatient hemodialysis and rehabilitation services (American Hospital Association, 1979, Table 5A). *Hospital Statistics* provides considerable detail on these data by such variables as number of beds, ownership, type, geographical region, and medical school affiliation (American Hospital Association, 1979, Tables 3, 5–9, 12, 13).

Utilization of Hospital Services

Turning to utilization of hospital services, patient-perspective data are provided by the HIS. For 1978, there were 14.0 reported discharges per 100 persons from short-stay hospitals* (National Center for Health Statis-

---

*Note that the HIS definition of a "short-stay hospital" differs from that of the AHA. The HIS defines it as "one in which the type of service provided . . . is general; maternity; eye; ear, nose and throat; children's; or osteopathic; or it may be the hospital department of an institution" (National Center for Health Statistics, 1979c, p. 55). The AHA defines short-stay as a hospital in which average length of stay is less than 30 days or over 50% of patients are admitted to units where length of stay is less than 30 days (American Hospital Association, 1979, p. xviii).

tics, 1979c, Table 15). This amounts to about 30 million discharges. The average reported length of hospital stay was 7.9 days, representing a slight downward trend from the early 1970s; 10.4% of all persons were hospitalized one or more times. Further breakdowns by age and sex are also given (National Center for Health Statistics, 1979c, p. 4, Tables 15–17).

The National Center for Health Statistics also provides provider-perspective hospital-utilization data through the Hospital Discharge Survey (HDS). The Center points out that because of "differences in collection procedures, population sampled, and definitions," the results from the HIS and the HDS are not entirely consistent (National Center for Health Statistics, 1979a, p. 1). For 1977, the HDS reported about 36 million discharges, excluding newborn infants, from nonfederal short-stay hospitals. The discharge rate per 100 population reported by the HDS is 16.9, in contrast to the rate of 14 reported by the HIS. The average length of stay was 7.3 days. Other classes of data provided by the Hospital Discharge Survey are utilization by various hospital characteristics and morbidity, discussed above, and an analysis of surgery.

The other major source of hospital utilization data is the American Hospital Association. In addition to the annual *Hospital Statistics*, "Hospital Indicators" appears monthly in *Hospitals*, the *Journal of the American Hospital Association*. For 1979, the 7,015 AHA-registered hospitals, with a total of 1.4 million beds, reported 37.2 million admissions, an occupancy rate of slightly over 75%, and an average daily census of 1.04 million (American Hospital Association, 1979, Table 3). In the same year, the 5,935 hospitals that the AHA classifies as nonfederal short-term admitted 34.6 million patients to their 980,000 beds. The occupancy rate was 73.5% and the average daily census was just over 700,000. *Hospital Statistics* contains voluminous data on these variables and many others, including fiscal parameters, by hospital type, size, ownership, geographical location, and the like. "Hospital Indicators" covers similar parameters, and also publishes special studies. An advantage of "Hospital Indicators" is its frequency of appearance.

Certain provider-perspective hospital utilization data also appear in *Health Resources Statistics*, a National Center for Health Statistics data source published on an annual/biennial basis and *Health: U.S.*, which has appeared annually since the mid-1970s. The NCHS counts hospitals in a slightly more comprehensive manner than does the AHA (National Center for Health Statistics, 1979a, p. 303). It also compiles hospital utilization data slightly differently.

Of course, it should be pointed out that, in addition to publishing provider-perspective hospital utilization data, *Hospital Statistics*, "Hospital Indicators," and *Health Resources Statistics* are the major sources of hospital census data.

Conclusion

In the United States, a great deal of data concerning the population, its health, and how it uses the health care delivery system are collected. As we have seen, not all of these data are consistent with one another. This lack of consistency may result in part from a lack of coordination of data-collection efforts. Furthermore, there is the obvious gap between the provider perspective and the patient perspective on the counts of events. One effort to introduce coordination to the collection of health data is the Cooperative Health Statistics System.

The Cooperative Health Statistics System (CHSS) operates under the specific legislative authority of Section 306(e) of the Public Health Service Act.* The CHSS was established by Congress for the purpose of producing comparable and uniform health information at the national, state, and local levels. States participating in the system designate a state agency to administer or be responsible for the administration of the statistical activities within the state under the system. Operating under guidelines prescribed by the Secretary of the Department of Health and Human Services, the statistical activities under the system are to produce uniform and timely data and assure health data users appropriate access to such data. The National Center for Health Statistics assists states participating in the system by means of: (1) contracts and grants in the development and implementation of the Cooperative Health Statistics System, (2) short-term training, and (3) technical assistance. Research, development, demonstrations, and evaluations of the system are undertaken and supported by NCHS.

Nevertheless, there are criticisms of the federal statistical collection, reporting, and analysis system. A study of it by the Congressional Office of Technology Assessment found "federal data collection activities . . . to be overlapping, fragmented, and often duplicative" (Office of Technology Assessment, p. iii).† In brief, the report recommended that a "strengthened coordinating and planning unit within [HHS]" be established that "would embody three basic characteristics: sufficient authority to impose decisions on agencies; the necessary statistical and analytical capabilities to conduct activities requiring technical expertise and judgment; and adequate resources to build a viable core effort" (Office of Technology Assessment, p. 55).

*This paragraph was supplied by the office of Ruth Hanft, Deputy Assistant Secretary of the USDHHS for Health Research, Statistics and Technology, 1980.

†This report is especially valuable to students of the federal data system and its users. It not only describes the existing data collection activities and the way they are organized and supervised, but also presents and analyzes all of the statutory authorities establishing them.

Regardless of the problems with the system, however, we do know a great deal about health, disease, and illness in the United States, and about the functioning of the U. S. health care delivery system. There are gaps in our knowledge, to be sure; some of them will be filled if the provisions of the National Health Resources Planning and Development Act (P. L. 93–641, Sect. 1513, b, 1) relating to data are carried out. These requirements, which call for the mandatory national collection of data on population health status, health care delivery system utilization, effects of the health care delivery system on health, health care delivery resources, and environmental and occupational exposure factors relating to health, will if met constitute the biggest step forward in health data assemblage since the organization of the Vital Statistics System. By 1980, however, little movement forward had occurred, although the act was passed in 1974. Despite these problems with the data themselves, however, what we need to remember above all is that data mean little until they are put to use.

References

American Hospital Association. *Hospital Statistics*, for the years 1975 and 1978. Chicago, 1976 and 1979.

Andersen, R. "Health Status Indices and Access to Medical Care." *American Journal of Public Health, 68*, 458, 1978.

Balinsky, W., and Berger, R. "A Review of the Research on General Health Status Indexes." *Medical Care, 13*, 283, 1975.

Bergner, M., et al. "The Sickness Impact Profile: Validation of a Health Status Measure." *Medical Care, 14*, 57, 1976.

Bureau of the Census. *Statistical Abstract of the United States: 1979*. Washington, D.C.: Department of Commerce, USGPO, 1979.

Bush, J. W., et al. "Health Indices, Outcomes, and the Quality of Medical Care." In Yaffe, R., and Zalkind, D., Eds., *Evaluation in Health Services Delivery*. New York: Engineering Foundation, 1975.

Center for Disease Control. *Morbidity and Mortality Weekly Report Annual Summary, 1978*. Vol. 27, No. 54, September 1979.

Grove, R. D., and Hetzel, A. M. *Vital Statistics Rates in the United States: 1940–1960*. Washington, D.C.: National Center for Health Statistics, USDHEW, 1968.

Hanft, R. Personal communication, December 21, 1979.

Jonas, S. "Physician Visits." *American Journal of Public Health, 64*, 204, 727, 1974. (Letters)

Kaplan, R. M., et al. "Health Status Index: Category Rating versus Magnitude Estimation for Measuring Levels of Well-Being." *Medical Care, 17*, 501, 1979.

Kessner, D. M., et al. *Infant Death: An Analysis by Maternal Risk and Health Care*. Washington, D.C.: Institute of Medicine, National Academy of Sciences, 1973.

Koran, L. "The Reliability of Clinical Methods, Data and Judgments." *New England Journal of Medicine*, 293, 695, 1975.

Morris, J. N. *Uses of Epidemiology*. Baltimore: Williams and Wilkins, 1964.

National Center for Health Statistics. "Origin, Program and Operation of the U. S. National Health Survey." *Vital and Health Statistics*, Series 1, No. 1, August 1963.

————. "National Ambulatory Medical Care Survey: Background and Methodology: United States—1967–1972." *Vital and Health Statistics*, Series 2, No. 61, April 1974a.

————. "The National Ambulatory Medical Care Survey: Symptom Classification." *Vital and Health Statistics*, Series 2, No. 63, May 1974b.

————. "Current Estimates from the Health Interview Survey: United States—1973." *Vital and Health Statistics*, Series 10, No. 95, October 1974c.

————. "Serum Uric Acid Values of Youths 12–17 Years: United States." *Vital and Health Statistics*, Series 11, No. 152, August 1975.

————. "Limitation of Activity Due to Chronic Conditions: United States—1974." *Vital and Health Statistics*, Series 10, No. 111, June 1977.

————. *Health Resources Statistics: Health Manpower and Health Facilities*, 1976–77. Hyattsville, Maryland: DHEW Pub. No. (PHS) 79–1509, USGPO, 1979a.

————. "Physician Visits: Volume and Interval Since Last Visit—United States—1975." *Vital and Health Statistics*, Series 10, No. 128, April 1979b.

————. "Current Estimates from the Health Interview Survey: United States—1978." *Vital and Health Statistics*, Series 10, No. 130, November 1979c.

————. "Utilization of Short-Stay Hospitals: Annual Summary of the United States, 1977." *Vital and Health Statistics*, Series 13, No. 46 March 1980a.

————. "Provisional Statistics, Births, Marriages, Divorces, and Deaths for 1979." *Monthly Vital Statistics Report*, 28, No. 12, March 14, 1980b.

————. "The National Ambulatory Medical Care Survey." *Vital and Health Statistics*, Series 13, No. 44, April 1980c.

————. "Final Natality Statistics, 1978." *Monthly Vital Statistics Report*, 29, No. 1, Supp., April 28, 1980d.

Ninth Revision International Classificaton of Diseases, Adapted for Use in the United States. Hyattsville, Maryland: National Center for Health Statistics, USDHHS, 1979.

Office of Health Resources Opportunity. *Health Status of Minorities and Low Income Groups*. Washington, D.C.: DHEW Pub. No. (HRA) 79–627, USGPO, 1979.

Office of Technology Assessment. *Selected Topics in Federal Health Statistics*. Washington, D.C.: USGPO, 1979.

P. L. 93–641. Health Planning Resources and Development Act of 1974. Washington, D.C.: U.S. Congress.

Rosen, G. *A History of Public Health*. New York: MD Publications, 1958.

Sackett, D. L., et al. "The Development and Application of Indices of Health: General Methods and a Summary of Results." *American Journal of Public Health*, 67, 423, 1977.

Worthington, N. L. "Expenditures for Hospital Care and Physicians' Services: Factors Affecting Annual Changes." *Social Security Bulletin*, November 1975, p. 3.

4

Health Manpower

Ruth S. Hanft

Introduction

With this chapter, we begin our consideration of the personnel and institutional inputs to the health care delivery system in the United States, with emphasis on physician manpower. The health care industry is labor-intensive; consequently, the education and use of health manpower is a critical variable in determining the distribution, efficiency, economy, and cost of the industry and its products. Manpower is of course not a variable standing on its own: financing, organization and delivery of health services, regulatory requirements, biomedical research, and consequent technological developments all affect the size and use of the health manpower pool.

The health care field has enjoyed a long period of expansion, with continuous growth in funding of services and programs from both the private and public sectors (see Chapter 10). Until the mid-1970s, it was not really necessary to make hard choices among programs because more money always seemed to be available and resources were relatively unconstrained. Moreover, since World War II, both the number and types of health care workers have increased greatly. Because of the open-ended flow, until recently, of third-party payments for certain types of health services, relatively few observers of the system raised questions concerning efficiency, efficacy, and cost-effectiveness, or considered the cost implications of adding new types of personnel, new technology, or new services.

Overall, the health industry is labor-intensive. Many new health services, particularly high-technology services, require large manpower inputs; as a result, they significantly affect costs. Furthermore, physicians, who are the centerpiece of the health care delivery system, create a major portion of the demand for their own services (Fuchs and Kramer; Reinhardt; Wennberg and Lapenas), as do certain other types of health manpower. Increases in the manpower pool and the development of new types of manpower tend to increase the total supply of services—more physical therapists mean that more physical therapy services will be available. Since health manpower creates its own demand, by prescribing the use of services for patients, increases in supply may well increase the demand for services. The traditional constraints of the economic market do not operate in the health field (Fuchs; see also Chapter 10).

In the late 1970s, a number of health manpower problems were being discussed in government, by the public, and among experts in the field (Graduate Medical Education National Advisory Committee; Health Resources Administration; Institute of Medicine, 1978; Subcommittee on Health and the Environment). The problems discussed included the following:

- How large a manpower pool is needed? Are we actually producing, for example, too many physicians?
- Why is the manpower to hospital-bed ratio higher in the United States than it is in any other industrialized country?
- How can the distribution of manpower by both specialty and geography be improved? Is intervention necessary?
- How many primary care physicians are needed? How many specialists? What is a primary care physician?
- Should the trends toward further specialization of professional and allied health manpower be encouraged or halted?
- Will "physicians' extenders" (e. g., physicians' associates and clinical nurse practitioners) be substitutes for physicians or will they be used instead to expand and enhance services and possibly add to health sector costs? Or will a growth in the number of physicians foreclose use of new professions?
- Should the methods of financing health professional education be altered? Should the government continue to subsidize the education of high-earning professionals when it subsidizes other professions only minimally?
- What are the implications of the United States' medical students studying abroad?

Mick has noted that a number of these problems have been with us for some time. In this chapter, we will deal with some of these questions and discuss the available information that can be used in answering them.

Types of Health Workers

For 1978, the National Center for Health Statistics recorded over 6.7 million active workers in the health field, a growth of 2.3 million in 8 years as shown in Table 4.1 The total does not include the large but unknown

Table 4.1

Persons Employed in the Health Service Industry, According to Place of Employment: United States, 1970–1978
(Data are based on household interviews of a sample of the civilian noninstitutionalized population.)

Place of employment	Year								
	1970[1]	1971	1972	1973	1974	1975	1976	1977	1978
	Number of employed persons in thousands								
Total	4,246	4,741	5,043	5,303	5,554	5,865	6,122	6,328	6,673
Offices of physicians	477	559	602	612	595	607	641	677	753
Offices of dentists	222	243	277	295	292	327	325	321	360
Offices of chiropractors	19	21	26	27	28	30	27	29	- - -
Hospitals	2,690	2,906	3,026	3,148	3,269	3,394	3,568	3,645	3,781
Convalescent institutions	509	609	682	730	798	884	945	949	1,009
Offices of other health practitioners	42	43	46	58	65	60	68	75	83
Other health service sites	288	360	384	433	507	563	548	632	687

[1]April 1, derived from decennial census; all others are July 1 estimates.
Note: Totals exclude persons in health-related occupations but who are working in nonhealth industries (as classified by the U.S. Bureau of the Census), for example, pharmacists employed in drug stores, school nurses, nurses working in private households.
Source: National Center for Health Statistics, *Health United States, 1979.* Washington, D.C.: USDHEW, 1979, Table 47. (See Appendix I, A–9.)

number of housekeeping, kitchen, and maintenance personnel who work
in the health care industry, primarily institutions. The range of skills
required in the industry is vast and overlaps those of many other industries. The sites of employment in the industry are also numerous; they
include hospitals, nursing homes, private offices, ambulatory health care
centers of various types, health maintenance organizations, research laboratories and foundations, patients' homes, elementary and secondary
schools, colleges and universities, manufacturing plants, hospital supply
companies, pharmaceutical companies, prisons, custodial institutions, and
ships. Of growing concern has been the expansion of physician manpower,
largely because of the role of the physician in stimulating the demand for
services and hence ancillary manpower. Each physician is estimated to
produce $250,000–$300,000 in demand (Reinhardt).

In terms of mode of functioning, health care providers may be divided
into three major groups: independent practitioners, dependent practitioners, and supporting staff, the lines separating the three groups being rather
unclear at times. This model is similar to that described by Eliot Friedson
in *Professional Dominance: The Social Structure of Medical Care*, New
York: Atherton Press, 1970, especially Chapter 5. The independent practitioner group consists of those health care providers allowed by law to
deliver a delimited range of services to any persons who want them,
without supervision or authorization of the practitioner's work by third
parties. Among the independent practitioners are physicians (osteopathic
and allopathic), dentists, chiropractors, optometrists, and podiatrists.

The dependent practitioner group is allowed by law to deliver to persons a delimited range of services, often of a particular type specified by
law, under the supervision and/or the authorization of independent practitioners. The dependent category includes nurses; psychologists; social
workers; pharmacists; physicians' assistants; dental hygienists; and speech,
physical, and occupational therapists.

However, in certain situations, in relation to certain patients, many of
the workers in these occupations may and can assume the role of independent practitioner. The definition of the line between the independent and
dependent groups is the source of many conflicts at present. There has
been a growing demand for independent practice status, particularly in the
nursing profession. The Rural Clinics Act (P. L. 95–210) reduced the
supervision required of nurse practitioners and physicians' assistants for
reimbursement of services under Medicare and Medicaid.

Supporting staff, rather than providing a range of services to patients,
carry out specific work tasks authorized by and under the supervision of
independent and/or dependent practitioners The work of supporting staff
may or may not be regulated by laws directly pertaining to them, but if
there are not special laws, they work under the legal sanctions provided for

their supervisors. This group includes clerical, maintenance, housekeeping, and food-processing workers, research workers, administrators, recordkeepers, nurses' aides, dental assistants, and technicians, primarily laboratory and radiological. In certain situations, some of these persons may assume the role of dependent practitioner; the struggles over status and responsibility between certain categories of supporting staff and dependent practitioners sometimes mirror those between independent and dependent practitioners.

In 1978, the largest categories of health workers were as follows: nursing and related services, 2.6 million; physicians, 424,000; dentists and allied services, 247,000; technicians and technologists; 498,000; pharmacists, 136,000 (see Table 4.2). Most health care workers are female, but most physicians, dentists, other independent health care practitioners, administrators, and other persons in policy-making positions are male (Navarro, 1975). This is changing regarding health policy positions, however. For further detail on types and roles of nurses and physicians in the United States health care system, see Chapters 5 and 6.

Compared with other nations, the United States is amply supplied with health workers. The United States has one of the highest physician-population ratios in the world, although the ratios in Belgium, Sweden, and France have been increasing rapidly as well. The U.S. physician-population ratio has increased substantially since 1970 and is expected to exceed 240 per 100,000 population by 1990 (Graduate Medical Education National Advisory Committee, p. xv; Stambler). The types of health manpower in the United States are also more varied than elsewhere—in the independent category, for example, osteopaths, podiatrists, and optometrists are virtually unknown in most other countries. The number and variety of allied manpower categories is also unique to the United States. In contrast, other nations have experimented more widely with substitutes for physicians—for example, the *feldsher* (Sidel, 1968); barefoot doctor (Sidel, 1972; Wang); and other types of auxiliaries (Fendall). With the development of the physicians' assistant/nurse practitioner mid-level health worker (see Chapter 5), the U.S. is beginning to move in the direction of physician substitutes (Scheffler et al., 1979).

Training of Health Manpower

The sites for health manpower training are numerous. Allopathic and osteopathic physicians, dentists, veterinarians, optometrists, pharmacists, podiatrists, and nurses are all trained in both independent and university-based colleges and professional schools. Nurses are also trained in hopitals, although nurse training in hospitals is declining. These various schools are found in both the public and private sectors, with a growing trend toward

Table 4.2

Persons 16 Years of Age and Over Employed in Selected Health-related Occupations: United States, 1970–1978
(Data are based on household interviews of a sample of the civilian noninstitutionalized population.)

Occupation	Year								
	1970[1]	1971	1972	1973	1974	1975	1976	1977	1978
	Number of persons in thousands								
Total, 16 years and over	3,103	3,443	3,621	3,806	3,973	4,169	4,341	4,517	4,753
Physicians, medical and osteopathic	281	309	328	344	346	354	368	403	424
Dentists	91	99	107	105	100	110	107	105	117
Pharmacists	110	113	126	123	127	119	123	138	136
Registered nurses	830	772	801	823	904	935	999	1,063	1,112
Therapists	75	92	115	109	132	157	159	178	189
Health technologists and technicians	260	289	315	330	371	397	436	462	498
Health administrators	84	115	118	137	150	152	162	175	184
Dental assistants	88	90	94	114	107	126	122	123	130
Health aides, excluding nursing	119	144	148	170	186	211	229	234	270
Nursing aides, orderlies, and attendants	718	866	912	942	959	1,001	1,002	1,008	1,037
Practical nurses	237	345	343	358	349	370	381	371	402
Other health-related occupations[2]	210	209	214	251	242	237	253	257	254

[1]Based on the 1970 decennial census; all other years are annual coverages derived from the Current Population Survey.
[2]Includes chiropractors, optometrists, podiatrists, veterinarians, dietitians, embalmers, funeral directors, lens grinders and polishers, dental lab technicians, lay midwives, and health trainees.
Source: National Center for Health Statistics, *Health United States, 1979.* Washington, D.C.: USDHEW, 1979, Table 48. (See Appendix I, A–9).

public schools and university-based institutions. In the past 15 years, most of the expansion of medical and osteopathic schools has come through state university institutions and the expansion of nursing programs through states and locally supported community colleges (see also Chapter 5).

As of 1979, there were 112 fully accredited allopathic medical schools in the United States (American Medical Association, Section II). There were an additional 13 allopathic medical schools with provisional accreditation. Allopathic medical school accreditation is carried out by the Liaison Committee on Medical Education, an agency jointly sponsored by the American Medical Association and the Association of American Medical Colleges. Although the number of U.S. medical schools increased sharply between 1960 and 1980 (there were 85 schools in 1960), and most schools have significantly enlarged their class size, the rate of growth has dropped sharply with the increasing concern over the predicted oversupply of physicians (see below).

The schools had over 46,000 full-time faculty and almost 63,000 students, a student to full-time faculty ration of 1.4 to 1. There were also over 95,000 part-time faculty. (The very low student to full-time faculty ratio is one of the reasons why medical education is so expensive. On the other hand, medical school faculty are involved to at least some degree in the teaching of about 170,000 other health science students.) Teaching for medical students was done in almost 1,600 separate clinical facilities, having about 540,000 beds and reporting 536 million outpatient visits and 284 million emergency room vists. (The visit figures do *not* correlate at all with those reported to the American Hospital Association; see Chapter 7.) For the 16,527 spaces allotted to medical students entering in the fall of 1978, there were 36,636 applicants. The applicant-to-acceptance ratio of 2.2 was down from its high of 2.8 in 1973–1975.

The average minimum curriculum time was 37 months, usually spread over 4 years. For 1977–1978, the total revenues for the 112 fully accredited schools was $4.3 billion. Of that total, 57% percent came from various government sources (American Medical Association, Table 23), down from 65% in 1976–1977.

Many of the schools that train health professional manpower have multiple functions. In medicine, for example, most schools are also centers of major biomedical research activities; are responsible for training both Doctors of Medicine (M.D.s) and basic scientists (Ph.D.s); and are involved in the training of graduate physicians at the internship, resident, and fellowship (subspecialty) levels. Faculty of medical schools also instruct nursing, dental, and other students. In addition, their own or affiliated teaching hospitals provide patient care services. Some of these hospitals are tertiary care centers for a region or a state or multiple states.

They are often the sole source of care for large indigent populations (Freymann, Section IV; Institute of Medicine, 1976).

The number of schools and hospitals engaged in health professional education and their graduates increased substantially during the decade and a half from 1965 to 1979 (Table 4.3). More than 1,600 schools in the United States provide health professions education, of which over 1,300 are for nurses.

Individual health professional schools on university campuses were being tied together into academic health science centers (Freymann, Chapter 26; Pellegrino, 1973) until the mid-1970s. The university position of vice-chancellor for health sciences, to whom deans of the individual schools would report, was created. These combinations are designed to facilitate the sharing of faculty and services, to reduce duplication in the basic science curriculum, and to provide unified management of the school and hospital. In some institutions, students in the different disciplines

Table 4.3

Graduates of Health Professions Schools and Number of Schools, According to Profession: United States, Selected Years, 1950–1977 Estimates and 1980–1990 Projections (Data are based on reporting by health professions schools.)

Year	Profession				
	Medicine	Osteopathy	Dentistry	Optometry	Pharmacy
Number of graduates					
1950	5,553	373	2,830	961	- - -
1960	7,081	427	3,290	364	3,497
1970	8,367	432	3,749	445	4,747
1975	12,714	698	4,937	806	6,886
1977	14,393	964	5,324	1,027	7,908
1980	16,086	1,069	5,150	998	7,455
1990	18,318	1,669	5,400	1,067	7,469
Number of schools					
1950	79	6	42	10	- - -
1960	86	6	47	10	76
1970	103	7	53	11	74
1975	114	9	59	12	73
1977	122	11	59	13	72
1980	121	13	60	12	72
1990	121	13	60	13	72

Source: National Center for Health Statistics, *Health United States, 1979.* Washington, D.C.: USDHEW, 1979, Table 54. (See Appendix I, A–9.)

receive some of their clinical training together, in an effort to provide team teaching and greater efficiency in the provision of services. These efforts met with some success (Pellegrino, 1975), but this trend has slowed.

Allied health manpower is trained in 4-year colleges, community colleges, proprietary technical schools, hospitals, and on-the-job training programs (McTernan and Hawkins). There is no accurate count available of the number of institutions or programs training allied health manpower. Degrees in the allied health field range from certificates of completion of less than a year of training for certain technicians and L.P.N.s to associate degrees, baccalaureate degrees, master's, and, in some cases, Ph.D. degrees.

Many health workers receive training in institutions not regarded as health professional schools. Often programs are started without regard to national or local health manpower needs, thus leading to an oversupply of certain categories of technician and therapist. People are even trained for nonexistent jobs or taught skills too narrow to be transferable. This occurred in some training programs for local residents associated with Neighborhood Health Centers funded by the Office of Economic Opportunity. Community colleges in the last 15 years have proliferated training programs in a wide variety of health and health-related fields without undertaking market research surveys.

In the professions, training can extend for many years beyond the college degree and even the first professional degree. In some programs in surgery and the subspecialties of medicine, training is as long as six or seven years past the M.D. degree. In many of the professional and allied fields, the trend has been to extend the length of training. In the professions, the postgraduate trainee is also a provider of services.

In 1978, a Work Group on the Education of the Health Professions of the National Center for Health Services Research identified a series of policy issues in health professions education that, in their view, could be subject profitably to research (Magraw et al.). They concluded that research should:

- Address relationships between what is learned in health professions education and the effect of professional intervention on the care of individual patients and the health status of the American people;
- Examine health services and the health status of people in different regions and cultures in relation to variations in health professions education and practice;
- Address the lack of attention to preventive health measures in health professions education and professional practice and by the public;
- Address the effect of educational programs aimed at diminishing professional and disciplinary insularity on practice patterns and, subsequently, on the health status of the populations served;

- Identify contributions of education and practice to professional behavior and their effect on health services, health status, and relief from discomfort;
- Relate financing and reimbursement policies for education and practice to the educational system, practice patterns, and health status;
- Provide a better understanding of how health services research can influence changes in education, practice, health status, and relief from discomfort. (pp. 543–545)

Foreign Medical Graduates

The manpower pool was augmented until 1976 by foreign-born and foreign-trained physicians and nurses. The United States no longer is a major importer of physician manpower from abroad. The Health Professions Educational Assistance Act of 1976 (P.L. 94–484) ended this trend. Between 1965 and 1973, 66,757 foreign medical graduates entered the United States, while there were 76,041 new graduates of American medical schools (Stevens, 1975). In 1974, 10,038 United States medical graduates and 6,485 foreign medical graduates were licensed to practice medicine. With the sharp reduction in the inflow of foreign medical graduates, serious house-staff personnel problems were created for some hospitals (Friedman; United Hospital Fund; Way et al.; Weinstein).

The use of foreign medical graduates (FMGs) provoked considerable debate (Butter; Friedman; Kleinman et al., 1974, 1975a, 1975b; Saywell et al.; Stevens et al.). Concern had been expressed in a number of reports about the dependence of the United States health care system on FMGs, the "brain drain" on underdeveloped nations, and the quality of the education of FMGs (Natonal Advisory Commission on Health Manpower; National Board of Medical Examiners; Association of American Medical Colleges).

Another trend, which began on a small scale in the 1920s, is now causing growing concern: U.S. students studying medicine abroad (Meskauskas et al.; Mulvihill and Rosner; Relman; Stillman et al.; Stimmel and Smith; Stimmel et al.; Stimmel and Benenson; Weinberg and Bell). Until the mid-1970s, most U.S. students studying medicine abroad attended university medical schools, most of whose students were their own country's nationals. One independent proprietary medical school at Guadalajara in Mexico served a predominantly U.S.-citizen student body, but it was almost unique. However, responding to the applicant crush of the mid-1970s, which had largely subsided by the end of the decade, a number of new foreign proprietary medical schools, catering primarily to U.S. citizens, were established (Bloom). They are located in Puerto Rico, other Caribbean islands, and Mexico. The adequacy of the undergraduate training and the ability of their students to obtain residency training are in question. Yet mechanisms to limit licensure of less than adequately trained physicians who happen to be U.S. citizens have proved difficult to develop in practice. The resolution of this situation, which will only aggravate the coming oversupply of physicians, is not yet in sight.

Costs of Education in the Health Professions

The cost of education in the eight major health professions exceeds that of virtually every other profession. The Institute of Medicine (1974) studied these costs at the request of Congress in 1973. No further studies have been conducted. The average annual cost per student by profession in 1973 is shown in Table 4.4. The costs increased by 30% or more between 1973 and 1979. Part of the reason for the high cost of education is the training process itself, which includes not only instruction but also research, patient care, and community service essential for education. Indeed, the health professions are the only ones for which the training institutions must themselves deliver the professional product in order to carry out the education—that is, a medical school must practice medicine as a school, teaching its students through that practice, whereas no law school practices law as a school, even though individual faculty members may do so.

No definite studies have been undertaken to estimate the cost of the postprofessional degree training, but these costs are also thought to be high. In the health professions, postdoctoral training is carried out in osteopathy, dentistry, medicine, and podiatry through internships and residencies. The costs of training include the stipends or salaries and fringe benefits paid to the residents, as well as faculty costs. Furthermore, many observers of the education process believe that additional health care costs are incurred through extra procedures and diagnostic tests that are part of

Table 4.4

Average Annual Cost per Student, for Education in Selected Health Professions, 1972–1973

Medicine	$12,650
Osteopathy	8,950
Dentistry	9,050
Optometry	4,250
Pharmacy	3,250
Podiatry	5,750
Veterinary medicine	7,500
Nursing	
Baccalaureate	2,500
Associate	1,650
Diploma	3,300

Source: Institute of Medicine, *Costs of Education in the Health Professions*. Washington, D.C.: National Academy of Sciences, 1974.

the educational process; these require additional equipment and allied health manpower. The patient care services provided by the graduate trainees offset these costs. Approximately 84% of house-staff time is spent in patient care (Institute of Medicine, 1976). No national cost figures are available on the training of allied health manpower.

Unlike the situation for any other profession, the public sector is now preeminent in the support of health care provider education, mainly the state government. Substantial increases in federal government support began in the late 1960s, but this support began to decline in the mid-1970s. Beginning in 1979, the Administration proposed to terminate capitation support, that is, grants based on the number of students (Office of Management and Budget). In addition, the federal government served as a catalyst for the creation of a number of new types of health manpower, particularly physician and dental extenders of various types. It also indirectly encouraged the proliferation of allied manpower through research support and the introduction of new sophisticated technologies, which require various types of technician skills (Altman and Blendon).

Until the 1960s, the federal government provided little direct support for the training of health manpower, which was regarded as a state and private responsibility. The federal government began to support the education of health professionals directly through institutional grants to the health professional schools in 1963 (Subcommittee on Health and the Environment). The support grew, and in 1971 the federal government began to provide capitation aid to educational institutions for eight health professions: medicine, osteopathy, dentistry, nursing, podiatry, pharmacy, optometry, and veterinary medicine. The federal government also supports graduate medical education and allied health manpower training in the Veterans' Administration, military, and other federal hospitals. In the late 1970s both concept and size of capitation support for the professions underwent extensive review, particularly in Congress. As indicated, in the early 1980s, there was a great deal of interest in the federal government in terminating capitation.

The government also indirectly supports the training of health manpower—both professional and allied—in hospital-based programs through the reimbursement formulas of Medicare and Medicaid (Institute of Medicine, 1976). The major indirect support for the training of physician manpower and allied health manpower comes from third-party payments to hospitals. Hospital-based training programs include the training of interns and residents, diploma nurses, and a variety of technicians. The costs of these programs are included as part of hospital costs or charges paid through patient care revenues and thus they have been hidden.

Until the 1972 Social Security Act amendments, reimbursement for hospital-based training programs was essentially open-ended, since the original reimbursement mechanisms made Medicare and Medicaid "uncontrollable" expenditures. The 1972 amendments gave the Social Security Administration more authority to determfine the "reasonableness" of reimbursements. The amendments also allowed Medicaid to deviate from the Medicare method of reimbursement of hospitals. In accordance with this legislative change, the Social Security Administration began to classify hospitals into groups and to put a ceiling on the amount paid for routine hospital costs, including graduate training costs (P. L. 92–603, Sec. 223). At the same time, Blue Cross began to question some training costs, particularly in hospitals in Pennsylvania and Michigan, and to cut back the level of support. State rate-regulation commissions began to take a hard look at these costs as well. The New York commission has limited payment for residencies. The magnitude of hospital costs that can be attributed to the education of health professionals and allied health manpower is unknown.

Tuition, except in nursing and podiatry, meets only a very small proportion of the cost of health sciences education, smaller than for any other professionals' education. There are no tuition charges for internship and resident training. As would be expected, tuition in the private institutions is substantially higher than in the public colleges and universities (Institute of Medicine, 1974). In all types of institutions, however, tax-levy money pays a significant proportion of the total costs.

Issues in Health Manpower

The major issues in health manpower under public and governmental discussion, mainly physician manpower, fall into two different categories: the size of the health care manpower pool and how it should be distributed by specialty and geographical area.

Health care manpower is but one major factor in the mix of resources that produces health services. Although the discussion that follows treats health care manpower as a separate issue, the readers should recognize that changes in the organization and delivery of services and in their financing affect the size and distribution of the health care manpower supply (Davis). In addition, an increasing proportion of experts in the field (Anderson; McKeown; Fuchs, Chapter 2) are concluding that an increase in health services (and manpower) may have only marginal effects on health. (See Chapters 2 and 15.) It may well be more crucial to turn our attention to income support, environmental protection, housing, improved nutrition, and community health services, rather than personal health services.

Size of the Health Manpower Pool

The health industry has expanded exponentially over the past 30 years, as pointed out above. The supply of physician manpower is of particular concern (Fordham; Graduate Medical Education National Advisory Committee; Health Resources Administration; Holden). The proportion of the GNP consumed for health has increased rapidly, as has the manpower employed. Without external constraints, these trends could continue. The nature and magnitude of the expenditures and the nature of the medical care cost inflation are such that artificial constraints on expenditures are beginning to be imposed. The role of the physician in generating cost and expenditures has led to efforts to determine what total supply should be. (See Chapter 10.)

To determine rationally the size of the physician manpower pool, some measure of need or demand for services is necessary (Institute of Medicine, 1976), but need and demand alone cannot be the base for determining manpower. Patterns of practice vary (Wennberg and Gittlesohn), productivity varies (American College of Surgeons; Schoenfeld et al.), and supply affects demand (Lave et al.; Reinhardt; Roddy). One can alternatively try to rely on the force of an economic market to regulate the size of the pool, regulate supply, or do some of both. This is, in general, what has been tried to date; it has not been too effective (see Chapter 10). If market mechanisms were effective, the manpower pool would expand or contract, as it does in other sectors of the economy, in relation to changes in supply and demand. The market mechanisms, however, falter because of lack of consumer information; artificial licensure and certification barriers; the nonprofit nature of most of the hospital sector; the ability of the provider to influence the demand for services; rapid changes in technology; and consumer expectations (Fuchs; Reinhardt). Only for allied health workers do market forces exercise some constraint.

The increase in physician specialization has serious cost implications (Worthington; Wennberg and Gittelsohn; Wennberg and Lapenas). For example, dermatologists will demand and receive a higher price for treating a rash than a family practitioner will demand; more rashes will be treated, but no improvement in health status will necessarily result. There is considerable uncertainty in medical practice as to effectiveness of procedures and their use (Wennberg and Lapenas). The United States and Canada have the highest population–surgery rates in the world. Data show that where there is a high surgeon-to-population ratio, there is a high surgery rate (American College of Surgeons; see also Chapter 7).

Through the 1960s, there was a widespread opinion that the United States faced a serious physician shortage (Surgeon General's Consultant

Group on Medical Education; Peterson and Pennell; National Advisory Commission on Health Manpower; Carnegie Commission on Higher Education; Johnson). However, another view, increasingly adopted, identified the problem not in terms of absolute supply of physicians, but rather in terms of what they do, what specialties they are in, and where they are geographically located (Fein; Castleton; Senior and Smith; Navarro, 1974). Current projections, as indicated earlier, are that physician-to-population ratios will double by 1990 (Health Resources Administration; Stambler).

Western European countries are experiencing the same problems. Some of these nations are beginning to limit entrance into their medical schools. Sweden, Finland, Belgium, Germany, and France have all experienced rapid increases in expenditures and their economists have reached similar conclusions to those of their U. S. counterparts. However, only some of these nations—Sweden, Canada, and Finland—can control medical school entry; the U. S., with its decentralized state-private education system, exerts much less central control.

Some of these nations also exert control on total expenditures and hence on fees and incomes for physicians. The U. S. system of financing care is also decentralized, divided among federal, state, and private sources. Without a limit on expenditures, the factors of expanded physician supply and the ability of physicians to generate demand for their own and ancillary services exacerbate cost problems.

What effect will adding more physicians have on costs and utilization of services? Will more physician services or medical services create improved health outcomes? What has happened to physician productivity? (With rising incomes, the number of hours worked by physicians per week has decreased.) These same questions can be raised about most of the specialties and subspecialties and many types of allied manpower. The answers, of course, have implications for determination of the total manpower pool and costs.

If a rational plan for the development of an optimal physician manpower pool were to be developed, the following types of informaton would be needed (Kramer and Roemer; Wennberg and Lapenas; Institute of Medicine, 1974; Graduate Medical Education National Advisory Committee):

● Data on health care needs cannot easily be measured, but adequate health care utilization data and national epidemiological data would be useful.

● Functional analysis of tasks to provide health care services, and analysis of how these tasks could be distributed within the health manpower pool. Productivity data.

- Effects of different organizational models on the use of health manpower.
- Cost implications of manpower pools of different sizes and distributions.
- Effects of substitution of capital (machinery) for labor and analysis of whether in the health care industry new capital requires expansion of manpower rather than substituting for it in a significant proportion of cases.
- The relationship of manpower distribution to health outcomes (Lave et al.; Institute of Medicine, 1976).
- Financing and reimbursement policy.

Data in all of these areas are limited and currently inadequate to develop optimal manpower numbers. A major study of physician productivity at the University of Southern California was completed in 1979, as were projections by the Graduate Medical Education Advisory Council (not published at the time of this book's writing). In fact, either dollar constraints or arbitrary numbers limitations, rather than rational planning, may well set the size of the manpower pool for the late 1980s and early 1990s.

Distribution of Physician Manpower by Geography

In the middle to late 1970s, great attention was devoted to the issues of specialty and geographic distribution (Hudson and Nourse). The geographic distributon of practicing physicians is uneven (see Table 4.5). In 1976, in South Dakota there were fewer than 81 practicing physicians per 100,000 population. In New York and Massachusetts, the practicing physician-to-population ratio exceeded 185 per 100,000, far greater than that of the nation as a whole, which was about 144 per 100,000. Part of the difference can be explained by the location in the high physician-to-population ratio states of major tertiary-care medical centers, serving patients who reside out of state. However, the most important source of these differences lies in the complex set of factors that make some areas of the country particularly attractive to physicians and others particularly unattractive.

Comparing physician-to-population ratios for areas as large as states can blur the magnitude of the geographic inequities in physician distribution within states by averaging out high- and low-distribution areas. These disparities can be truly enormous. For example, a study of the variation in physician-to-population ratios among counties in Maryland showed a range of physician concentraton from 308 per 100,000 population to 30 per 100,000 population between the most physician-rich and physician-poor counties in that state (Alexander and Bowden).

In 1979, the Secretary of the DHEW designated as having physician

Table 4.5

Active Patient-Care Physicians, Civilian Population, and Physician-to-Population Ratios, 1976

State	Civilian population July 1, 1976 (× 1,000)	MDs per 100,000 population	DOs per 100,000 population	Total physicians per 100,000 population
TOTAL	212,296	137	7	144
Alabama	3,640	89	0	89
Alaska	357	79	1	80
Arizona	2,243	141	17	158
Arkansas	2,099	88	1	89
California	21,234	172	1	173
Colorado	2,535	153	10	163
Connecticut	3,106	178	1	179
Delaware	576	131	9	140
D.C.	693	359	1	360
Florida	8,326	139	10	149
Georgia	4,912	108	2	110
Hawaii	831	147	3	150
Idaho	824	90	3	93
Illinois	11,191	135	3	138
Indiana	5,295	100	3	103
Iowa	2,869	97	14	111
Kansas	2,283	112	9	121
Kentucky	3,390	105	1	106
Louisiana	3,815	106	0	106
Maine	1,059	113	18	131
Maryland	4,099	169	1	170
Massachusetts	5,797	186	3	189
Michigan	9,090	121	28	149
Minnesota	3,962	143	1	144
Mississippi	2,331	82	0	82
Missouri	4,750	122	23	145
Montana	747	105	2	107
Nebraska	1,541	113	1	114
Nevada	600	109	4	113
New Hampshire	818	135	2	137
New Jersey	7,306	142	13	155
New Mexico	1,152	106	10	116
New York	18,057	198	3	201
North Carolina	5,370	112	0	112
North Dakota	631	96	1	97
Ohio	10,675	125	12	137
Oklahoma	2,734	99	17	116
Oregon	2,326	141	8	149
Pennsylvania	11,852	140	17	157
Rhode Island	922	162	9	171
South Carolina	2,778	95	0	95
South Dakota	680	78	3	81
Tennessee	4,193	117	1	118
Texas	12,331	113	7	120
Utah	1,223	134	1	135
Vermont	476	162	6	168
Virginia	4,887	122	1	123
Washington	3,556	138	5	143
West Virginia	1,820	104	4	108
Wisconsin	4,607	117	4	121
Wyoming	386	90	2	92

Source: AMA Distribution of Physicians in the U.S., 1976, American Osteopathic Association. (See Appendix I, A–9.)

shortages areas in which the physician-to-population ratio was less than 1 primary-care physician for 4,000 people. More than 1,667 areas were so designated; more than 36 million people live in them.

In the past several years, efforts have been made to alter the geographic imbalances. The data on factors that influence geographic distribution are not clear, however. The following factors have contributed to the imbalances:

• The content of the training programs at the undergraduate and graduate medical education levels, including the site of clinical training (Mason; Weber).
• The selection of medical students; where they were raised; and their interests (Balinsky; National Center for Health Services Research).
• The social and cultural amenities of given geographic areas (Sloan; Steinwald and Steinwald).
• For location choice, the peer contact available in different areas, including the existence of medical schools, area health education centers, and contact with other physicians, particularly through organized group-practice arrangements.
• Geographic disparities in fees for the same services.

Study of economic influences has just begun. Data on physicians' income are not available geographically or in small regions, but fee differences are available. Analyses of physician fee levels shows that high prevailing charges and high fees tend to correlate with high physician-to-population ratios (Institute of Medicine, 1976). There is some evidence that shifts in physician distribution are correlated with shifts in the geographic distribution of relative per capita income (Clark and Koontz).

To encourage physicians to locate in underserved areas, the federal government is supporting two major programs (Comptroller General; Mullan), the National Health Service Corps and Area Health Education Centers (P. L. 92–157, 1971). The first is designed to place physician and nonphysician health manpower in areas designated as health manpower scarcity areas. This endeavor was greatly strengthened by provisions of H. R. 94–484 (1976). By 1979, almost 2,000 National Health Service Corps physicians were deployed in underserved areas. Area health education centers are designed to provide peer contact, continuing education, and remote-site training in rural areas. Since these programs are relatively new, it is somewhat early to assess their impact. Yet anecdotal reports from North Carolina report success (Health Resources Administration). Some additional anecdotal, as yet undocumented, reports indicate that with the increased supply of physicians, geographic spillover is beginning. The states of Colorado, Vermont, and New Hampshire now indiciate that they have few geographic gaps in distribution. Recent data show that board-certified physicians are moving into nonmetropolitan areas (Schwartz and Newhouse).

Primary Care

The concept of the physician who would coordinate the full range of services for the patient and perhaps the family emerged as a leading health manpower issue of the 1970s (Institute of Medicine, 1978; Scheffler et al., 1978). A major effort is underway to increase the ratio of primary care physicians to specialists.

There is a perceived imbalance of physicians between primary care and certain specialties, if primary care is defined as general internal medicine, pediatrics, and family practice. The imbalance is between primary care and general surgery and subspecialties in medicine and pediatrics (Institute of Medicine, 1976; Roddy). There is little agreement as to what the right ratios are, and international data show that specialty ratios vary widely from country to country (see Table 4.6; these data are available only every 10 years.)

Table 4.6

Physician Distribution by Contact and Specialty Areas, Selected Countries, 1970

Country	Total Physicians	General and Family Practice, Internal Medicine, Pediatrics[a]		Specialist Physicians		Others	
		N	%	N	%	N	%
Canada	31,166	15,557	49.9	9,556	30.7	6,053	19.4
England & Wales	59,791	29,304	49.0	18,217	30.5	12,270	20.5
France	68,000	48,408	71.2	19,592	28.8	—	—
German Fed. Rep.	105,976	74,067	69.9	25,597	24.1	6,312	6.0
Israel	7,281	5,386	73.9	2,029	27.9	168	2.3
Japan	117,195	52,904	45.1	43,400	37.1	20,891	17.8
Netherlands	16,292	6,632	40.7	4,401	27.0	5,259	32.3
New Zealand	3,232	1,648	51.0	919	28.4	665	20.6
N. Ireland	2,015	1,097	54.4	807	40.1	111	5.5
Norway	5,361	3,942	73.5	1,674	31.2	6	.1
Scotland	6,769	4,255	62.9	2,168	32.0	346	5.1
S. Africa	10,912	8,925	81.8	1,943	17.8	44	.4
Sweden	10,950	8,568	78.2	4,039	36.9	—	—
Switzerland[b]	8,890	3,578	40.3	2,140	24.1	3,382	38.0
USA	323,203	150,932	46.7	152,537	47.2	19,734	6.1
USSR	577,300	239,300	41.5	212,500	36.8	125,500	21.7

Source: World Health Statistics Annual, 1970, vol. 3. Geneva: World Health Organization, 1974.
[a]Includes subspecialties of internal medicine and pediatrics.
[b]Some multispecialty physicians are included in more than one category.

Compared to other developed countries, the United States has fewer primary physicians and more specialists per population.

Current U.S. data (Table 4.7) show that there has been little increase in primary-care specialties as a proportion of total physicians since 1970, despite major efforts to increase the proportion.

Complicating the problem is the lack of a firm agreement on the definition of primary care or the distribution of tasks among health professionals, including physicians. For example, the AMA regards obstetricians and gynecologists as primary-care providers; the Institute of Medicine (1976) does not. There is extensive literature on the definitional problems (Alpert and Charney; Draper and Smits; Jonas, 1973; Parker; Petersdorf, 1975; Silver and McAtee; Hudson and Nourse; Kirkham; Ruby et al.). Definitional problems and overlap exist among the specialties and the various professional organizations, with little agreement as to the use of specialists, subspecialists, and generalists for a wide range of conditions—fractures, rashes, emotional upsets, childbirth, and other. Even less agreement exists as to the transfer of certain functions from physicians to other manpower, such as nurse-midwives and clinicians. (See also Chapter 6, on primary care.)

The 1978 Institute of Medicine study avoids defining such care in terms of types of professionals. Primary care is defined (Institute of Medicine, 1978) as: ". . . accessible, comprehensive, coordinated and continual care provided by accountable providers of health services. It is generally recognized as the first level of personal health services. . . . where initial professional attention is paid to current or potential health problems. Frequently primary care is associated with care of the 'whole person' rather than care for an illness." (p. 2).

The definition of primary care and who is a primary-care physician has obvious implications for medical education at the undergraduate level, numbers of residency programs by specialty, federal and state manpower training support, and the roles of nurse practitioners and physicians' assistants. There is growing evidence that some form of primary care is provided by surgeons, obstetricians, and the subspecialties in medicine and pediatrics (Mendenhall et al.; American College of Surgeons; Aiken et al.)

Even though consensus has not been reached as to the definition of primary care and who is to provide it, public policy actions have been taken to stimulate "primary-care training." Since graduate medical education is critical in altering specialty distribution, the support available to the different specialty training programs is important. It is more difficult to support ambulatory-care-oriented graduate medical education programs in primary-care specialties than programs in other specialties. The reasons include the benefit packages under insurance programs and the way outpatient hospital services are reimbursed under private health insurance programs, Medicare, and Medicaid (Institute of Medicine, 1976).

Since 1971, the federal and state governments have tried to ameliorate specialty imbalance. In the area of increased primary-care training, the federal government provided special project grant support for family practice residencies (P. L. 92–157, 1971); general internal medicine; and pediatrics (P. L. 94–484). Some state governments are providing direct appropriations for training in primary care. In addition, the National Health Service Corps scholarships give preference to candidates in primary care. The structure of the scholarship program allows only three years for residency training before service is required—too short a time period for surgical and subspecialty training.

Congressional testimony by the AMA based on 1975 residency data indicated that changes were beginning to occur in the distribution of residency positions (Nesbitt). These data show increases in filled positions in primary-care residency positions—defined by the AMA as internal medicine, pediatrics, family practice, and obstetrics and gynecology—and a decline in surgical residencies. However, the data include obstetrics and gynecology and subspecialty training in internal medicine and pediatrics. Subsequent data have not clarified the actual trends, since many residents in internal medicine and pediatrics continue residencies or fellowships in the subspecialties.

While there will be a substantial increase in physician-to-population ratios in this decade (Graduate Medical Education National Advisory Committee; Stambler), there are no current control mechanisms to assure that the increases will provide better ratios in primary care, however defined. An extensive debate continues as to whether the medical profession can exert the internal discipline to provide more equitable geographic and specialty distributions of physicians without direct federal government intervention (Aiken et al.; Angrist; Fordham; Holden; Louria; Petersdorf, 1978).

Several recent reports have recommended that commissions be established to determine the number of residency positions needed, by specialty (Institute of Medicine, 1976; Macy Foundation). The Graduate Medical Education Advisory Council established by the Secretary of DHEW in 1977 sought to determine the number of physicians needed by specialty and was expected to issue its final report in 1981 (Graduate Medical Education Advisory Council). The role of the Health Systems Agencies (see Chapter 12) in manpower distribution is unclear. For many of the agencies the first priority is control of facilities and other capital expansion.

Table 4.7

Professionally Active Physicians (M.D.s), According to Primary Specialty: United States, Selected Years 1970–1977
(Data are based on reporting by physicians.)

Primary specialty	Year					
	1970	1972	1974	1975	1976	1977
	Number of physicians					
Professionally active physicians	304,926	315,522	325,567	335,608	343,876	359,515
Primary care	115,505	120,876	124,572	128,745	134,051	139,248
General practice[1]	56,804	54,357	53,152	53,714	54,631	54,361
Internal medicine	41,196	47,343	51,143	53,712	57,312	61,278
Pediatrics	17,505	19,176	20,277	21,319	22,108	23,609
Other medical specialties	17,127	16,282	17,220	18,743	18,702	19,656
Dermatology	3,937	4,166	4,414	4,594	4,755	4,844
Pediatric allergy	388	379	423	439	469	485
Pediatric cardiology	471	505	521	527	537	563
Internal medicine subspecialties[2]	12,331	11,232	11,862	13,183	12,941	13,764
Surgical specialties	84,545	89,666	92,123	94,776	97,416	100,059
General surgery	29,216	30,518	30,672	31,173	31,899	32,014
Neurological surgery	2,537	2,716	2,824	2,898	2,959	3,049
Obstetrics and gynecology	18,498	19,820	20,607	21,330	21,908	23,038

Ophthalmology	9,793	10,318	10,621	11,011	11,326	11,483
Orthopedic surgery	9,467	10,216	10,861	11,267	11,689	12,223
Otolaryngology	5,305	5,563	5,509	5,670	5,788	5,910
Plastic surgery	1,583	1,770	2,075	2,224	2,337	2,509
Colon and rectal surgery	663	645	655	655	667	652
Thoracic surgery	1,779	1,899	1,909	1,960	2,020	2,131
Urology	5,704	6,201	6,390	6,588	6,823	7,050
Other specialties	87,749	88,698	91,652	93,344	93,707	100,552
Anesthesiology	10,725	11,740	12,375	12,741	13,074	13,815
Neurology	3,027	3,438	3,791	4,085	4,374	4,577
Pathology	10,135	10,881	11,274	11,603	11,815	12,260
Forensic pathology	193	187	192	186	203	206
Psychiatry	20,901	22,319	23,075	23,683	24,196	24,689
Child psychiatry	2,067	2,242	2,384	2,557	2,618	2,877
Physical medicine and rehabilitation	1,443	1,503	1,557	1,615	1,665	1,742
Radiology	10,380	11,772	11,485	11,417	11,627	12,062
Diagnostic radiology	1,941	2,055	3,054	3,500	3,794	4,236
Therapeutic radiology	855	920	1,060	1,161	1,202	1,305
Miscellaneous[3]	26,082	21,641	21,405	20,796	19,139	22,783

[1]Includes general practice and family practice.

[2]Includes gastroenterology, pulmonary diseases, allergy, and cardiovascular diseases.

[3]Includes occupational medicine, general preventive medicine, aerospace medicine, public health, other specialties not listed, and unspecified specialties.

Note: Federal and nonfederal active M.D.s in the 50 states and the District of Columbia are included. Physicians not classified, inactive physicians, and physicians with unknown address in the United States are excluded. For 1977 this includes 17,953 physicians not classified, 28,231 physicians inactive, and 10,946 physicians with unknown address.

Source: National Center for Health Statistics, *Health United States, 1979.* Washington, D.C.: USDHEW, 1979, Table 51. (See Appendix I, A–10.)

The state of the art of manpower planning in terms of total numbers and distribution by function, specialty, and geography is still primitive. Fine tuning of manpower and its distribution is decades off.

Trends in manpower in the industry have been toward greater specialization of both professional and allied health manpower (Freymann, Chapters 5, 11, 12; Health Resources Administration; Stevens, 1971). While the recent debate has focused on the imbalances of specialists and generalists in medicine, these same trends exist in the allied health field, with a proliferation of new technician and nursing categories and new allied health professions. (See also Chapter 5.) The nation rarely heard of an oncologist (specialist in cancer) or an inhalation therapist 20 years ago. Functions previously performed by one person are assigned to more than one. With every new technological development, one or several new allied health titles are born, as are physician specialties. As cost constraints continue, attention will be focused on allied manpower as well

Problems in Medical Education

The problems in the medical education process and in the educational institutions are linked to the problems in health manpower distribution and the delivery of services, particularly the distribution of physicians by specialty and geography, and costs. The medical education community and the public have been engaged in a serious debate regarding the role of medical schools in producing physicians. Much of this debate can be found in testimony related to Health Manpower Legislation presented in 1974 and 1975 (Subcommittee on Health) before the Congress in the Health Manpower Hearings and in the discussions between the professional associations and the DHEW. The positions and arguments change little over time. The issues being debated include the medical schools' responsibility for training primary-care physicians; the medical schools' responsibility for graduate medical education programs; the appropriate curricula and training sites for the development of primary-care physicians; the medical schools' possible role in improving the supply of physicians in underserved areas; and constraining the rise in health care costs. Leading figures in medical education expressed serious concern over the changing relationship between government and the medical schools (Cooper, 1978; Rogers). Pleas were made to government for understanding and flexibility and to the schools for creativity, resourcefulness, and responsiveness.

The medical school, the orientation of its curriculum, and the sites used for training are the critical components of health professions education. The training of the physician as generalist or specialist; the inpatient or outpatient orientation of the training; a curriculum related to prevention and public health; social and economic factors; team teaching; and team practice all influence the way the physician practices, where he practices, and how he uses other services (Jonas, 1979).

Medical education evolves slowly and the changes it does make are only gradually reflected in the health care delivery system because of the length of the education process. The education of a physician takes from 10 to 15 years after graduation from high school. To affect the choices of physicians regarding specialty and geography, intervention would be needed at the college, medical school, residency, and practice levels.

Historical Factors

Historically, several major trends influenced the current orientation of medical schools. The Flexner Report, originally published in 1910, was very significant (Flexner, 1960). Flexner is credited by some with initiating the modern medical education system (Cooper, 1979; Ebert). David Banta, among others, has pointed out that Flexner was not an initiator as much as he was a summarizer, catalyzer, and publicizer of change. Nevertheless, it is the so-called Flexnerian model that is followed by most American medical schools today. This model has five principal requirements (Richmond):

1. That a minimum of 2 years of undergraduate college work be required for admission to medical school;
2. That a 4-year curriculum be employed, with 2 years in the basic medical sciences, followed by 2 years of supervised clinical work on both inpatient and outpatient hospital services;
3. That regular laboratory teaching exercises be included;
4. That a high level of quality of instruction be maintained through the use of full-time faculty; and
5. That the medical schools be within the framework of the universities. (p. 3)

These five elements reflect only some of the many recommendations that were made by Flexner (Jonas, 1979, Chapter 8); they reflect in particular the model of medical education that had been developed at the Johns Hopkins University School of Medicine since its opening in 1893. One result of the Flexner Report was a sharp decline in the number of proprietary medical schools, which had been very prominent until that time, as well as in the preceptorship-apprenticeship orientation of clinical medical education.

Following World War II, the federal government decided to give financial support to biomedical research in the medical schools, rather than in the science departments of parent universities. This decision was strongly influenced by the adamant opposition of the American Medical Association to direct federal aid to medical education. Supporting biomedical research in medical schools was one way that the federal government could indeed support medical education without appearing to do so directly. This approach had the effect of orienting the medical schools and their faculties toward research (Strickland, Chapters 3 and 4). The availability of research grants to support faculty salaries allowed the medical schools to expand the scope of faculty capabilities in specialties and subspecialties.

The technological breakthroughs achieved in the 1940s, 1950s, 1960s, and 1970s, combined with the growing desire of World War II veterans to enter specialty training, changed the emphasis of graduate medical education toward greater specialization and training in highly sophisticated hospital settings.

State legislatures expected their medical school hospitals to be the source of tertiary care and skilled care for large regions or whole states, as in the cases of the Universities of Colorado, Washington, Indiana, Iowa, and Mississippi. Both before and after the implementation of Medicare and Medicaid, the states also expected the public medical school hospitals to care for their indigent populations. The university-owned and university-associated hospitals of many private medical schools found, as populations shifted from the city to suburbs, that they were located in low-income areas and were the principal source of outpatient and inpatient care for large low-income populations.

Need for Community Exposure

By and large, medical schools and their teaching hospitals are located in large cities, offering few opportunities for clinical training in rural areas. Because of the hospital-based, specialty-oriented nature of graduate medical education and teaching hospitals (Mumford), undergraduate and graduate medical students get little exposure to office-based or group practice. One of the problems in altering specialty and geographic distribution of physicians and in providing primary-care training is the need to develop nonhospital-based training and training in small communities, with close and adequate supervision of the trainees by medical school faculty (Petersdorf, 1975). Several experiments in the 1970s aimed to train undergraduate and graduate students in office-based sites, community hospitals, and small communities (Breisch; Steinwald and Steinwald). Some examples include the University of Indiana statewide system; the University of Illinois extensions in Rockford and Peoria (Evans et al.); the University of Washington WAMI (Washington, Alaska, Montana, Idaho) system; the George Washington University HMO; and preceptor-training programs, such as the one at Dartmouth. A number of medical schools developed programs designed to train physicians to deal with the very serious health care delivery system problem of cost-containment (Hudson and Braslow).

There has been a growing trend toward a new type of medical school with the emergence of new state medical schools. These newer schools, for example, Eastern Virginia, the University of Illinois at Rockford, University of South Alabama, and the University of Nevada, rely more on decentralized community hospitals, outpatient settings, and use of preceptorships than do the older schools with strong tertiary-care hospital affiliations. Objectives-based curriculum design is a major element of the programs in new medical schools at Southern Illinois University (Silber et al.); the University of Illinois at Urbana-Champaign(Sorlie); and the University of Missouri at Kansas City (University of Missouri at Kansas City). In the early 1980s, the Texas College of Osteopathic Medicine, at Forth Worth, another new school, took the lead in developing a fundamentally health- and prevention-oriented curriculum along the lines proposed by Jonas in 1979 (Texas College of Osteopathic Medicine). Federal intervention through project grants under the Health Professions Education Act of 1971 for family medicine and primary care; state support for primary care; and the priority given in the National Health Service Corps scholarships provide incentives for these changes. Strong disincentives, however, continue to exist in third-party reimbursement systems for the support of primary care and outpatient training (Institute of Medicine, 1976; National Center for Health Services Research).

Health sciences education functions, particularly in medical schools, are just one of a number of activities. Medical schools and, to a lesser extent, other professional schools perform multiple functions of education, research, patient care, and community service. The missions are mixed and the internal and external actions affecting one functon has ripple effects on the others.

During the 1940s, 1950s, and early 1960s, the influx of money for biomedical research, combined with technologic advances, spurred the trend toward specialization. The 1960s saw an interest in patient care and community service, spurred by reimbursement from Medicare and Medicaid. However, the differentials paid to specialists under these programs provided further incentives for specialization. Yet the federal government's OEO program highlighted and stimulated the need for primary care and primary-care training.

The flow of reimbursement that continued through the 1970s and its impact on physician earnings created a disincentive for physicians to embark on biomedical research careers. With the leveling of biomedical research and the reduction in training grants, this trend is accelerating (Office of Management and Budget).

The 1960s saw entry of the federal government into health sciences education, to stimulate an expanded supply of physicians and in the 1970s to address issues of geographic and specialty distribution (Health Resources Administration). A regulatory revolution also began in the 1970s, affecting all aspects of medical school activities. Health planning agencies began looking at capital investment for patient-care facilities. Medicare and Medicaid placed limits on hospital reimbursement at all sites, including medical school teaching hospitals, affecting the ability of medical-school-affiliated hospitals to support residencies and teaching physicians. Biomedical research funds declined in real dollars, affecting medical school financing of faculty and training of M.D.s for research careers. Federal support of education shifted from general support to support for specific projects, such as primary-care training and curriculum changes.

Conclusions

The trends in the 1980s in terms of public policy are uncertain. The impact of public and private activities during the last 30 years are also uncertain, although some comments can be made with reasonable certainty.

The health manpower supply has expanded rapidly in the past 30 years, in response to increased expenditures for health care and new technology. Combined with this expansion, an accelerating trend toward specialization developed. In the past several years, concern has grown regarding inequities in distribution of manpower by specialty and geography and the influence and cost of the training process for health professional manpower; these concerns continue.

A major public policy discussion is taking place regarding the following: the size of the manpower pool and whether its growth should be constrained; a change in the balance between primary-care manpower and specialty manpower; greater equity in the geographic distribution of health professional manpower; the role of training in influencing specialty and geographic distribution; and the role of the public and private sectors in effecting change. The sources of support of undergraduate and graduate medical education are being reevaluated, as are the sources of support for biomedical research and patient care. The constraints on economic resources and the inflation in the medical care sector of the economy require more analysis of choices in the health manpower field, but are more closely related to choices in support of all aspects of health care and social programs.

References

Aiken, L. H., et al. "The Contribution of Specialists to the Delivery of Primary Care." *New England Journal of Medicine, 300,* 1363, 1979.

Alexander, C. A., and Bowden, G. R. *Physician Manpower in Maryland, 1973.* Baltimore: University of Maryland School of Medicine, 1974.

Alpert, J., and Charney, E. *The Education of Physicians for Primary Care.* Washington, D. C.: Bureau of Health Services Research, USDHEW Pub No. (HRA) 74–3113, Autumn, 1973.

Altman, S. H., and Blendon, R., Eds. *Medical Technology: The Culprit Behind Care Costs?* Washington, D. C.: Office of Health Research, Statistics, and Technology. DHEW Pub. No. (PHS) 79–3216, USGPO, 1979.

American College of Surgeons and the American Surgical Association. *Surgery in the United States: A Summary Report of the Study on Surgical Services to the U.S.* Chicago, 1975

American Medical Association. "Medical Education in the United States, 1978–79." *Journal of the American Medical Association,* Vol. 243, No. 9, March 7, 1980.

Anderson, O. W. *Health Care: Can There Be Equity?* New York: Wiley, 1972.

Angrist, A. A. "Now Too Many Physicians!" *New York State Journal of Medicine,* January 1979, p. 15.

Association of American Medical Colleges. "Graduates of Foreign Medical Schools in the United States: A Challenge to Medical Education." *Journal of Medical Education, 49,* 809, 1974.

Balinsky, W. L. "Distribution of Young Medical Specialists from Western New York." *Medical Care, 12,* 437, 1974.

Banta, H. D. "Medical Education: Abraham Flexner—A Reappraisal." *Social Science and Medicine, 5,* 655, 1971.

Bloom, M. "The 'Other' Medical Schools"; "Coming Home." *Medical World News,* May 28, June 11, 1979.

Breisch, W. F. "Impact of Medical School Characteristics on Location of Physician Practice." *Journal of Medical Education, 45,* 1068, December, 1970.

Butter, I. *Foreign Medical Graduates: A Comparative Study of State Licensure Policies.* Rockville, Maryland: National Center for Health Services Research. DHEW Pub. No. (HRA) 77–3166, 1976.

Carnegie Commission on Higher Education. *Higher Education and the Nation's Health.* New York: McGraw-Hill, 1970.

Castleton, K. B. "Are We Building Too Many Medical Schools?" *Journal of the American Medical Association, 216,* 1989, 1971.

Clark, L. J., and Koontz, T. L. "Analysis of the Impact of the Hill-Burton Program on the Distribution of the Supply of General Hospital Beds and Physicians in the United States, 1950–1970." Paper delivered at the annual meeting of the American Public Health Association, November 1973, San Francisco, California.

Comptroller General. *Progress and Problems in Improving the Availability of*

Primary Care Providers in Underserved Areas. Washington, D. C.: General Accounting Office, Pub No. (HRD) 77–135, Aug. 22, 1978.

Cooper, J. A. D. "Academic Medical Centers and Government: An Indispensable Partnership." *Journal of Medical Education, 53*, 998, 1978.

————. "Testimony Submitted by the Association of American Medical Colleges to the Subcommittee on Labor-Management Relations, Committee on Education and Labor, U.S. House of Representatives." Washington, D.C.: Association of American Medical Colleges, July 19, 1979, p. 2.

Davis, K. "Financing Medical Care: Implications for Access to Primary Care." In Andreopoulos, S., Ed., *Primary Care, Where Medicine Fails*. New York: Wiley, 1974.

Draper, P., and Smits, H. "The Primary-Care Practitioner—Specialist or Jack-of-All-Trades." *New England Journal of Medicine, 293*, 903, 1975.

Ebert, R. H. "The Medical School." *Scientific American, 229*, No. 3, 138, 1973.

Evans, R. L., et al. "The Community-Based Medical School: Reactions at the Interface between Medical Education and Medical Care." *New England Journal of Medicine, 288*, 713,1973.

Fein, R. *The Doctor Shortage*. Washington, D. C.: Brookings Institute, 1967.

Fendall, N. R. E. *Auxiliaries in Health Care: Programs in Developing Countries*. Baltimore: Johns Hopkins Press, 1972

Flexner, A. *Medical Education in the United States and Canada*. The Carnegie Foundation for the Advancement of Teaching, 1910. Reprinted, Washinton, D.C.: Science and Health Publications, 1960.

Fordham, C. C. "Public Policy and Health Manpower." *Science, 204*, 459, May 4, 1979.

Freymann, J. G. *The American Health Care System: Its Genesis and Trajectory*. New York: Medcom Press, 1974.

Friedman, E. "FMGs, Hospitals, P.L. 94–484, and the Future." *Hospitals*, June 16, 1979, p. 74; July 1, 1979, p. 58.

Fuchs, V. *Who Shall Live?: Health Economics and Social Change*. New York: Basic Books, 1974.

Fuchs, V., and Kramer, M. J. "Determinants of Expenditures for Physicians' Services in the United Stastes 1948–1968." Washington, D. C.: USDHEW Pub. No. (HSM) 73–3013, December 1972.

Graduate Medical Education National Advisory Committee (GMENAC). *Interim Report*. Washington, D.C.: DHEW Pub. No. (HRA) 79–633, USGPO, 1979.

Health Resources Administration. *A Report to the President and Congress on the Status of Health Professions Personnel in the United States*. Washington, D.C.: DHEW Pub. No. (HRA) 78–93, USGPO, 1978.

Holden, W. D. "A Perspective of Physician Manpower." *New England Journal of Medicine, 300*, 493, 1979.

Hudson, J. I., and Braslow, J. B. "Cost Containment Education Efforts in United States Medical Schools." *Journal of Medical Education, 54*, 835, 1979. (See also five additional papers in same issue.)

Hudson, J. I., and Nourse, E. S., Eds. "Perspectives in Primary Care Education." *Journal of Medical Education*, 50, Part 2, December 1975.

Institute of Medicine. *Costs of Education in the Health Professions*. Washington, D.C.: National Academy of Sciences, 1974.

——————. *Medicare-Medicaid Reimbursement Policies*. Washington, D. C.: National Academy of Sciences, 1976.

——————. *A Manpower Policy for Primary Health Care*. Washington, D. C.: National Academy of Sciences, 1978.

Johnson, R. L. "Physician Shortage Threatens Health Proposals." *Hospitals, J.A.H.A.*, July 1, 1972, p. 53.

Jonas, S. "Some Thoughts on Primary Care: Problems in Implementation." *International Journal of Health Services*, 3, 77, 1973.

——————. *Medical Mystery: The Training of Doctors in the United States*. New York: W. W. Norton, 1979.

Kirkham, F. T. "Issues in Primary Care: The 1976 Annual Health Conference: New York Academy of Medicine." *Bulletin of the New York Academy of Medicine*, 2nd. Ser., 53, 1977.

Kleinman, J. C., et al. "Physician Manpower Data: The Case of the Missing Foreign Medical Graduates." *Medical Care*, 12, 906, 1974.

Kleinman, J. C., et al. "Postgraduate Training and Work Experience of Non-ECFMG Certified Physicians in the U.S." *Medical Care*, 13, 305, 1975a.

Kleinman, J. C., et al. "A Reply to Stevens, Goodman and Mick." *Medical Care*, 13, 445, 1975b.

Kramer, C., and Roemer, R. "Health Manpower and the Organization of Health Services" Institute of Industrial Relations: University of California at Los Angeles, 1972. Mimeographed.

Lave, J. R., et al. "Medical Manpower Models: Need, Demand and Supply." *Inquiry*, 12, 97, June 1975.

Louria, D. B. "Coping with the Approaching Doctor Glut." *New England Journal of Medicine*, 300, 1047, 1979.

McKeown, T. *The Role of Medicine: Dream, Mirage, or Nemesis*. London: The Nuffield Provincial Hospitals Trust, 1976.

McTernan, E. J., and Hawkins, R. O., Eds. *Educating Personnel for the Allied Health Professions and Services*. St. Louis, Missouri: C. V. Mosby, 1972.

Macy Foundation. *Physicians for the Future: Report of the Macy Commission*. New York, 1976.

Magraw, R. M., et al. "Health Professions Education and Public Policy: A Research Agenda." *Journal of Medical Education*, 53, 539, 1978.

Mason, R. "Medical School, Residency, and Eventual Practice Location: Toward a Rationale for State Support of Medical Education." *Journal of the American Medical Association*, 223, 49, 1975.

Mendenhall, R. C., et al. *Practice Profiles in 24 Specialties*. Los Angeles: University of Southern California School of Medicine, Division of Research in Medical Education, 1979.

Meskauskas, J. A., et al. "Performance of Graduates of Foreign Medical Schools on the Examinations of the American Board of Internal Medicine." *New England Journal of Medicine, 297,* 808, 1977.

Mick, S. S. "Understanding the Persistence of Human Resource Problems in Health." *Health and Society, 56,* 463, 1978.

Mullan, F. S. M. "The National Health Service Corps." *Public Health Reports,* Supplement to July–August 1979 issue. (Also has seven additional articles and a bibliography.)

Mulvihill, J. E., and Rosner, F. "Americans Studying Medicine Abroad." *New York State Journal of Medicine,* April 1979, p. 774.

Mumford, E. *Interns: From Student to Physician.* Cambridge, Massachusetts: Harvard University Press, 1970.

National Advisory Commission on Health Manpower. *Report.* Vols. I and II. Washington, D. C.: USGPO, 1967.

National Board of Medical Examiners. "Evaluation in the Continuum of Medical Education." *Report of the Committee on Goals and Priorities of the NBME.* Philadelphia, 1973.

National Center for Health Services Research. *Financing Graduate Medical Education.* Hyattsville, Maryland: USGPO, 1979.

National Center for Health Statistics. *Health: United States, 1979.* Washington, D.C.: USDHEW, 1979.

Navarro, V. "A Critique of the Present and Proposed Strategies for Redistributing Resources in the Health Sector and a Discussion of Alternatives." *Medical Care, 12,* 721, 1974.

————. "Women in Health Care." *The New England Journal of Medicine, 292,* 398, 1975.

Nesbitt, T. Testimony before Subcommittee on Health, Committee on Labor and Public Welfare. U.S. Senate, Washington, D. C., November 18, 1975.

Office of Management and Budget. *U.S. Budget—1981.* Washington, D. C.: USGPO, 1980.

Parker, A. W. "The Dimensions of Primary Care: Blueprints for Change." In Andreopoulos, S., Ed., *Primary Care: Where Medicine Fails,* pp. 15–77. New York: Wiley, 1974.

Pellegrino, E. D. "The Regionalization of Academic Medicine: The Metamorphosis of a Concept." *Journal of Medical Education, 48,* 119, 1973.

————. "The Academic Role of the Vice President for Health Sciences: Can a Walrus Become a Unicorn?" *Journal of Medical Education, 50,* 211, 1975.

Petersdorf, R. G. "Issues in Primary Care: The Academic Perspective." *Journal of Medical Education, 50,* Part 2, p. 5, December 1975.

————. "The Doctors' Dilemma." *New England Journal of Medicine, 299,* 628, 1978.

Peterson, P. Q., and Pennell, M. Y. "Physician-Population Projections 1961–1975: Their Causes and Implications." *American Journal of Public Health, 53,* 163, 1963.

P. L. 92–157. *Amendments to Title VII of the Public Health Service Act.* U.S. Congress, Washington, D.C.

P. L. 92–603. *National Health Planning and Resources Development Act of 1974.* U.S. Congress, Washington, D. C.

P. L. 93–641. *Social Security Act Amendments of 1972.* U.S. Congress, Washington, D.C.

P. L. 94–484. *Health Professions Educational Assistance Act of 1976.* U.S. Congress, Washington, D.C.

P. L. 95–210. *Rural Clinics Act of 1977.* U.S. Congress, Washington, D.C.

Reinhardt, U. *Physician Productivity and the Demand for Health Manpower.* Cambridge, Massachusetts: Ballinger, 1975.

Relman, A. S. "Americans Studying Medicine Abroad." *New England Journal of Medicine,* 299, 887, 1012, 1978.

Richmond, J. *Currents in American Medicine: A Developmental View of Medical Care and Education.* Cambridge, Massachusetts: Harvard University Press, 1969.

Roddy, P. C. "Need-Based Requirements for Primary Care Physicians." *Journal of the American Medical Association,* 243, 355, 1980.

Rogers, D. E. "On Preparing Academic Health Centers for the Very Different 1980's." *Journal of Medical Education,* 55, 1, 1980.

Ruby, G., et al. "Definitions of Primary Care." Washington, D. C.: Institute of Medicine, 1977. Photocopy.

Saywell, R. M., et al. "A Performance Comparison: USMG–FMG Attending Physicians." *American Journal of Public Health,* 69, 57, 1979.

Scheffler, R. M., et al. "A Manpower Policy for Primary Health Care." *New England Journal of Medicine,* 298, 1058, 1978.

Scheffler, R. M., et al. "Physicians and New Health Practitioners: Issues for the 1980s." *Inquiry,* 16, 195, 1979. (This paper has an extensive bibliography.)

Schoenfeld, H. K., et al. "Numbers of Physicians Required for Primary Medical Care." *New England Journal of Medicine,* 286, 571, 1972.

Schwartz, W., and Newhouse, J. *A Study Report: Do Board Certified Specialists Diffuse? Facts and Theory.* Santa Monica, California: Rand Corporation, 1979.

Senior, B., and Smith, B. A. "The Number of Physicians as a Constraint on Delivery of Health Care." *Journal of the American Medical Association,* 222, 178, 1972.

Sidel, V. W. "Feldshers and Feldsherism." *New England Journal of Medicine,* 278, 934, 981, 1968.

————. "The Barefoot Doctors of the People's Republic of China." *New England Journal of Medicine,* 286, 1292, 1972.

Silber, D. L., et al. "The SIU Medical Curriculum: Systemwide Objectives-Based Instruction." *Journal of Medical Education,* 53, 473, 1978.

Silver, H. K., and McAtee, P. R. "A Descriptive Definition of the Scope and Content of Primary Health Care." *Pediatrics,* 56, 957, 1975.

Sloan, F. "Economic Models of Physician Supply." Ph.D. dissertation, Harvard University, 1968.

Sorlie, W. E. *A Word About SBMS-UC*. Urbana-Champaign, Illinois: University of Illinois, 1979.

Stambler, H. V. "Health Manpower for the Nation—A Look Ahead at the Supply and Requirements." *Public Health Reports, 94*, 3, 1979.

Steinwald, B., and Steinwald, C. "The Effect of Preceptorship and Rural Training Programs on Physicians' Practice Location Decisions." *Medical Care, 13*, 219, 1975.

Stevens, R. *American Medicine and the Public Interest*. New Haven, Connecticut: Yale University Press, 1971.

————. "Physician Migration Reexamined." *Science, 190*, 440, 1975.

Stevens, R., et al. *The Alien Doctors*. New York: Wiley, 1978.

Stillman, P. L., et al. "Students Transferring into an American Medical School." *Journal of the American Medical Association, 243*, 129, 1980.

Stimmel, B., and Benenson, T. F. "United States Citizens in Foreign Medical Schools and the Future Supply of Physicians." *New England Journal of Medicine, 300*, 1414, 1979.

Stimmel, B., and Smith, H. "Career Choice and Performance on State Licensing Examinations of 'Fifth Pathway' Students." *New England Journal of Medicine, 299*, 227, 1978.

Stimmel, B., et al. "Clinical Performance and Specialty Choice of COTRANS Students." *Journal of the American Medical Association, 241*, 139, 1979.

Strickland, S. P. *Politics, Science and Dread Disease*. Cambridge, Massachusetts: Harvard University Press, 1972.

Subcommittee on Health. *Health Manpower Legislation, 1975*. Washington, D.C., USGPO, 1975.

Subcommittee on Health and the Environment. *Current Health Manpower Issues*. Washington, D.C.: Committee Print 96–IFC–34, USGPO, 1979.

Surgeon General's Consultant Group on Medical Education. Report. *Physicians for a Growing America*. Washington, D.C.: Public Health Service, USDHEW, 1959.

Texas College of Osteopathic Medicine. *Design of the Medical Curriculum in Relation to the Health Needs of the Nation*. Fort Worth, Texas, 1980.

United Hospital Fund. *Foreign Medical Graduates in New York City*. Proceedings of the Health Policy Forum. New York, June 1978.

University of Missouri at Kansas City. *The Academic Plan for the School of Medicine*. Kansas City, Missouri, 1979.

Wang, V. L. "Training of the Barefoot Doctor in the People's Republic of China: From Prevention to Curative Service." *International Journal of Health Services, 5*, 475, 1975.

Way, P. O., et al. "Foreign Medical Graduates and the Issue of Substantial Disruption of Medical Services." *New England Journal of Medicine, 299*, 745, 1978.

Weber, G. I. *An Essay on the Distribution of Physicians Amongst Specialties*. Washington, D.C.: USDHEW Pub. No (OS) 171–71, 1973.

Weinberg, E., and Bell, A. I. "Performance of United States Citizens with Foreign Medical Education on Standardized Medical Examinations." *New England Journal of Medicine, 299,* 858, 1978.

Weinstein, B. M. "The Foreign Medical Graduate Issue and U.S. Hospitals." *Journal of the American Medical Association, 241,* 917, 1979.

Wennberg, J. E., and Gittlesohn, A. "Consumer Characteristics and Physician Choice as Determinants of Health Care Consumption." Burlington: University of Vermont, 1975. Mimeographed.

Wennberg, J. E., and Lapenas, J. D. "On Choosing the Numbers of Needed Physicians." Prepared for the GMENAC Panel on Geographic Variations. Washington, D. C.: Health Resources Administration, DHEW, January 1980.

Worthington, N. L. "Expenditures for Hospital Care and Physicians' Services: Factors Affecting Annual Changes." *Social Security Bulletin, 38,* 3 November 1975.

5

Nursing

Nancy Barhydt-Wezenaar

The development of the nursing profession, its history, its present status and problems, and its prospects for future change and growth are discussed with emphasis placed on their impact on the total health care system. The largest single category of health manpower consists of a wide range of health care providers that are grouped together under the single rubric, "nursing." The providers are distinguished by title, training, job description, salary, requirements for credentials, and educational background. They include the licensed practical nurse (L. P. N.) with one year of training in a hospital; the registered nurse (R. N.) with a 2-year associate degree or diploma from a hospital-affiliated school; the R. N. with a baccalaureate degree from a 4- or 5-year collegiate program; and the R. N. with a master's degree or doctorate, representing up to 9 years of training. Additionally there are nurses' aides, assistants, and nursing technicians, all with a variety of training programs and job descriptions whom patients, not knowing the fine distinctions, often call "nurse."

In nursing, which is both an art and a science, certain principles are applied in the delivery of quality health care to the sick and to the well. It involves highly complex relationships with a multitude of health care providers, increasingly depends on technology, and demands a high level of clinical decision-making. Nursing is equally concerned with the prevention of disease and conservation of health and uses a holistic approach. The profession as a whole has been engaged for many years in a struggle to broaden its role. According to Bonnie Bullough, 38 states have now amended their nurse practice acts to facilitate role expansion for registered nurses. She notes that several approaches are being used in these laws, including mandating new board regulations, expanding the definitions of nursing, increasing the power of physicians to delegate, and mandating the use of standardized protocols to guide the practice of nurses who are accepting new responsibilities (Bullough, 1976).

As is well known, the vast majority of nurses are women—in fact, as was pointed out in the previous chapter, the vast majority of all health workers

are women (Ehrenreich). However, most independent health professionals, as the term is used in the preceding chapter, and most administrators
are men. This fact lends an added significance to the conflict over "the
expanding role of the nurse."

Historical Development of Nursing*

The nursing profession, which was shaped by the apprentice system as an
arm of hospital administration rather than as a clinical department, developed during an era when relatively few women attended college (O. W.
Anderson). As early as the colonial period, women were serving as auton-
omous healers or general practitioners, as well as midwives (Ehrenreich).
Anne Hutchinson, the religious reformer, was a general practitioner, and
Harriet Tubman, the black leader who guided many slaves to freedom,
worked as both nurse and doctor. Practice by these female "lay" healers
was suppressed and outlawed when physicians established themselves as
the legal and official medical profession and relegated women to a subsidi-
ary position. During the mid-19th century, it was a rare woman indeed
who was accepted into medical school; those few who were, were excluded
from medical associations and from the male collegial referral system
(Kushner). Most women were left with only one career choice in health
care—nursing.

The evolution of the medical and nursing professionals was thus com-
plementary. Two distinct occupations emerged where there had once been
a single generalized "healer": nurses took on the responsibility for "caring";
physicians were concerned with "curing" and the technical functions. The
sexism pervading the health care delivery system in this country has its
roots in early 19th-century medicine. This division of labor also had economic implications: technology could be profitably used in private enterprise, caring could not. Thus the medical division of labor contributed to
the downgrading of the nurse (Ehrenreich).

During the Victorian era, hospital nursing was considered by many to be
a disreputable occupation; nurses were often depicted in the literature as
lewd, drunken, and dishonest (Kushner). Florence Nightingale (1820–
1910) deserves a great deal of credit for encouraging "well-bred" young
women to emancipate themselves from their subservient role in the home
by providing scientifically based nursing at the hospital. However, these

*A useful history of the nursing workforce in the United States is found in
Kathleen Cannings and William Lazonick's "The Development of the Nursing
Labor Force in the United States: A Basic Analysis," *International Journal of
Health Services*, 5, 185, 1975.

lowly paid women, forced to do menial tasks, were simply freed from one straitjacket only to be strapped into another (Bullough, 1975). Nightingale did, however, suggest that nurses, like doctors, be required to take examinations and be licensed. State licensure throughout the United States was finally achieved in 1923, on a voluntary basis, at least, but it did not remove the stigma of "women's work." In the disciplined environment of the nursing school, nurses were taught the traditional feminine qualities, submissiveness and obedience. This conventional existence, complete with a set of social values—curfew, dress rules, lights out—did not support individual initiative or self-confidence in nursing (Kushner).

Florence Nightingale's philosophy for those dedicated women perpetuated the "feminine mystique" in the nursing profession. Nurses were expected to treat doctors with wifely obedience, to devote a mother's loving care to patients, and to supervise hospital personnel with the condescension of the household manager dealing with maids, butlers, and grocery boys (Navarro). However, this stereotype is dying as a new breed of nurses emerges, aided by the women's movement and changes in the health care delivery system.

Nursing has come a long way toward the kind of independence that is a prerequisite for either competitive practice or a collaborative one. The introduction of the nurse practitioner into the health care system has caused much controversy in the nursing community as well as considerable confusion for the consumer of health services. This occurred because the nurse practitioner concept was implemented in a variety of settings and with many different types of formal training, ranging from 6-week certification programs to 2-year graduate programs. Nurses now are able to function more creatively. The end result of this creativity may well be to make the nurse's role separate from but equal to that of the physician, which would not only raise nurses' status but could also ultimately improve the quality of patient care.

In 1971, the AMA and the American Nurses Association (ANA) together established the National Joint Practice Commission; the Commission sponsored experimental joint practice or collaborative practices throughout the country. Additionally, nurse practitioners have joined joint practices with physicians in private offices. Acceptance has been slow, but the concept remains that the two professionals can jointly work out the best health care plan for the patient for whom both are responsible. "Professional turf" must be relinquished with true delegation of responsibility.

It appears that society has come of age and understands the significance of health and illness care. It not only demands the best in terms of quality and the widest range of services, but it also demands that such services be delivered by providers who are free, accountable, and unencumbered by constraints that counteract consumer interests (Mauksch).

Education Programs in Nursing

There are hundreds of training programs for nurses at all levels of proficiency in many different types of institutions, including hospitals, 2- and 4-year colleges, universities, and a wide variety of graduate programs. Of 25,365 full-time and 5,221 part-time nurses employed as faculty members in nurse education programs, 52% have been prepared on a master's or doctoral level, 36% at the baccalaureate level, 3% at the diploma level, and 1.5% at the associate degree level (Moses and Roth). Approximately 5,624 faculty members are employed in the training of licensed practical nurses. The United States Office of Education has recognized the National League for Nursing as the official accrediting agency for master's, baccalaureate, associate degree, diploma, and practical nursing programs (Walsh). For the nondegree nurse practitioner programs, the American Nurses Association has become the accrediting body.

Practical Nursing Programs

Practical nursing programs prepare men and women to give nursing care under the supervision of a registered nurse or a physician to patients who require less complicated nursing procedures (National League for Nursing, 1974–75). In more complex situations, the licensed practical nurse functions as an assistant to the registered nurse to release the professional nurses from "bedside" nursing level of care. Preparation for licensure as an L. P. N. is usually completed in a 1-year program, although programs range in length from 8 to 24 months (National League for Nursing, 1974–75). Each program establishes its own admission requirements; academic requirements as well as tuition and fees vary from state to state. Satisfactory completion of a state-approved program in practical nursing is required before the nurse is permitted to take the examination for licensure, given by the state Boards of Nursing. Licensed practical nurses are employed in a wide variety of health care facilities, including hospitals, extended care facilities, nursing homes, and clinics. The number of L. P. N.s is growing rapidly. There are 1,300 programs that prepare L. P. N.s in the United States; 39 of the programs are in New York State. More than 46,000 were graduated from schools of practical nursing in 1976 (Rowland).

Registered Nursing

Registration in nursing means licensure for nurses who have completed a higher level educational program than that needed for the L. P. N. All states had enacted legislation providing for voluntary registration by 1923 (Bullough, 1975); under this system a registered nurse was defined in terms of educational requirements met and examinations passed, not in terms of work tasks performed. Registration merely conferred the privilege of using the letters R. N. after one's name, much like contemporary

certification in other health care occupations (Chapter 14). The first mandatory licensing law, which did define a body of work, was not passed until
1938, in New York State.

Associate degree programs.   Among the available academic prepara-
tions for registered nursing is the community college offering an associate
degree program. First instituted in 1952, these programs continue to
proliferate as hospital programs slowly diminish (National League for
Nursing, 1976b). By 1975, the 618 associate degree programs accounted for
nearly one-half of all nursing education programs.

With some variations, a number of features are basic to the associate
degree programs. Most are conducted under the auspices of public, junior,
or community colleges. They vary in length from two academic years to two
calendar years, with the program of study combining nursing courses and
related college courses. The students must meet requirements of the
college to be admitted to the nursing program and on completion they are
granted the associate in Arts degree. The associate degree nursing programs prepare students to take state board examinations to become registered nurses. College credits earned in the associate degree programs
often can be applied toward a baccalaureate degree in nursing, should a
graduate decide to pursue further education (National League for Nursing,
1976b).

Registered nurses with associate-level degree work for the most part in
hospitals or other institutions as general-duty or staff nurses engaged in
giving direct care to the sick. They are sometimes referred to as "bedside"
nurses. Since these nurses give direct care to patients, they must possess
considerable technical knowledge and skill, and must understand the
scientific principles of nursing care. It should be noted, however, that
associate degree nurses are not prepared for teaching on a collegiate level
or for total patient management. Unfortunately, many nurses now carry
out the latter functions by default, since agencies and institutions place
these nurses in positions for which they are not fully trained. Consequently, institutions and health care providers are often not altogether happy
with the performance of the associate degree graduate, because they often
impose extra expense upon hospitals for remedial training programs (Lenberg, 1980).

A recent innovation in the education of nurses at the associate degree
level leads to an external degree in nursing. One example, authorized by
the New York State Board of Regents in 1971, is a degree program
approved by the State Department of Education in 1973. This program
makes it possible for candidates to earn an external degree with or without
formal in-residence courses; it is completed entirely on the basis of independent study. During the course of study, the student must take seven
high-quality, standardized examinations. If the student passes these ex-

aminations, a final Clinical Performance Nursing Examination is administered, in which nursing knowledge equal to that of students who complete the associate degree program in a collegiate institution must be demonstrated. The student is then qualified to take state board examinations for licensure as an R. N. The first class was graduated in 1974. The New York Board of Regents also has developed a program to grant an external bachelor of science degree in nursing (Lenberg, 1976).

Diploma programs. Another setting for preparation as a registered nurse is the school that awards its graduates a diploma in nursing. These schools, which may apply for accreditation by the National League for Nursing, are usually under the control of a hospital, although in some instances they are independently incorporated. The predominance of diploma programs has declined markedly in the past 15 years. In 1975, they accounted for only 30% of all nursing education programs, as compared with over 80% in 1960. The diploma programs suit qualified high school graduates who desire a program centered in a community institution that is identified with the care of patients. As opposed to the situation in a college-based program, both students who want an early opportunity to be with patients and health services personnel and those who want to prepare for beginning staff positions in hospitals and similar institutions find diploma programs attractive (National League for Nursing, 1976a).

The school of nursing may enter into cooperative relations with collegiate or other institutions to provide certain courses of study needed to meet the requirements for graduation. The nursing courses combine theory with practice, reinforcing learning through experience with caring for medical and surgical patients, mothers, children, and the mentally ill. According to the National League for Nursing or NLN, (1976a), graduates of accredited diploma programs in nursing:

1. Know basic scientific principles, and utilize them in planning and giving quality nursing care to people;
2. Recognize the indications of diseases and disabilities, and the psychological, social, and physical needs of patients;
3. Have the understanding and the skills necessary to organize and implement a plan of nursing care that will meet the needs of groups of patients and promote the restoration of health;
4. Are qualified to plan for the care of patients with other members of the health care team and to direct other members of the nursing team;
5. Are qualified for general duty nurse positions in the medical, surgical, obstetrical, pediatric, and psychiatric nursing areas of the hospitals and similar community institutions;

6. Need to be oriented to new work situations as beginning practitioners and to be given time and opportunity to become increasingly effective in the practice of nursing.

Graduates of a school offering a program approved by a state board of nurse
examiners are eligible to take the state examination for licensure to practice
as registered nurses.

Baccalaureate Degree Programs

A baccalaureate degree program in nursing prepares graduates for the
general practice of professional nursing. The first collegiate school was
founded in 1909. In this program the student earns a B. S. degree and also
becomes eligible to take a state licensing examination. The program must
include all learning experiences required to prepare the student to practice
professional nursing in all environments where health care is offered and in
any setting where the need for nursing care manifests itself (Ozimek). A
baccalaureate degree program prepares the beginning practitioner of professional nursing as a generalist, capable of providing health care to persons, families, and groups in a variety of settings through the utilization of a
nursing process that incorporates both scientific and humanistic concepts.
Moreover, it provides an educational base upon which graduate study for
specialization as a clinician, teacher, administrator, or researcher in nursing may be built. The program emphasizes intellectual skills such as
problem-solving, critical thinking, and decision-making, as well as interpersonal and technical skills.

In these 4-year programs, the nursing major is concentrated in the last 2
years and is built upon a broad general education in natural and social
sciences. The nursing major focuses on the entire life span and total health
care needs of persons and families, rather than solely on an individual and
an acute episode of illness. Emphasis is on prevention, teaching, intervention, restoration, and rehabilitation (Ozimek).

There are those who support the concept that no conclusive evidence
suggests that a 4 to 5-year education program at the baccalaureate level
produces a better nurse than does the 3-year diploma program. The
transferring of nurse education from a hospital to a campus aids the nurses'
general education, but dilutes the essential part of the education and direct
contact with patients (Reichow and Scott).

Advanced Education Programs

Advanced education consists of "sequences of professional courses aimed
at developing specialized qualifications characterized by formal academic
recognition of completion, such as the awarding of a degree" (Bullough and
Bullough, 1977).

Graduate programs. Graduate programs in nursing education prepare the registered nurse for more complex practice as a clinical specialist, a nurse practitioner, a nursing administrator, or a teacher. Many nurses prepare for such positions by completing a course leading to a master's degree. One well-known area of study at this level is public health. Most baccalaureate undergraduate programs prepare their students for beginning level staff positions in public health agencies, but those who hold a master's degree provide the backbone of nursing administration in public health departments at state and local levels throughout the country.

Doctoral level work. Doctoral level work in nursing offers preparation for careers in research, teaching, and educational administration (Abdellah). Increasingly, these highly qualified nurses are engaging in both basic and clinical research—particularly the latter, where the objectives are for improved clinical practice and quality patient care. Several major assumptions are basic to the doctoral program. They are:

1. Nursing is a legitimate and important field of graduate study in which faculty and students search to verify nursing knowledge regarding the sciences and modes of caring. A special focus is placed on ways to apply this knowledge to promote, improve, and sustain human health.
2. Doctoral programs will provide an intellectual climate to formulate and test knowledge and skills relevant to the different dimensions of nursing.
3. No academic discipline has come into being without substantive research related to identifying, defining, and refining its knowledge base.
4. Doctorally prepared nurses are a national asset, an excellent investment for health protection and maintenance of people.
5. The health care systems are undergoing drastic changes and need scholars who will identify new pathways in health care services.

Several critical issues have been identified: (1) federal and state funds are limited and doctoral education is expensive; and (2) how to prepare a sufficient number of well-qualified deans for the complex and large university schools of nursing.

The Doctorate of Nursing Science is a practice-oriented professional degree; the research-oriented academic degree is the Ph. D. Currently, there is some indication that the Ph. D. is favored. There is a greater interest in the Midwest in doctoral programs than anywhere else in the country (Leininger).

Continuing Education Programs

Continuing education (C. E.) for nurses is defined as "formalized learning experiences or sequences designed to enlarge the knowledge or skills of practitioners. As distinct from advanced education, continuing education tends to be more specific, of generally shorter duration, and may result in certification or completion of specialization, but not formal degrees" (Bullough and Bullough, 1977).

Continuing education is an increasingly important aspect of professional life, both for active nurses and for returning inactive nurses. State nursing associations and selected interest groups have set up committees to deal with the many problems involved in ensuring that C. E. programs maintain certain standards. One such committee, appointed by the Midwest Continuing Educational Professional Education for Nurses (MCEPEN), had as its objectives the identifying of local C. E. needs and the setting up of mechanisms for planning and coordinating C. E. efforts in their area (Forni and Bolte).

One of the current issues in regard to C. E. is whether it should be mandatory for continued licensure. While one state had enacted such legislation as of 1980 (California) and several others were considering doing so, nursing leaders were divided on this question. Other important issues are how the costs of presenting high-grade programs can be met, whether and by what standards credits should be given for various offerings, how to obtain uniformity in quality of programs, and how to secure adequately trained faculty. (Similar questions obtain for continuing education for virtually all categories of health professional.) A criticism of continuing education providers is that they frequently fail to measure and evaluate the results of the C. E. program, and that the C. E. program unit (C. E. U.) becomes merely an attendance record (Reichow and Scott).

Continuing education does not necessarily have to take place in a classroom setting. For example, one psychiatric nurse practitioner working in a mental health center in a small town taped conferences with a group of outpatients, added comments and questions to the tapes, and mailed them to a more experienced clinician in a distant city. The clinician evaluated and returned the tapes with comments and recommendations in time for the practitioner to have them before the next meeting with the group (Lego).

Nurse internship programs are developing to help new graduates bridge the gap between being a student and being an independent practitioner. Because of the differences in preparation of nurses coming from three distinct types of nursing education programs, internship programs may also be integrated into undergraduate curricula. One such experiment, in which the investigator dubbed the course "Technoterm," has been reported in detail (Treece).

In-service education programs. Programs that are administered by an employer and are "designed to upgrade the knowledge and skills of employees for their functioning in that agency" are referred to as in-service education programs. Both active and inactive returning nurses benefit from these courses, which are usually given in the work setting. Many hospitals and other care agencies employ a full-time in-service education director.

Issues in nursing education. There is a great deal of concern regarding education for all those who are licensed to practice nursing. There are strong feelings among many educators that education should take place in institutions of higher education and that the official recognition given to the graduates of associate degree programs should be as "technical nurses," as distinguished from "professional nurses." There are indications that the minimum preparation for professional nursing practice should be at the baccalaureate degree level, and the minimum preparation for "technical nursing practice" should be at the associate degree education level. Currently, examinations for accepted nursing practice are available only for the L. P. N.s and professional nurses, with little differentiation between graduates of 2-, 3-, or 4-year programs. Graduates of associate degree programs are eligible to take the same examination and obtain the same licensure as graduates from the 4- to 5-year baccalaureate programs. Upon successful passing of these examinations, both become known as R. N.s. Few employing agencies make any clear distinction between the different levels of preparation the nurses have received. Often there is preference given to the graduate of a program that provided the student with greater clinical experience; this is usually the diploma program. However, there is a movement to eliminate the diploma programs. It is projected that by 1985 such programs will either be extinct or will account for only 1% of the new admissions (Diers). The elimination of diploma programs may appear contrary to the expressed needs to close the gap between academia and employers (Reichow and Scott).

Federal Government Support for Nursing Education

The first federal support program for nonmilitary nursing education, developed to meet war needs, lasted from July 1941 to July 1943. It provided funds for refresher courses for inactive nurses, grants for teachers and other nursing personnel, the preparation of nurses for advanced administrative positions, and increased enrollment in nursing schools (Bullough and Bullough, 1974). The United States Cadet Nurse Corps, which was directly related to the military, provided nursing students with free education and uniforms, as well as a small monthly stipend for a maximum of 30 months. In return, the students had to promise to serve in the armed forces or in a critical civilian nursing capacity after graduation.

Broad federal support for nursing education became available under the Nurse Training Act of 1964 (P. L. 88–581), which aimed to increase the number of nurses capable of providing quality nursing care. Federal assistance programs authorized direct support for students, operating expense money for nursing schools, funds for construction of nursing education facilities, and support for demonstration projects to improve nurse training. The Act allowed hospital training programs and schools of nursing to raise educational standards, expand facilities, and reorganize curricula to implement the developing new philosophies in nursing education and to provide expanding career ladders (Bullough and Bullough, 1974). Open curriculum, independent study, and self-paced learning are all curriculum innovations designed to encourage people to enter nursing and to be free to change career goals without penalty. The Health Manpower Act of 1968, Title II, broadened the programs for all three major types of schools of nursing. The Nurse Training Act of 1971 further expanded federal aid in the form of capitation grants to schools of nursing for the purpose of increasing enrollments and providing advanced education for certain categories of nurses and nursing practitioners. The 1971 Act, with continuing resolutions through 1978, also made grants to schools in financial distress as well as special project grants for new nurse-training programs (Report to the Congress). At the end of the 1970s, the Carter Administration tried several times without success to terminate federal support for nursing education.

In a study conducted in 1978 by the U.S. Health Resources Administration (DHEW), the average cost per student per year for nursing education in the diploma programs was found to be $4,334; in associate degree programs, $4,349; and in baccalaureate degree programs, $10,231. These identified costs take into account the tuition, fees, and books, and allow for the different lengths of training (Moses and Roth).

Data on Nurses
Supply of Nursing Personnel

The ratio of nurses to population has increased steadily from 249 per 100,000 in 1950 to 500 per 100,000 in 1979. In contrast, during the same period the physician-to-population ratio went from 141 to 150 per 100,000 (USDHEW, 1979). In 1977 there were 1,401,633 registered nurses holding current licenses to practice in the United States. Of that total, 70% were employed in nursing (45% full-time), 3% were seeking nursing employment, and the remaining 27% were not seeking employment in nursing at the time of a survey conducted by the *American Journal of Nursing* (Moses and Roth). It is significant that so many qualified R. N.s (about 400,000) do not work in nursing; clearly shortages of nurses in many areas could be at least partly dealt with by attracting inactive nurses back to work—even if only on a part-time basis during the childbearing years—by providing refresher courses and continuing education as needed (Moses and Roth).

The R. N. population is still predominantly female. It is estimated that only 26,991 of the 1,401,633 nurses licensed to practice in 1977 were men. The median age of the nurse population was 39.8 years; the median family income was $19,889. The average salary for nurses was significantly lower in the South Atlantic states and the east southern central and west north central areas of the country than in the country as a whole. It was significantly higher in the Pacific area (Rowland).

The U.S. Public Health Service claims that 20% of the present supply of nurses, or an additional 150,000 nurses, will be needed during the next decade to provide the nation with adequate numbers to deliver safe, effective nursing care. Any change in the education requirements or licensure that threatens to reduce the number of competent nurses will be contrary to public interest (Rowland).

Distribution of Nursing Personnel

The geographic distribution of nurses in the United States is uneven. New York had the largest number of active registered nurses in 1976, followed by California. In general, the New England states had the highest nurse-population ratios while the south-central states had the lowest. The District of Columbia had the highest registered nurse ratio—673 nurses per 100,000 population—followed by Massachusetts with 640 per 100,000. Arkansas had the lowest nurse-population ratio with 190 per 100,000 population (Moses and Roth).

Work Settings

In 1977, approximately 75% of all R. N.s and L. P. N.s were employed in hospitals, nursing homes, and related institutions (Rowland). Hospitals employed 16% more nurses than they did in 1972, while nursing homes and extended care facilities had a 42% increase over 1972. The greatest increase in employment of nurses between 1972 and 1977 was in those areas involved in the care of noninstitutionalized persons (nurses employed in public health agencies and community health settings). Only 5% of nurses were employed in administrative positions, 5% were in teaching, 15.5% were in supervisory positions, while 64% were on a staff level.

It appears that the pattern of employment corresponds directly to the level of education preparation. Approximately 75% of the employed nurses whose highest education preparation was on the associate degree level were working in hospitals, while only 30% of the master's-prepared nurses were in hospitals. Of those holding diploma certification, 61% worked in hospitals, as did 60% of those with baccalaureate degrees. It appears that master's- and doctorate-level prepared nurses are more heavily concentrated in the nursing education areas; 42% of the master's degree graduates and 72% of the doctoral graduates are employed in education (Moses and Roth).

The proportion of nurses working in private duty (one nurse working full-time taking care of one patient on a private-pay basis) has declined steadily over the years. In 1962, 12% of employed nurses were working in private duty; this figure declined to 9.7% in 1966 to 5% in 1972. One reason for this decline was the growth of intensive-care and special care units, making it less necessary for the seriously ill or postoperative patient to employ a "special" nurse. These units have also created a demand in the hospital for highly trained, clinically specialized nursing personnel. Increased salary commensurate with the advanced training needed have made these positions competitive (Moses and Roth), and they have siphoned off nurses from private duty.

A national survey conducted by the American Nurses Association showed that the majority (67%) of nurses were educated on the diploma level; 11% were educated in associate degree programs; 17.5% were educated on the baccalaureate level; and 4% were on a master's or doctoral degree level. Of the 978,324 employed nurses sampled, an estimated 77% hold associate degrees or diploma certification and 18.5% hold a master's or doctoral degree. There were 165,979 nurses involved in some form of continuing education, 78% enrolled part-time and 21.7% full-time (Moses and Roth).

Nursing Research and Quality Assessment

Because nursing has traditionally been a practice profession, nurses and nurse educators have stressed its clinical aspects. Therefore, the earliest research studies—those done in the 1920s and 1930s—were either time and motion studies or those that concentrated on nursing techniques or procedures. Studies conducted during the 1940s were concerned with various aspects of nursing education. It was not until programs for nursing education were established within the framework of colleges and universities that nurses could be adequately prepared to do research. From the 1950s onward, the growth of collegiate education for nurses and the support of national nursing leaders, national nursing organizations, and government at various levels have made research a major movement in the profession (Notter). It is important to note that, whereas in the past most courses in research methods (for nurses) were limited to persons studying at the master's or doctoral level, such courses are now included in the curricula of all 4- and 5-year programs and in curricula of some of the other types of nursing education programs also.

Nursing research is now taking on new directions as the profession attempts to develop a valid system for assessing the role and functions of the nurse. In addition, the clinical expertise of nurses is being utilized in research activities that are developing systems of evaluating the quality of patient care. The American Nurses Association has established standards for practice and recommends the use of the nursing audit as one tool for measuring the quality of care delivered by nurses (Carter et al.). Such audits are accepted practice in most institutions and health agencies (Report to the Congress).

In *A Methodology for Monitoring the Quality of Nursing Care,* by Jelinek et al. (1974), the quality of care given is assessed by monitoring a set of nursing activities. These activities are components of the nursing process and include assessing the patient's needs and problems, formulating a plan of nursing care, implementing the plan of care, and evaluating the patient's progress, as well as the achievement of nursing goals. These components constitute the basis against which the quality of nursing care is measured.

The political and economic climate affecting nursing care delivery is such that the time has come for nursing administration to use empirical data obtained through evaluation research. Integration of nursing research from the level of a conceptual framework for a particular study to the level of more general theory and ultimately to that of a unified body of nursing knowledge has not been pursued to any large extent, nor have there been widespread efforts on the part of those doing nursing research to relate individual studies to one another and thereby build a larger context for reference. This has contributed in the past to fragmentation of knowledge and confusion about a perspective for nursing research (Donaldson). For the continued growth, significance, and utility of the discipline of nursing, researchers must place research within the context of the discipline. Theories must also be viewed in terms of the basic structural conceptualization of the discipline. The responsibilities for revising and clarifying structural conceptions, the very framework of the discipline, rests with nurse researchers. This means lessening the preoccupation with the process of nursing and pedagogy and placing more emphasis on content (McClure).

Components for Change

Nurse Practitioners: Role and Conflict

The impetus behind the development of the nurse practitioner has been cogently expressed by Fuchs:

> While most of the country goes around shaking its head about the doctor shortage, I am impressed by the existence of considerable waste. The waste is evident when you see so many physicians spending so much of their time at tasks that could be performed as well or better by someone with considerably shorter, more specialized training. The pediatrician providing well baby care, the gynecologist attending normal delivery, internists treating common colds are just a few of the examples of this phenomenon.

As early as 1943, Frances Reiter, the nursing educator, used the term "nurse clinician" to describe a superior kind of nurse, distinguished by the depth of her clinical knowledge and by her ability to form interdependent working relationships with physicians and other health care providers. Reiter proposed that the nurse clinician or clinical nurse specialist be prepared at a graduate level. One of the distinguishing characteristics of this clinical nurse specialist is the high degree of discriminative judgment the nurse uses in assessing nursing problems when determining priorities of care (Kinsella).

Since this early definition, some confusion has arisen over titles, for over the years many new terms arose for the "nurse practitioner." Primary care nurse, primary care nurse clinician, family nurse practitioner, clinical nurse practitioner were titles that began to be used interchangeably around the country. The term "nurse practitioner" was first used in a demonstration project at the University of Colorado in 1965. The purpose of the program was to prepare professional nurses to give comprehensive well-child care in an ambulatory care setting and to provide a research base for future changes in traditional collegiate nursing programs (Kalisch). Since that time the nurse practitioner concept has gained considerable attention in health professional circles as well as among consumer and legislative groups (Andrus). For the purpose of this chapter, the clinical nurse specialist and the nurse clinician are nurse practitioners with training at the master's degree level. Titles such as "primary care nurse practitioner" or "family nurse practitioner" will be applied to nurses in clinical practice (defined below) who do not necessarily have graduate degrees. The generic term, however, is "nurse practitioner," N. P.

The nurse may be prepared for the expanded role in several ways. Formal training may range from 6-week certification programs to 2-year graduate programs. Currently, most training programs are at the post-R. N. level, involving either programs leading to a certificate or full-time graduate work leading to an advanced degree. The concept of the nurse practitioner has been defined in different ways (National League for Nursing, 1979)

1. A registered nurse who has been trained by a physician "on the job" in physical assessment;
2. A registered nurse who had a short course in physical assessment given by a school of nursing or a school of medicine;
3. A graduate of a baccalaureate program that includes physical assessment;
4. A graduate of a master's program that includes physical assessment.

Although some early programs stress assisting the physician in performing routine medical tasks, emphasis has shifted dramatically in many education programs. In many cases, nurse practitioner curricula now focus on the aspects of patient care that come under the discipline of nursing such as psychosocial aspects of care, health education, and counseling.

All these professionals learn history-taking, physical assessment, interpretation of laboratory procedures, and selected aspects of clinical medicine (including diagnosis and treatment); they also gain an understanding of the utilization of community resources needed to deal with patients' total health care needs (Ross).

The first training programs prepared individuals to assist in meeting primary care health needs (Murray and Ross). According to the NLN, these programs had been considered (1) a means of controlling costs by introducing lower-paid health care providers into the system and (2) an answer to distribution problems by training individuals who would function in geographic areas that were short of physicians. As the scope of these programs expanded, new trends in many basic nursing programs emerged. For example, physical assessment skills are currently being taught in baccalaureate and master's programs and an increasing number of baccalaureate curricula are placing an emphasis on primary care. Many health policy makers have projected that as a result of the nurse practitioner movement, nurses will soon become recognized as the nation's major group of primary care specialists (Kalisch).

Although the provision of a formal academic education to prepare nurses for their expanded role is somewhat new, the role itself has a long history. The public health nurse, the nurse midwife, the private duty nurse, the frontier nurse in the hills of Kentucky (Kirk et al.), and the nurse anesthetist have long functioned well beyond the limits traditionally considered to constitute nursing practice, especially when physicians were not readily available (Lees). Nonetheless, an aura of newness surrounds the expanded role; there is an impression that a revolutionary process is taking place (Lees).

The term "expanded role" as applied to the N. P. refers to the nurse's potential for performing functions not traditionally considered within his/her domain. Direct patient care by nurses goes beyond the technical activities traditionally assigned to nursing. In the past, nurses usually found themselves primarily accountable to the physician and the institution, and only secondarily accountable to their patients.

Numerous reports from professional organizations and governmental agencies on the numbers and kinds of N. P. programs have been published (Report to the Congress; Sultz and Zielezny, 1976, 1980). These programs offer courses in child care (with such titles as "Pediatric Nurse Practitioner" or "Pediatric Nurse Associate"); in adult care (with such titles as "Adult Health Care Practitioner" or "Medical Nurse Associate"); and in maternal care (with such titles as "Nurse-Midwife," "Midwife-Family Nurse Practitioner," or "Ob-Gyn Nurse Practitioner").

The following outline summarizes the skills that all such programs aim to teach:

Collection of the data required for making nursing judgments
1. Obtaining a comprehensive health history.
2. Performing and recording a physical examination and assessing the patient's mental status.
3. Obtaining appropriate laboratory and X-ray studies.

Application of clinical judgment from data base
1. Recognizing and identifying major departures from normality on the basis of observation made during history-taking and physical examination.
2. Preparing a complete write-up of the health history and physical examination as well as formulating a problem and planning for management.
3. Analyzing and interpreting laboratory data in the management of common episodic and chronic illnesses.
4. Recognizing, appropriately assessing, and prescribing and/or managing treatment programs according to the established pro-

tocols mutually developed by the nurse practitioner, the physician, and/or the pharmacist.

5. Referring or consulting with another member of the health care team when indicated.
6. Interpreting to the patient and/or relatives the symptoms, disease, treatment, and prognosis appropriate to each patient.
7. Providing counseling, anticipatory guidance, and appropriate health education to the patient regarding the particular disease entity.
8. Recommending preventive health measures when appropriate.
9. Coordinating care by correlating pertinent clinical and social information from a variety of sources.

A positive result of the nurse practitioner movement has been a move toward greater autonomy for nurses. This trend led to the passage of the Rural Health Clinics Act of 1977, which for the first time allowed nurses to be reimbursed under Medicare for their services through certified rural health clinics (Sullivan et al.). The impact of the nurse practitioner movement on the health care delivery system and on the discipline of nursing, and the acceptance of the role will rest on this law and future determinations of how these practitioners will be reimbursed and regulated (National League for Nursing, 1979).

It is estimated that in 1978 there were 12,000 nurse practitioners in the United States (Moses and Roth). According to the American Nursing Association's former executive director, Eileen Jacobie, one of the greatest barriers to their expanded role is "attitudinal" (Kushner). The physician often is reluctant to relinquish functions because having another individual make decisions under the general cover of the physician's license could increase liability in the case of malpractice litigation. By the same token, the nurse often is reluctant to take on increased responsibilities and accountability. The male-female role caricature, a barrier to role expansion, has been called the doctor-nurse game (Bullough, 1975). Nurses have been making diagnostic decisions for years but have protected themselves with elaborate games. The object of the game is to make the doctor feel in control at all times. Nurses make recommendations so that they appear to have been initiated by the physician. If the N. P. is to function effectively, this game must be given up, a sad prospect for certain players on both sides.

The nursing profession has always valued the qualities of tact, gentleness, and patience. However, in order to be effective, nurses who move into the expanded role must also be self-assertive and decisive. The pri-

mary care nurse practitioner must communicate directly rather than obli-
quely with the physician and other members of the health care team.
Indeed, the present trend is to educate nurses to become competent and
more independent practitioners, rather than obedient handmaidens
(Rothenberg). Relationships may become strained if physicians do not
accept the judgments of the self-assertive and competent nurse.

Two important concepts inherent in the expanded role are "forseeabil-
ity" and accountability to the patient (Anderson et al.). "Foreseeability"
means that the N. P. has adequate scientific preparation to predict with
considerable accuracy the outcome and consequences of her acts. Accountability entails the N. P.'s recognition of responsibility for his or her
actions.

As pointed out above, physicians who work with this new type of
practitioner often experience an identity crisis (Bullough, 1975). The
physician as principal provider is legally responsible for many of the
traditional steps in the diagnosis and therapeutic process. As portions of
the conventional role are relinquished, difficulties are often experienced in
trusting another health worker's data base and decision-making (Bates).
The physician has been taught in medical school that any good doctor does
his or her own history and physical. Often it is difficult to share the
decision-making process and to accept and trust the judgments and decisions of others. Physicians are often sensitive to the potential for competition that the existence of the nurse practitioner implies (Burrows and
Traver; Pickard). Although dissatisfied with their own professional roles,
nurses have not been willing to give up any professional turf to auxiliaries
(Weiler 1975, 1979).

There has been a widespread trend toward developing protocols that
can be used by N. P.s as well as by P. A.s (physicians' assistants; see below)
for diagnosis and treatment of minor acute diseases and other well-defined
conditions. However, disease protocols have limited value in that they do
not always take into account every possible variation and have too rigid and
binding an approach.

The clinical work of various types of N. P. has been extensively evaluated (Lawrence). For example, in an internal medicine clinic, "nurse care
was judged to be adequate in dealing with 98 per cent of old problems
(defined by the physician) and 85 per cent of new problems (detected by
the nurse)" (Spector et al., p. 1234). A pediatric nurse practitioner program
was studied and found satisfactory (Yankauer et al.). A Canadian study
found that for randomly allocated patients, the quality of care provided by
nurse practitioners was similar to that provided by physicians in a primary
care practice (Sackett et al.; Spitzer et al.) A study undertaken in a university hospital medical clinic randomly allocated a small group of patients

with chronic diseases between an experimental nurse practitioner clinic and the regular medical clinic. They found that there were no differences in deaths or severity of disease between the two groups of patients, and that the nurses did better in terms of patient satisfaction and reduction of disability (Lewis et al.).

In another carefully regulated experiment using N. P.s, it was found that physician time per patient was reduced by 92% and average visit costs were 20% less (Scheffler). A major national review showed that N. P./P. A. substitution for physicians in primary care would be cost-effective while maintaining, possibly even improving, the quality of care (Record et al.). Research findings appear to indicate that the nurse practitioner has demonstrated that he or she fully fulfills a role intensely needed by society (Mauksch). In addition, data indicate that 75%–80% of all primary care can be provided in any given primary care setting and met by appropriately trained nurse practitioners. The N. P. has proven to be an efficient coordinator of an individual's or family's health care needs (Chambers; Chambers and West). Patients and clients, once they have had contact with the N. P., appear to have confidence in the N. P. and rate this provider equal to or preferable to other health care providers.

In a recent study, 57% of N. P. employers indicated that the extension of health services is the most significant contribution of the N. P.; another 40% considered improvement in the quality of care provided to be their most significant effect (Sullivan et al.). In another study, supervising physicians rated N. P.s as either good or excellent in the performance of 85%–90% of tasks. When both groups worked in similar settings, N. P.s were considered to require less supervision than P. A.s (Greenfield et al.).

The N. P.'s role has quickly become appreciated by the public. However, the nursing profession itself has had a more difficult time with acceptance. Not only did it refuse initially to accept this role, but it also failed to recognize the paramount importance carried by the N. P. movement for nursing (Rogers). Nursing students are now being educated to become risk-takers, to develop autonomy based on competence, to act as patient advocates, and to assume responsibility for self-growth in continued learning. The problems of instituting widespread use of N. P.s of various kinds thus seem much more related to history, attitudes, psychology, economics, and male-female role definition than they do to the technical content of the N. P.s' work and the quality of their performance.

A recent study prepared under contract to DHEW's Health Care Financing Administration evaluated an experimental physician-extender reimbursement program (National League for Nursing, 1980). The average bill was $8.13 when the service was performed by a nurse practitioner, compared with $16.48 when done by a physician. With data such as these, it is not surprising that as of 1980 DHEW was funding 102 of the 200 nurse practitioner training programs throughout the country. During that year, between 1,000 and 1,300 nurse practitioners were expected to complete programs in 67 schools of nursing and 6 medical schools.

Nurses today are better educated than previously. The ANA's official policy, as of 1980 not yet accepted by the National League for Nursing, is that by 1985 all persons entering training should work toward a baccalaureate degree as the minimum qualification to become an R. N. Currently, the National League for Nursing believes all nurse practitioners should have master's degrees. Whatever their qualifications to replace or become colleagues of primary care physicians, nurses today are moving in the direction of independence. According to Bonnie Bullough, Women's Liberation came along at the right time for nurses (Mauksch).

The Physicians' Assistant

One proposed solution to the (now nonexistent) health manpower shortage (see Chapter 4) has been the development of programs to train an additional health care provider called the physicians' assistant or associate (P. A.). The educational preparation for the physicians' assistant seems to vary even more than that for the clinical nurse practitioner. Programs range from eight weeks to five years. Eugene Stead, of the Duke University Physicians' Assistant Program, one of the originators of the concept, described the intended role of physicians' assistants (1966):

> The Physicians' Assistant is seen as a new category within the structure of the health field, designed to provide a career opportunity for men functioning under the direction of doctors, with greater capabilities and growth potential than informally trained technicians. As the title implies, these individuals will be trained to assist the doctor in his clinical or research endeavors in such a way as to facilitate better utilization of available physicians and nurses. Graduates of the program at Duke are viewed as the individuals capable of performing responsibly and reliably certain of the skills currently practiced by doctors, nurses, and technicians. (p. 1108)

The role of the physicians' assistant differs from that of the nurse in that P. A.s do not make nursing diagnoses or do bedside nursing care (Estes). Other differences are:

1. P. A.s work for an individual physician, who assumes responsibility for the validity of all activities.
2. They work in several physical locations depending on the doctor's needs, over a workday whose length coincides with that of the doctor.

3. They carry out data-gathering and treatment functions, using the tools of the physician—the stethoscope, the ophthalmoscope, the sigmoidoscope, and so on.

The P. A. is responsible first to the physician and then, through the physician, to the patient. The role and function are personally defined by the employing physician (Stead).

Masculine pronouns are often used in descriptions of P. A.s and their training. This is due in part to the origins of the P. A.: P. A. programs were designed to take advantage of and provide useful, interesting careers for medics returning from the Vietnam War in the 1960s, who were, of course, mostly male.* Women are now admitted into P. A. programs, but the male orientation often prevails.

The National Academy of Sciences has developed three classifications of P. A.s. The Type A assistant is capable of approaching the patient, collecting historical and physical data, and organizing and presenting data so that the physician can visualize the medical problem and determine appropriate diagnostic and therapeutic steps. The Type B assistant, while not equipped with the general knowledge and skills relative to the whole range of medical care, possesses exceptional skill in one clinical specialty or, more commonly, in a certain technical procedure within such a specialty. The Type C assistant is capable of performing a variety of tasks over a whole range of medical care under the supervision of a physician, although he does not possess the level of medical knowledge necessary to integrate findings. He is comparable to the practical nurse. Type A is qualified to act as the primary patient contact, Type B is characterized as the "assistant specialist," and Type C resembles the Type A assistant in the range of supporting services, but his formal training is more limited in depth and breadth (Estes).

Education of the P. A. The P. A. receives formal education within one of the three basic programs (Perry, 1977):

1. The Medex program, originally designed for military corpsmen, requires 12–15 months of study. This usually involves 3 months of

---

*At the Annual Meeting of the American Public Health Association in Atlantic City in November 1972, there was a panel presentation on new health care delivery developments in Canada. One speaker's topic was nurse practitioners and their use. A questionner asked if there were P. A. programs as well in Canada. The answer came back: "We don't need to have P. A. programs. We have had no Vietnam War with the large number of returning medics to use and provide for. We need only nurse practitioner programs" (Jonas).

intensive didactic work followed by a preceptorship with a practicing physician for 9–12 months. The student, upon completion of the program, receives a certificate (Kane).

2.   University-medical-center-based program. This program consists of a 2-year training period beginning with 9–12 months of didactic material followed by 12–15 months on various clinical rotations. The student receives a certificate and/or a baccalaureate degree.

3.   College or university program in a non-medical school. This program requires about 2 years of training, beginning with 9–12 months of didactic work followed by 10–15 months of clinical rotations. The program results in a certificate or an associate's or baccalaureate degree.

The P. A. was developed around five fundamental functions, which establish the parameters of P. A. practice. They are (Detmer):

1.   To elicit a comprehensive health history
2.   To perform a comprehensive physical examination
3.   To perform simple diagnostic laboratory determinations
4.   To perform basic treatment procedures for common illnesses
5.   To make appropriate clinical responses to commonly encountered emergency care situations.

Of the 1,250 P. A.s who were graduated prior to 1975, 23% were in family practice; 22% in general medicine; 15% in internal medicine; 5% in pediatrics; and 2% in Ob/Gyn (Aschenbrenner and Horowitz; Perry, 1978). In 1976, there were 5,000 P. A.s who had completed training programs (USDHEW, 1976). The highest concentration of P. A.s exists in the southern and Pacific regions of the United States (Lawrence; Perry, 1978).

For the physician assistant, the American Medical Association House of Delegates in 1971 adopted standards, which were implemented by the AMA Council on Medical Education. The P. A.s are unified under several national organizations. In contrast, the nurse practitioners are without a separate organization but are part of the American Nurses Association. The physicians' assistant is seen as being somewhere in the middle of the conflict between the medical and nursing professions (Greenfield et al.).

Both P. A.s and N. P.s have demonstrated that they can "extend" the role of the physician in the delivery of health care. Certain aspects of their duties do overlap. The N. P. assumes some responsibilities as an associate of the physician who provides primary and follow-up health care to patients. The degree of independence or interdependence varies, but the nurse is independent as a licensed professional when functioning within the scope of nursing. Physicians' assistant training programs prepare P. A.s to assume a dependent position under supervision by the physician. However, there is no specific or clear definition of "supervision"—it can be direct, with the physician on site, or it can be indirect, with a connection by telephone or other electronic means to the physician with whom the P. A. works.

The overlapping and indistinct lines of work distribution between N. P.s and P. A.s is an area needing more examination. There is a great deal of potential and actual conflict between the two groups, who seem to be fighting over the same turf (Bullough, 1975). In fact, the struggle is really three-sided, with the physicians involved as well: both the P. A.s and the N. P.s are struggling to move from the dependent to the independent health-care provider group, against the resistance of the physicians. Unfortunately, as often happens in cases of parallel struggle against the same adversary, the P. A.s and N. P.s sometimes dispute with each other harder than either disputes with the physicians. The fact that most of at least the earlier generation of P. A.s are men and can earn salaries considerably higher than nurses who have a great deal more training contributes significantly to the rivalry and animosity, where it does exist. It should be noted, however, that there are instances in which P. A.s and N. P.s work very well together.

In reality, it is as hard to see real differences between the work of P. A.s (at least, Type A physicians' assistants) and N. P.s as it is to see differences between their work and the majority of tasks carried out by most primary care physicians. These difficult conflicts must be resolved; if they are not, in the end only the patients—and the taxpayers—will suffer.

Trends in Nursing

The National Health Planning and Resources Development Act of 1974 (P. L. 93–641) established a national network of local planning agencies called Health Systems Agencies (see Chapter 13). One of the major provisions and priorities of the Act is the training and increased utilization of nurse practitioners. Designating N. P.s as important providers of primary care, the Act included them in the category of physicians' assistants and in some cases physician extenders (National League for Nursing, 1974).

The changing roles of health care professionals have created serious concern about possible shortages of nurses in the traditional roles (O. W. Anderson; Keaveny and Hayden). According to NLN research data from the late 1970s, the nursing shortage is "real" and is apparently intensifying. A recent HEW report projected that in 1985 the aggregate supply of nurses will be roughly equal to aggregate requirements. However, the NLN cites studies showing close to total employment among the nation's nurses who consider themselves as active in the nursing profession, as well as a zero growth rate and declining admissions in nursing education. There will be widespread local shortages and forecasts that a serious national shortage is likely to develop during the 1980s. The study further pointed out that graduations of new nurses have reached a plateau and will in all likelihood decline in the following years. There are indications that nursing education has entered a phase of retrenchment (National League for Nursing, 1980).

Admissions to R. N. programs have not grown significantly since 1974. In 1978, the first decline in admissions since the 1960s was recorded. An ANA study indicates that about 26,000 more nurses left the employed pool than returned. Additions to the actual nursing supply in 1977 were, therefore, considerably less than the sum of newly licensed and reinstated nurses. Unemployment rates for new licensees reached a record low of 2% in 1977. NLN studies reveal that nearly two-thirds of 1977's new licensees found employment before graduation, while 29% found jobs within three months. According to the NLN, all indices point to an intensification of the shortage between 1976 and 1978. There are concerns that the supply of nurses has leveled off before expected and is probably destined to decline.

In 1980, the nursing shortage situation was summarized in *RN* magazine (Donovan):

- The ANA estimates that 30% of today's 1.4 million qualified, nonretired nurses are currently not working in the field—by choice (*RN* estimates the dropout rate at 40%). In fact, the unemployment rate for newly licensed RNs is estimated to be a record low, 2%.
- Forty percent of the nurses currently active are working only part time, according to ANA estimates.
- As far back as 1978, some cities were reporting nursing vacancies of 10% to 33%, according to recent NLN testimony.
- The patient population continues to rise—0.5% in 1978, according to the latest data from the American Hospital Association.
- The U.S. Department of Labor projects 240,000 more nursing jobs by 1985.
- Diploma schools are closing—fast. The NLN says 23 closed down in the 2-year period ending in October 1979.
- Applications to nursing schools went down 16% between 1977 and 1978, according to the NLN.
- Government aid to nursing students and to nursing education is threatened with stiff cutbacks. The secretary of HEW recently testified that such aid was unjustified.
- Bounties of $100 to $1,000 are being paid to fill nursing positions in cities as disparate as Chicago and Corpus Christi, Texas, according to the ANA.
- A recent National Association of Nurse Recruiters study reports that an average U.S. hospital with about 450 beds has about 72 full-time RN jobs open. The hospital will spend more than $62,000 to attract and hire these

nurses (an average of about $866 for each RN). And it will cost the hospital nearly $20,000 each year to replace the nurses, who leave at a rate of 31.7% per year.

Much has been written about the confusion regarding roles that exists within nursing itself. The changing roles of health care professionals have created serious concern about possible shortages of nurses in the tradition- al roles (O. W. Anderson). In the past, nursing education has placed much emphasis on the psychosocial aspects of patient care, whereas the physician has focused primarily on the pathophysiological aspects of illness. The trend today is toward educating both doctors and nurses to view the patient as a whole and unique individual within a complex social framework. The physical diagnosis component traditionally dominant in medical schools has now found its way into the curricula of N. P. programs at the bacca- laureate and master's degree levels. In these new educational programs, students are oriented toward providing care to patients, not service to institutions. They are educated to make more decisions, to take more responsibility, to become accountable for their actions. Unfortunately, upon graduation many nurses accept employment in institutional health care settings where the bureaucratic structure operates by means of hierar- chical restraints: obedience to rules and authority is valued more than independence and initiative. The resulting conflict between educational ideals and job realities—a kind of role-deprivation—may be the most significant reason why so many R. N.s are not active in nursing.

Nursing, a young profession, has come a long way in a little over 100 years. But there is much to be done. Nursing is at the crossroads of its development and its future will be determined by the commitments its professionals make and the attitudes they adopt. Nurses must decide who they are, which directions they will follow, and how they will interact with other health care professionals in determining the quality of patient care. Nursing not only has the right to share in the planning, delivery, and evaluation of health care, but also has the responsibility to do so. At present, securing this professional right and assuming this professional responsibility represent nursing's principal challenge.

References

Abdellah, F. G. "Doctoral Preparation for Nurses (A Continuation of the Dia- logue)." *Nursing Forum* 5 (3) 44–43, 1966.
American Nurses Association, Department of Statistics. Personal communication, 1980.
Anderson, J., et al. "The Expanded Role of the Nurse: Independent Practitioner or Physician's Assistant." *The Canadian Nurse*, September 1975, p. 34.

Anderson, O. W. *Toward an Unambiguous Profession? A Review of Nursing.*
    Health Administration Perspectives No. A6. Chicago: University of Chicago,
    1968.
Andrus, L. H. "New Teacher in Medical Education: The Family Nurse Practition-
    er." *Journal of Medical Education, 52,* 896, 1977.
Aschenbrenner, T., and Horowitz, S. "Working Papers." Bethesda, Maryland:
    Health Resource Administration, USDHEW, 1976.
Bates, B. "Physicians and Nurse Practitioners: Conflict and Reward." *Annals of
    Internal Medicine, 82,* 702, 1975.
Bullough, B. "Barriers to the Nurse Practitioner Movement: Problems of Women
    in a Woman's Field." *International Journal of Health Services, 5,* 225, 1975.
───────. "The Law and the Expanding Nursing Role." *American Journal of
    Public Health, 66,* 249, 1976.
Bullough, B., and Bullough, V. L. *The Emergence of Modern Nursing.* New York:
    Macmillan, 1974.
───────. *Expanding Horizons for Nurses.* New York: Springer Publishing Co.,
    1977.
Burrows, B., and Traver, G. A. "Nurse Practitioner Programs." *Annals of Internal
    Medicine, 80,* 268, 1974.
Carter, J., et al. *Standards of Nursing Care: A Guide for Evaluation.* New York:
    Springer Publishing Co., 1976.
Chambers, L. W. "Controlled Trial of Family Practice Nurse." *Medical Care, 15,*
    971, 1977.
Chambers, L. W., and West, A. "Assessment of the Role of the Family Practice
    Nurse in Urban Medical Practices." *Canadian Journal of Public Health, 69,*
    November/December 1978.
Detmer, L. M. "1975 Physicians Assistants—Education, Accreditation and Con-
    sumer Acceptance." Prepared for the Annual Group Health Institute of the
    Group Health Foundation. Chicago, Illinois, June 23, 1975.
Diers, D. "A Different Kind of Energy: Nurse-Power." *Nursing Outlook,* January
    1978, p. 51.
Donaldson, S. "The Discipline of Nursing." *Nursing Outlook,* February 1978, p.
    113.
Donovan, L. "The Shortage." *RN,* June 1980, p. 21.
Ehrenreich, B. "Where Women Work, The Health Care Industry. A Theory of
    Industrial Medicine." *Social Policy,* November/December 1975, p. 74.
Estes, E. H. Quoted in Carlson, C. L., and Athelstan, G. T. "The Physician's
    Assistant: Versions and Diversions of a Promising Concept." *Journal of the
    American Medical Association, 214,* 1857, 1970.
Forni, P. R., and Bolte, I. M. "Planning for Continuing Education." *American
    Journal of Nursing, 73,* 1912, 1973.
Fuchs, V. R. "Improving the Delivery of Personal Health Services." *Journal of
    Bone and Joint Surgery, 51,* 407, 1969.
Greenfield, S., et al. "Efficiency and Cost of Primary Care by Nurses and Physi-
    cians Assistants." *New England Journal of Medicine, 298,* 305, 1978.

Jelinek, R. C., et al. *A Methodology for Monitoring the Quality of Nursing Care*. DHEW Pub. No. (HRA) 74–25. Washington, D.C.: Government Printing Office, 1974.

Jonas, S. Personal communication. July 1, 1976.

Kalisch, B. J. "The Promise of Power." *Nursing Outlook*, January 1978, p. 42.

Kane R. "Adding a Medex to the Medical Mix." *Medical Care, 14*, 996, 1976.

Keaveny, T., and Hayden, R. "Manpower Planning for Nurse Personnel." *American Journal of Public Health, 68*, 7, 1978.

Kinsella, C. R. "Who Is the Clinical Nurse Specialist?" *Hospitals, J.A.H.A.*, November 1, 1973, p. 93.

Kirk, R. F. H., et al. "Family Nurse Practitioners in Eastern Kentucky." *Medical Care, 9*, 160, 1971.

Kushner, T. D. "Nursing Profession." *Ms. Magazine*, September 1973.

Lawrence, D. "Physician's Assistants and Nurse Practitioners." *Health and Medical Care Services Review, 1*, 2, 1978.

Lees, R. E. "Physician Time-Saving by Employment of Expanded-Role Nurses in Family Practice." *Canadian Medical Association Journal, 108*, 871, 1973.

Lego, S. "Continuing Education by Mail." *American Journal of Nursing, 73*, 840, 1973.

Leininger, M. "Doctoral Programs for Nurses: Trends, Questions, and Projected Plans," *Nursing Research, 25*, 3, 1976.

Lenberg, C. B. "The External Degree in Nursing: The Promise Fulfilled." *Nursing Outlook, 24*, 423, 1976.

————. Personal communication, 1980.

Lewis, C. E., et al. "Activities, Events and Outcomes in Ambulatory Patient Care." *New England Journal of Medicine, 280*, 645, 1969.

Martel, G. D., and Edmunds, M. W. "Nurse-Internship Program in Chicago." *American Journal of Nursing, 72*, 940, 1973.

Mauksch, I. "The Nurse Practitioner Movement—Where Does It Go From Here?" *American Journal of Public Health, 68*, 1074, 1978. (See related articles on pp. 1090 and 1097 of the same issue.)

McClure, M. "The Long Road to Accountability." *Nursing Outlook*, January 1978, p. 47.

Moses, E., and Roth, A. "Nurse Power: What Do Statistics Reveal About the Nation's Nurses." *American Journal of Nursing*, October 1979, p. 1745.

Murray, R. H., and Ross, S. A. "Training the Family Nurse Practitioner." *Hospitals, J.A.H.A.*, November 1, 1973, p. 93.

Navarro, V. "Women in Health Care." *The New England Journal of Medicine, 293*, 398, 1975.

National League for Nursing. *Health Policy Making in Action: The Passage and Implementation of the National Health Planning and Resources Development Act of 1974*. Papers by the NLN Summer Study Fellows in Public Policy. Pub. No. 41–1600. New York, 1974.

————. *Practical Nursing Career*, New York, 1974–75.

————. *Education for Nursing—The Diploma Way*. Pub. No. 16–1314. New York, 1976 a.

————————. *Associate Degree Education for Nursing.* Pub. No. 23–1309. New York, 1976 b.

————————. *Position Statement on the Education of Nurse Practitioners.* Pub. No. 11–1808. New York, October 1979.

————————. "Testimony Cites Intensifying Nurse Shortage." *NLN News, 28,* 1, 1980.

Notter, L. E. *The Essentials of Nursing Research.* New York: Springer Publishing Co., 1974.

Ozimek, D. *Initiating a Baccalaureate Degree Program in Nursing—Asking the Essential Questions.* New York: National League for Nursing, Pub. No. 15–1536, 1974.

Perry, B. "Physician's Assistant; An Overview of an Emerging Profession." *Medical Care, 15,* 12, 1977.

————————. "Analysis of Specialty and Geographic Location of Physicians' Assistants." *American Journal of Public Health, 68,* 1019, 1978.

Pickard, C. G. "Family Nurse Practitioners: Preliminary Answers and New Issues." *Annals of Internal Medicine, 80,* 267, 1974.

Record, J., et al. *Primary Care Staffing in 1990: Physician Replacement and Cost Savings.* New York: Springer Publishing Co., 1981.

Reichow, R., and Scott, R. "Study Compares Graduates of 2, 3, and 4 Year Programs." *Hospitals, J.A.H.A.,* July 16, 1976, p. 95.

Report to the Congress. *Nursing Training 1974.* USDHEW Pub. No. (HRA) 75–41. Rockville, Maryland: USDHEW, 1974.

Rogers, M. "Nursing Is Coming of Age Through the Nurse Practitioner Movement—A Con Position." *American Journal of Nursing, 75,* October 1975.

Ross, S. A. "The Clinical Nurse Practitioner in Ambulatory Care Service." *Bulletin of the New York Academy of Medicine, 49,* 393, 1973.

Rothenberg, J. S. "Nurse and Physician's Assistant: Issues and Relationships." *Nursing Outlook, 21,* 154, 1973.

Rowland, H. S. *The Nurses' Almanac,* Germantown, Maryland: Aspen Systems, 1978.

Sackett, D. L., et al. "The Burlington Randomized Trial of the Nurse Practitioner: Health Outcomes of Patients." *Annals of Internal Medicine, 80,* 268, 1974.

Scheffler, R. "The Employment Analyzation and Earnings of Physician Extenders." *Social Science and Medicine, 11,* 785, 1977.

Spector, R., et al. "Medical Care by Nurses in an Internal Medicine Clinic: Analysis of Quality and Its Cost." *Journal of the American Medical Association, 232,* 1234, 1975.

Spitzer, W. O., et al. "The Burlington Randomized Trial of the Nurse Practitioner." *New England Journal of Medicine, 290,* 251, 1974.

Stead, E. A. "Conserving Costly Talents—Providing Physician's New Assistants." *Journal of the American Medical Association, 198,* 1108, 1966.

Sullivan, J. A., et al. "The Rural Nurse Practitioner: A Challenge and Response." *American Journal of Public Health, 68,* 972, 1978.

Sultz, H., and Zielezny, M. *Longitudinal Study of Nurse Practitioners, Phase I.* Hyattsville, Maryland: USDHEW Pub. (HRA) 76–43, 1976.

————. *Longitudinal Study of Nurse Practitioners, Phase III.* Hyattsville, Maryland: USDHEW Pub. (HRA) 80–2, May 1980.

Treece, E. W. *Internship in Nursing Education: Technoterm.* New York: Springer Publishing Co., 1974

USDHEW. "The Training and Utilization of Assistants to the Primary Care Physician: An Overview." Washington, D.C. An unpublished working paper, Division of Medicine, January 1976.

————. "Nurse Training Act of 1975; Second Report to the Congress, revised March 15, 1979." Hyattsville, Maryland, 1979.

Walsh, M. E. *Why Nursing Education Programs Should Be Accredited.* New York: National League for Nursing, Pub. No. 14–1597, 1975.

Weiler, P. G. "Health Manpower Dialectic—Physician, Nurse, Physician's Assistant." *American Journal of Public Health,* 65, 8, 1975.

————. "Colleagues or Competitors?" *Medical World News,* July 9, 1979.

Yankauer, A., et al. "The Outcomes and Service Impact of a Pediatric Nurse Practitioner Training Program—Nurse Practitioner Training Outcomes." *American Journal of Public Health,* 62, 347, 1972.

6

Ambulatory Care

Steven Jonas, with Robert Greifinger

Introduction

Ambulatory care is a personal or combined health care service given to a person who is not a bed patient in a health care institution. Thus, the term "ambulatory care" covers all health services other than community health services and personal and combined services given to the institutionalized patient (see Chapter 2).

There are about four times as many visits to physicians on an ambulatory basis annually as there are hospital days of care (Givens, Table D). About 75% of the population makes a physician visit in a given year, while about 10% of the population is hospitalized one or more times. The majority of physician-patient contacts in the United States take place on an ambulatory basis.

There are two major categories of ambulatory care. One, by far and away the largest, is care given by private physicians in solo, partnership, or private group practice, on a fee-for-service basis. The other may be called "ambulatory care in organized settings." An organized setting here is taken to mean a locus of medical practice with an identity independent from that of the particular individual physician(s) working in it. This category includes hospital-based ambulatory services (primary clinics and emergency care); emergency medical services systems; health department clinics; Health Maintenance Organizations (HMOs); Neighborhood Health Centers (NHCs); organized home care; Community Mental Health Centers; industrial health services; school health services; and prison health services. In this chapter we will deal with the first six categories, which have a common base in a medical institutional setting. Organized home care is also discussed in Chapter 8. Community Mental Health Centers are dealt with in Chapter 9. Unfortunately, we do not have the space to deal with organized ambulatory services provided in nonmedical institutional settings.

126

Utilization of ambulatory care services varies with age, sex, region, and income. During 1977 the frequency of physician visits increased with patient age from an average of 4.1 visits per year for children under 17 years of age to 6.5 visits per year for people 65 years of age and over. Females had one visit per year more than males; black people had fewer visits than whites (USDHEW, 1979, p. 177).

Americans averaged 4.8 physician visits per person annually, including telephone contacts, but excluding inpatient visits. Among families earning less than $5,000 in 1977, the utilization rate was 5.8, compared with 4.8 for those earning over $25,000. This difference diminished beginning in the early 1960s, particularly since the enactment of Medicaid. The equalization of health services utilization among income groups has been due primarily to an increased visit rate among poorer people, rather than a decreased visit rate among higher-income persons. Between 1972 and 1977 there was an increase in per person contacts for lower income groups from 70.1% to 76.2%; the latter is a slightly larger percentage than that for middle income groups. Highest income groups average 1.6 visits more per year than do middle income groups. Racial differentials in utilization also decreased between 1972 and 1977 (USDHEW, 1979, p. 177). Although the trend toward equalization in utilization rates by race and income are encouraging, a caveat is important: the amount of medical care does not necessarily reflect the extent to which health needs are met. There are rather marked differences in health status by income groups, with higher morbidity among those with low income (USDHEW, 1979, pp. 37–39, Table I).

The several settings of ambulatory care tend to service different groups in the population, with different outcomes in utilization and quality of services provided. Dutton analyzed the impact of the several major forms of ambulatory care delivery on patients in Washington, D.C.:

> Sources used primarily by the poor—hospital outpatient departments, emergency rooms, and public clinics—contained important structural and financial barriers, and had the lowest rates of patient-initiated use. The prepaid system, in contrast, maximized patients' access to both preventive care and symptomatic care, and did not seem to inhibit physician-controlled follow-up care. The results suggest some perverse effects of fee-for-service payment: patients, especially poor patients, appeared to be deterred from seeking preventive and symptomatic care, while physicians were encouraged to expand follow-up services. Moreover, services in fee-for-service systems were distributed less equitably relative to both income and medical need than in the prepaid system. (p. 221)

Private Practice

The primary mode of organization of physicians in the United States (and, indeed, of most other health care providers who are licensed to practice independently, such as dentists, chiropractors, podiatrists, and optometrists) is what is called private practice. The physician in private practice provides a range of health care services limited only by the licensing laws of the state in which he or she may be operating as an independent entrepreneur. The physician, in effect, contracts directly with patients (although almost never in writing) to provide a set of services in return for payment of a fee. This arrangement is appropriately enough called the fee-for-service system. Physicians in private practice provide care on a fee-for-service basis in settings that include premises owned or leased by the physician, the patient's home (on rare occasions), or an institution. Under this arrangement, a patient hospitalized under the care of his or her private physician pays the hospital for all services other than physician care. The physician's fee is paid directly by the patient or by a third party on behalf of the patient. Thus, even when working in a hospital setting, the private practitioner's relationship to the patient remains that of an independent contractor. Physicians have a major say in setting fee levels, which are rarely subject to conventional competitive market forces, even when the fees are set and paid by a third party (Showstack et al.).

As of 1978, about 59% of all active U.S. physicians were in office practice (Gaffney and Glandon, Table 2). About 16% were house staff (interns and residents in training); 10% full-time hospital-based practitioners (including those in federal service); and the balance in non-patient-care positions. Recent data on the proportion of physicians in private practice are not available. However, as of the mid-1970s, of those in office practice outside hospitals, about 95% were in private practice, the balance working in prepaid group practices, federal service, public health centers, neighborhood health centers, and other organized settings (Warner and Aherne, derived from Table 23, 24, 34). Thus, taking into account all physicians who were in active practice, including hospital-based physicians but excluding house staff, about 80% were in private practice (Warner and Aherne, derived from Tables 23, 24, 34). While the proportion of physicians in private practice has presumably decreased somewhat with the expansion of prepaid group practice, it is clear that the dominant mode of physician organization in American medicine is private practice.

The majority of ambulatory patient visits are made to physicians in their private offices, as one would expect. The National Health Survey, counting from the patient side (see Chapter 3), reported that in 1975 about 75% of all visits to a physician were made to private practices, a total of about 690 million visits (Gentile, Table 16). The proportion of total ambulatory

physician visits made to hospital clinics or emergency rooms is slowly rising
over time (Gentile, p. 9), as is the proportion of total visits made to HMOs
(Health Maintenance Organizations). The proportion of home physician
visits fell from 9% in 1959 to 0.8% in 1975. Thus the proportion of total
visits provided by private fee-for-service physicians is gradually declining.

Although there are reasonably good measures of the number of private
practitioners and of the volume of their practices, we are less certain about
exactly what physicians do. Private practice is at once the most important
and the least studied sector of the U.S. health care delivery system. This is
not surprising, since private practitioners of any profession are somewhat
reluctant to have outside researchers looking into their work. Nevertheless, this situation is changing. Wolfe and Badgley (pp. 4–7) offered an
interesting picture of what is, in their estimation, the typical work-week of
a Canadian private family practitioner. A major study concerning the
organization, manpower supply, and practice of surgery was published in
the mid-1970s (American College of Surgeons and the American Surgical
Association). In the late 1970s, a major national study of the practice
characteristics, professional activities, and the classification of patient care
services was undertaken by the Division of Research in Medical Education
at the University of Southern California (Mendenhall, 1979; Mendenhall et
al., 1978a, 1978b).

There is still little idea about what the "doctor-patient relationship"
really consists of. It is not known what doctors really talk about with their
patients. There have been some studies of inter-doctor referral mechanisms (Shortell; American College of Surgeons and the American Surgical
Association, pp. 104–105). The decision-making methods in private practice are not well understood and the ability to measure the quality of care in
that setting is limited (see Chapter 14). Also, little information is available
about the business aspects of private practice. Physicians, interestingly
enough, are subject to a number of occupational health hazards (*Medical
World News,* Aug. 20, 1979). Among them are a higher cancer death rate
among radiologists; higher hepatitis-B rate; a TB rate double the national
average; and higher rates for suicide, airplane crash, accidental death, and
alcoholism. Stress is a special problem. Physicians are "highly prone to
midlife crisis" (*Medical World News,* June 25, 1979). Special causes of
stress in physicians are professional and leisure-time pressures, the threat
of malpractice litigation, the perceived necessity to practice "defensive
medicine," the fear of violent crime, and the pressures of engaging in peer
review (Mawardi).

As of 1978, about 80% of all physicians in office practice classified
themselves as being in a specialty other than general or family practice
(Gaffney and Glandon, Table 2). Thus, American medical practice is heavily specialized. Among physicians in active office practice, the highest

proportions specialize in general internal medicine (about 14%), general surgery (about 9%), obstetrics and gynecology (about 7%), and pediatrics (about 6%). In all, about 26% of physicians were in a medical specialty or subspecialty (internal medicine, cardiology, dermatology, etc.), about 32% in a surgical specialty or subspecialty (general surgery, neurosurgery, orthopedics), about 23% in "other" specialties (psychiatry, radiology, pathology, etc.). Over 80% of all patient visits to office-based physicians were to specialists (Gaffney and Glandon, Table 30). This high degree of specialization remains one of the major problems confronting American medicine (Terris, 1973; White, 1974).*

Patients, particularly those who use the private sector and thus can pick their own points of entry, face a bewildering array of physicians from whom to choose. The question has not been studied on a national scale, but many patients using the private sector seem to have what might be called a "group practice in the head," having, perhaps, "my" internist, "my" psychiatrist, "my" neurologist, "my" allergist, "my" surgeon, "my" obstetrician-gynecologist, and so on. (Fortunately, only a few patients have "my" pathologist, choosing to go to him or her at the appropriate moment, but you never can tell.) This means that when a new symptom (something a patient feels or experiences) or a new sign (something a patient or other observer notices objectively) appears, it is the patient, usually an untrained observer, who evaluates its meaning and picks an entry-point in the spectrum of specialists. Unfortunately for many patients, few members of the particular "group practice in the head" know each other; thus, communications between them are poor.

Specialists tend to concentrate on their own organ or organ system, and it is easy for the whole patient to get lost in a tangle of organs. The forest is indeed obscured by the trees. Patients may well suffer because there is no trained individual who can: (1) see them as a whole person; (2) put together a variety of complaints into one clinical picture; (3) guide the patient through an intelligent utilization of specialists' knowledge; and (4) establish an organized means for communication among specialists. This is not an argument against specialization per se; the tremendous expansion of medical knowledge requires such specialization, at least for a certain proportion of the profession. It is an argument for a more rational approach to the organization of specialists (White, 1973; Aiken, et al.; Relman, 1979). Aspects of the problems of specialization are also discussed in Chapter 4.

---

*A particularly erudite and detailed history of the development of specialization in American medical practice is presented by Rosemary Stevens in her book, *American Medicine and the Public Interest* (New Haven, Connecticut: Yale University Press, 1971).

An important feature of the private practice sector in the United States is that the majority of physicians see patients both on an ambulatory basis in their own offices and as hospital inpatients. (There is a small percentage of doctors who do not have hospital appointments, but the magnitude is unknown. Most of them are probably in urban areas.) In most other countries, physicians either see ambulatory patients only or work full-time in hospitals. The unusual American arrangement offers some significant advantages. For conditions for which one physician is technically competent to provide both ambulatory and inpatient care, as in many medical specialties, there is continuity of physician care for the hospitalized patient. For surgical conditions, in many cases the nonsurgical physician who referred the patient for surgery will participate in the preoperative and postoperative phases of care in the hospital, or at least will follow his or her hospitalized patient.

As of 1977, the average American physician spent about 50 hours per week working (Gaffney and Glandon, Table 16), the rural physician working slightly longer hours than his or her urban counterpart, for about 47 weeks per year (Gaffney and Glandon, Tables 11 and 19). About 90% of this time is spent in direct patient care (Gaffney and Glandon, Tables 16 and 21). During this time, the average American physician provides about 130 visits per week—92 in the office and 37 in the hospital (Gaffney and Glandon, Tables 30, 34, and 36). The range is rather broad, from about 55 visits per week for psychiatrists through approximately 110 for surgeons to 150 for pediatricians and 180 for general practitioners. For all specialties, rural physicians see about 35% more visits than urban physicians (Gaffney and Glandon, Table 33). The average American physician made about 36 hospital visits per week, ranging from about 44 for rural physicians to about 34 for urban physicians (Gaffney and Glandon, Table 37). Internists made the highest average number of hospital visits per week (about 45), and psychiatrists, the fewest (about 17). These figures confirm that the American physician does both hospital and nonhospital work, with nonhospital work predominating. They also portray him or her as being rather busy. For this level of work, the average physician's income, as reported by himself for 1978, was around $63,000, ranging from a high of $76,000 for surgeons to a low of $49,000 for psychiatrists (Gaffney and Glandon, Table 68.)

Ambulatory Services in Organized Settings

Hospital Ambulatory Services

Introduction. The institutional center of the American health care system is the hospital (see Chapter 7). For a variety of historical reasons (see Freymann, Chapter 3), the majority of American hospitals focus the bulk of their efforts and activities on patients who are acutely ill and confined to bed. Hospitals have also had to deal with a variety of other types of patients, however. Among them are those who do not immediately require admission to a bed. These patients are called "outpatients," as opposed to "inpatients."

Outpatients may require either immediate treatment for an acute and often serious illness or injury, or care for a more routine matter calling for medical attention, but not necessarily immediately. Very often the services required by the latter type of patient are very similar to those needed by patients who attend private practitioners' offices. Although there are some exceptions, the patients needing immediate attention go to one of the two major divisions of hospital ambulatory services: the "Emergency Unit," or the "Clinics." Increasingly, hospital staffs and administrations are confused as to the differences in role and function of the two divisions, and they and the patients themselves have trouble deciding who should go where for what.

Historically, it apparently has been easier for hospitals to determine that emergency services should be provided than that clinic services should be. One reason for this is that insurance carriers are more likely to reimburse hospitals for emergency services than for clinic services. About 90% of community hospitals in the United States (4,830 in 1978) have emergency units (American Hospital Association, 1979, Table 12A). (Community hospitals are, by the American Hospital Association definition, "non-federal, short-term, general, and other special hospitals." See Chapter 7.) The original intended function of emergency units was to take care of people acutely ill or injured, particularly with life-threatening or potentially life-threatening problems that require immediate attention, personnel, and/or equipment not found in private practitioners' offices, and, potentially, to provide prompt hospitalization. Most hospitals have found it desirable or necessary to provide such services.

Historically, on the other hand, two kinds of hospitals have paid the most attention to clinic services; those located in areas where patients could not or would not attend private practitioners' offices for more routine care, usually for economic reasons (Roemer, 1971); and/or those that have teaching programs. Only about 30% of community hospitals (1,658 in 1978) have clinics (American Hospital Association, 1979, Table 12A). It is probably not coincidental that emergency outpatient services, particularly for critically ill patients, are not among those services that private physicians can easily provide in their own offices, whereas the type of service provided in clinics can usually be given by the private physician, economic considerations aside.

In the 19th century, clinic service was part of the functions of most hospitals serving the poor in urban areas (Freymann, Chapters 3, 4). Until the late 19th century, hospitals were relatively uncommon in the United States. In 1875, there were fewer than 200 of them (Stevens, p. 52). A building boom then took place and, by 1909, there were 4,359 hospitals with a bed capacity of 421,000. Local government hospitals were established for the sole purpose of taking care of the poor, as both inpatients and outpatients; care of the sick poor was separated from the general custodial functions provided by the poorhouse/workhouse system for persons not self-sufficient for all reasons. (For additional material on the history of hospitals, see also Chapter 7.) Nonprofit "voluntary" hospitals were also established, at least in part, to fulfill charitable purposes. One way they did so was by providing free clinic care to the poor. However, the voluntaries, which were much more important in setting the style for the organization of medical practice than were the local government hospitals, established clinics on their premises only grudgingly, since they were likely to be used by nonpaying patients.

Dispensaries. So uninterested were the voluntaries in providing clinic services within the hospital walls that their corporations often established related but physically separate institutions to carry out that function. They were called "dispensaries" (Davis and Warner; Rosenberg). There were nonaffiliated charitable dispensaries, as well as local government ones. Dispensaries were an important factor in urban medical care at one time (Rosenberg, p. 33). In 1900, there were about 100 in the U.S.; in New York City alone in that year, dispensaries provided facilities for more than 800,000 visits. However, they were poorly staffed, poorly financed, and viewed with displeasure by private practitioners, who saw them as competing for patients. Most of them had disappeared by the 1920s (Rosenberg, p. 49).

Hospital clinics. Clinic services started growing in the voluntary hospitals themselves in the latter part of the 19th century. By 1916, 495 hospitals had clinics, in many cases serving an educational as well as a charitable function (Roemer, 1975a). However, the clinics certainly shared the second-class status of the dispensaries. When, for example, a clinic was built onto the archetypal 19th-century voluntary hospital, the Johns Hopkins in Baltimore, it was added at the back (Freymann, p. 56). This typified the approach. As Freymann says (p. 200): "It was and still is an appendix tacked on the periphery of the bed-filled tower that soaks up the pride and wealth of the community. The ambulatory services huddle at the nether end of the pecking order. . . ."

In considering problems of hospital ambulatory services, it should be kept in mind that they vary in type and are found in several categories of hospitals. Most of the literature on hospital ambulatory care in the United

States deals with university and other teaching hospitals and thus probably presents a distorted picture. In community hospitals, excluding Veterans' Administration hospitals (about which we also know little), approximately 65% of emergency department visits and 50% of clinic visits take place in hospitals not affiliated with medical schools (American Hospital Association, 1979, derived from Tables 3 and 8). Still, medical-school-affiliated hospitals do set a great deal of the hierarchical tone in the United States, and thus it is useful to look at what goes on in them.

In 1965, the then Director of the Massachusetts General Hospital described the scene cogently in terms that still largely apply (Knowles):

> Turning to the outpatient department of the urban hospital, we find the stepchild of the institution. Traditionally, this has been the least popular area in which to work and, as a result, few advances in medical care and teaching have been harvested here for the benefit of the community. Ever since the day of the Flexner report, university hospitals have treated outpatients and outpatient departments as if they all had the plague. Heads of departments and professors have never toiled in these vineyards, preferring the prostrate inpatient with florid disease and the convenience of multiple test results for obvious reasons: the situation was easier to grasp, diagnosis and treatment were simpler, and all the not-so-easy to settle social and mental diseases were screened out or not admitted. Similarly, the practicing, part-time, and courtesy staff were given the outpatient labor assignment while the full-time department men (academicians) were given two rewards: they were (1) excused from going to the outpatient department and (2) given choice of times for visiting the wards filled with inpatients. Those on the "inside" saw inpatients; the "outs" worked with the "outs." (p. 70)

Most clinics today play their historical role of caring for the poor, although little "free" care remains. At best, patients have some third-party coverage; at worst, they are faced with a means-test-related sliding fee scale. Then, despite their second-class status, clinics do have a teaching function for medical students and house staff. Finally, many clinical researchers have found the outpatient clinics to be a useful place to work. Since the teaching and research functions are not often designed with the needs of patient care in mind, their presence can lead to organizational problems resulting in confusion and conflict. During the 1970s the American Hospital Association began to take some interest in clinic reform (American Hospital Association, 1973). A promising development is the substitution of medical group practice, sometimes on a prepaid basis, for hospital clinics (Block). This movement has received considerable support from the Robert Wood Johnson Foundation.

Clinic organization and staffing. The best way of organizing outpatient clinics to provide opportunities for teaching and research—especially in view of the way contemporary medical education is structured—is to have a large number of disease-, organ-, or organ-system-specific clinics (Freymann, p. 255). The typical contemporary teaching hospital has three groups of clinics: medical, surgical, and other. The medical clinic group, which may or may not have a "general medical clinic" approximating the function of the general internist, includes cardiology, neurology, dermatology, allergy, gastroenterology, and so on. Patients may stay in one or more specialty clinics for long periods of time, particularly in the typical situation in which the general medical clinic is small or nonexistent and specialty clinics admit patients directly, as "walk-ins" or on referral from the emergency room or inpatient service, rather than on referral from a general clinic. The surgical clinic group includes general surgery, orthopedics, urology, plastic surgery, and the like. Since surgical care is usually more episodic than is medical care, patients are not as likely to remain in these clinics for long periods of time. The third group includes pediatrics and the pediatric subspecialties, obstetrics-gynecology and its subspecialties, and other specialties such as rehabilitation medicine.

Teaching hospital clinics are staffed by four categories of physicians. Voluntary attending staff may draw clinic duty as part of their obligation to the hospital in return for receiving admitting privileges. Full-time inpatient physicians, usually more junior ones, may be assigned, generally to carry out teaching, supervisory, and research functions. House staff, usually residents but occasionally interns, may be assigned to clinics on a rotating basis. In most teaching hospital clinics, the stress is on teaching and research rather than patient care. Since house staff are usually rotated frequently between various subspecialty clinics for teaching purposes, patients with stable conditions coming to a subspecialty clinic, say, once every three months, may see a different physician each time. Finally, for very busy clinics, hospitals may hire outside physicians on a sessional or salaried basis, exclusively to work in the clinics. They are usually not part of the regular hospital staff, do not participate in the educational program, and are truly what Knowles calls the "outs."

Most hospital outpatient departments are open all day on weekdays, but many individual clinics, particularly when they are highly subspecialized, meet once or twice a week. Some teaching hospitals have over 100 different specialty and subspecialty clinics. Thus, a hospital-based physician working in the usual hospital clinic organization can concentrate on diabetes, peripheral vascular disease, or stroke in his or her teaching and/or research. This is advantageous to the provider who has a focus confined to a particular disease or condition. It may also be advantageous to the patient who has a single disease problem of a rather complex or unusual nature.

Three kinds of patients face difficulties in using such clinics. First is the patient with the ordinary problem for which no specialty clinic exists; few hospitals, for example, have "sore throat" clinics. Second is the patient with a categorical disease, like diabetes, which, however, is uncomplicated. Going to a diabetes clinic, such a patient is likely to have to take a back seat to a diabetic patient who has complications. Third is the patient with multiple problems. These patients, often elderly, may end up attending diabetes clinic on Tuesday, stroke clinic on Wednesday, peripheral vascular clinic on Thursday, and cardiology clinic on Friday. (Fortunately, Monday is a free day.) This is distinctly disadvantageous for two major reasons: it necessitates multiple trips to the clinic and precludes looking at the patient as a whole person rather than as a collection of diseased organs and organ systems.

Thus the basic conflict in hospital ambulatory services is established, between the needs of specialty-oriented providers on the one hand and patients with either ordinary problems or several different problems requiring the care of specialists on the other. This situation is not new; neither is professional recognition of the situation and what ought to be done about it. In 1964, at a conference on "The Expanding Role of Ambulatory Services in Hospitals and Health Departments" held at the New York Academy of Medicine, Cecil Sheps, M.D., said:

As I sat through the sessions yesterday and today I had a persistent feeling of *deja vu*. I possess a book written by Michael M. Davis [*Clinics, Hospitals and Health Centers*, New York: Harper, 1927] and published in 1927. In it there is quoted a statement prepared in 1914 that describes the purpose of an out-patient department just as clearly as anything said at this conference; that the focus must be on the patient, that care must be organized around the patient, and that the hospital must take the community as its venue and not simply the patients who come to it (p. 148).

At the same conference, John Knowles, M.D., outlined his view of what comprehensive ambulatory care in the hospital setting would mean (Knowles):

Comprehensive medicine in this context means the coordination of all various caring elements in the community with those of the medical profession by a team of individuals representing all disciplines, with all the techniques and resources available to the physician and his patient. The aim of these individuals would be to provide total care—somatic, psychic, and social—to those in need, and to study and research the expanding social and economic problems of medical care with the intent of improving the organization and provision of health services (p. 73).

The goal of these proposals, still not achieved in many institutions, is primarily to make hospital clinics more responsive to community needs than they are now. An important effect of such changes would be the education of physicians who would perforce develop an entirely different view of hospital ambulatory services (Jonas, 1979, Chapter 12). It must be remembered that the essential difficulty is the contradiction between the needs of the majority of clinic patients to receive comprehensive care and the needs of the majority of the physicians staffing the clinics to carry out their teaching and research functions. At present, the latter requires a disease orientation and generally an orientation toward diseases for which the patient requires hospitalization at one point or another. If teaching and research were to be reoriented toward an emphasis on the more common rather than on the more uncommon, if hospitals were to define their roles and responsibilities in terms of community needs, the contradiction would be resolved straight away and hospital clinics would be on the road to first-class status (Jonas, 1973; Freymann, Chapter 18). In the late 1970s, a new federal initiative addressed the problem of providing comprehensive, community-oriented primary health care services in hospitals, on a demonstration basis (Bureau of Community Health Services, 1979b). Some results of this Hospital Affiliated Primary Care Centers Program should be available for examination in the early 1980s.

It must be borne in mind that these conflicts over clinic services affect only a minority of American hospitals, the 34% of hospitals that have clinics (American Hospital Association, 1979, Table 12A). Other problems, concerning emergency services, affect the majority of American hospitals, since about 80% of them have emergency departments, as do 90% of all community hospitals and over 95% of community hospitals with more than 200 beds (American Hospital Association, 1979, Table 12A).

Hospital emergency services. The hospital emergency unit serves a variety of functions. It does, of course, take care of critically ill and injured patients. In many hospitals, it serves as a secondary, well-equipped private doctor's office, in which staff physicians can see their own patients for whom more sophisticated care than that available in the doctor's own office is required. A third role is that of admitter of patients to the hospital (Kessler and Wilson). A fourth, increasingly important role is the provision of care to persons who are not injured or critically ill, who do not have or cannot reach a private physician, and/or who do not use the hospital clinic, if one exists, or another organized ambulatory service, or find that it is not open when needed (Kelman and Lane; Andrus; *Medical World News,* 1977).

Weinerman et al. defined three categories of patients presenting themselves to emergency units; nonurgent, urgent, and emergent (p. 1040).

Nonurgent is defined as: "Condition does not require the resources of an emergency service; referral for routine medical care may or may not be needed; disorder is nonacute or minor in severity." Urgent is: "Condition requires medical attention within the period of a few hours; there is possible danger to the patient if medically unattended; disorder is acute but not necessarily severe." Emergent is: "Condition requires immediate medical attention; time delay is harmful to patient; disorder is acute and potentially threatening to life or function." It should be borne in mind that these are professional definitions, from the point of view of the provider. Patients are not as likely to make these kinds of distinctions. Most patients presenting themselves for care to emergency departments are there because they feel that they need attention immediately, however their problem might be classified by a provider.

By the early 1960s, studies had shown that the proportion of patients in the nonurgent category had been on the increase since World War II (Weinerman and Edwards). A more recent review of data on categorical patient distribution showed that the average distribution by category among patients admitted to emergency departments is approximately 5% emergent, 45% urgent, and 50% nonurgent (Jonas et al.). There can be variations around these figures by type, role, and location of hospital (Torrens and Yedvab).

One problem faced by hospital emergency units is the "nonurgent" patient (Gibson, 1971). A variety of solutions has been proposed (Spencer, Chapter 1), ranging from virtually barring the door to nonurgent patients; to providing a sorting or triage system (Weinerman and Edwards; Beloff; Albin et al.) to screen for nonurgent patients and refer them to alternative sources of care after making certain that no acute illness is in fact present; to treating patients as they come, with equanimity (Hannas, 1975); to becoming a sort of community general clinic that happens to be open 24 hours a day (Satin and Duhl). The final word on this subject has not yet been written; rational solutions to the problem involve not only emergency departments but other sectors of the health care delivery system as well. What Weinerman and Edwards said in 1964 is still true today:

> The ultimate solution must be found outside the walls of the hospital. It must encompass an integrated system of medical care for the entire community assuring availability of appropriate medical care at all hours and to all classes of the population. When this dream is realized, the emergency service will again be appropriately named, and triage will no longer be necessary.

There are a variety of physician staffing patterns for emergency departments, but little survey work on the subject has been done since the study by Webb and Lawrence (1972). In teaching hospitals, it has been customary to staff emergency departments primarily with the least experienced members of the house staff, the interns. In many hospitals, they are being replaced with residents. Some teaching hospitals find that they cannot fully meet the service needs from house staff; they supplement them with full-time or sessional hired physicians, who, more often than not, occupy an "out" position similar in relation to the regular hospital staff to that of hired clinic physicians. An increasing number of teaching hospitals are assigning regular full-time staff to some responsibility in the emergency department.

The staffing situation is different in nonteaching hospitals. In those with light patient loads, members of the hospital attending staff may cover, in person or on call, on a rotating staff system. In certain states there are legal staffing requirements. An increasingly popular approach to the solution of this problem is the full-time emergency department group practice, which has taken a variety of forms (Hannas, 1971; Gersonde; *Medical World News*, 1974). To improve patient communications and flow, some ERs are adding "ombudsmen" or patient representatives (Lane and Evans).

There is a running controversy concerning categorization of emergency departments by level of service (Gibson, 1977a). In 1971, the AMA recommended that: "categorization [be] based on the capabilities to provide effective emergency medical care for those individuals in-house or brought to the hospital with severe or critical injuries or illnesses" (Gibson, 1977a, p. 97). Four categories, ranging from "comprehensive" to "basic" emergency service, were suggested. Although there is a great deal of logic to the concept (Harvey, 1973), and it is written into national and state laws and regulations, there has been a great deal of resistance to its implementation (Gibson, 1977a; Kippel; Weller; Hoffer). According to Gibson (1977a):

> . . . the strategy of categorization suffers from such severe planning, conceptual, and methodological deficiencies, both inherently and in the way it has been applied over the past sixty years, that it can no longer be regarded as a reasonable means of either assessing present emergency medical services or changing them for the better. No evidence exists that a single community has changed utilization patterns of hospital emergency departments as a result of categorization. Many communities, in fact, have found categorization to be a hostility-generating process that is so destructive of interfacility consensus that they have not been able to implement the results. (p. 98)

Nevertheless, categorization still has its strong supporters (*Medical World News*, 1978, p. 72), and the book is still open on the question.

The organization of hospital ambulatory services. There are at least as many modes of organization of hospital ambulatory services as there are types of hospitals, and, in the United States, that is many indeed. We will examine, briefly, one of the major patterns of organization, that found in a typical teaching hospital with both an emergency unit and clinics. In many such hospitals, there are three vertical organizational lines: one for the medical staff, one for the nursing staff, and one for business administration, support services, and hotel operations. (The latter includes housekeeping, dietary, and maintenance. It is interesting to note that "hospital" and "hotel" both derive from the same Latin word.) Sometimes these vertical lines meet in the director's office; sometimes they never meet; occasionally they are well integrated.

This organizational structure is reflected in the ambulatory services. Generally, each medical department is responsible for physician services in its own clinics. The pattern may extend to the emergency unit as well, or it may be the primary responsibility of one department, say, surgery. Alternatively, physician staffing in the emergency unit may be entirely the responsibility of a separate entity, an Emergency Department, which may stand on its own, may be part of a Department of Ambulatory Services or Community Medicine, or may be attached to the office of the hospital's director. In teaching hospitals, Departments of Ambulatory Services, when they exist, may exert some control over emergency unit physicians, but only rarely do they have any true control over clinic physician staffing.

The Nursing Department generally controls the nursing services for both clinics and emergency units, sometimes designating an Associate or Assistant Director of Nursing for Ambulatory Care. Likewise, the hospital's administration runs the clerical and other support services, often through an associate or assistant administrator or director.

This tripartite approach works well as long as one is not particularly interested in establishing one coordinated *program* in ambulatory care. When there is not one person, or office, in charge of all the resources required to provide ambulatory services, it is very difficult indeed to mount such a unified program (Jonas, 1973). If one wishes to provide ambulatory services of a comprehensive nature in which the patient, rather than the disease or injury, is the focus (as discussed above), coordination of physician, nursing, and support services under unified leadership is essential.

Hospitals around the country are wrestling with this problem. Its resolution will require major changes in the way in which hospitals are administratively structured, and those structural changes will in turn require major changes in the way people think and feel. With a few exceptions, hospitals are not used to mounting coordinated *programs*, but rather to delivering *services*, each component putting in its piece more or less as it sees fit. To establish an ambulatory care program with a single director having ultimate responsibility for the whole means that the medical, nursing, and support services each must surrender some sovereignty, something each is loath to do. Furthermore, even if a *functionally decentralized* program in ambulatory care could be developed, offering coordinated, comprehensive care to patients, other problems would be created. Does one end up with duplicated departments of medicine, pediatrics, surgery, nursing, and clerical services for inpatient and outpatient services for the very important functions of hiring, firing, discipline, quality control, setting patient-care policies, education, research, and the like? This question is still being debated. However, many of the problems are created by the present contradictions evident in the role and work of hospitals, as discussed above, among service, teaching, and research. Resolution of these contradictions along the lines of Freymann's "mission-oriented hospital" (1974) would solve many problems, as will be further discussed in the next chapter.

Emergency Medical Services

Emergency medical services are those provided to victims of accidents and acute, overwhelming illnesses on an immediate basis, in an effort to preserve life and/or diminish to the extent possible the degree of potential temporary and/or permanent disability suffered by the victim. Virtually all patients entering the emergency medical services system are in the "emergent" or "urgent" category (see p. 137).

As pointed out by Ruth Roemer et al., in a detailed treatment of the history and major problems of this service sector, the emergency medical service (EMS) has three principal components: (1) ambulance services and emergency prehospital care; (2) emergency medical care provided at the hospital; and (3) disaster medical services. In this section, we are focusing on (1). In federal legislation, 15 components of a functioning emergency medical services system are identified (Hoffer): provision of manpower, training of personnel, communications, transportation, facilities, critical-care units, use of public-safety agencies, consumer participation, accessibility to care, transfer of patients standard medical-record keeping, consumer information and education, independent review and evaluation, disaster linkage, and mutual-aid agreements. A principal goal has been to provide for the whole nation a set of coordinated emergency care dispatch centers, using the 911 uniform emergency telephone number.

Ambulance services are the key linkage in transporting victims of accidents and acute, overwhelming illnesses safely and quickly to an appropriate emergency medical facility and in rendering indicated first aid at the site and in transit (Gibson, 1973). They are seriously deficient in many parts of the United States. Historically, ambulance services developed from a for-profit enterprise established by funeral directors. In this system, sometimes the same vehicle has been able to serve more than one purpose, on occasion consecutively. Since ambulance services tend to be unprofitable, funeral directors have gradually abandoned this service, leaving it for communities to provide (*Medical World News*, 1970). However, in many communities there is an absence of defined responsibility for ambulance services. The deficiencies in emergency services in many communities are particularly disturbing, given that traumatic injuries are among the leading causes of death in the productive age groups (National Academy of Sciences, National Research Council). Many of these deaths could be prevented if high-quality emergency services were readily available (National Conference on Cardio-Pulmonary Resuscitation and Emergency Cardiac Care).

Ambulance services must be able to respond quickly to calls. The vehicles must be appropriately designed and they must be adequately staffed and organized so that the patient is taken to the most appropriate hospital emergency department. The success of an emergency medical services system is dependent upon a series of communication links, including victim and ambulance service, dispatcher and ambulance, and ambulance and hospital (Gibson, 1971, 1973).

Any viable EMS requires adequate financing, manpower, equipment, and facilities, with strict standards for each, and the willingness of professions, agencies, institutions, and units of local government to work together and coordinate their resources (Hanlon; Gibson, 1974). A concise history and consideration of the policy issues in the development of EMSs has been presented by Gibson (1977b), who sees serious problems in the program (1977a). Some solutions have focused on upgrading facilities, equipment, and/or personnel. Two pieces of federal legislation have been important. The National Highway Traffic Safety Act of 1966 contained performance criteria for EMSs and required the states to submit EMS plans. The Emergency Medical Services System Act of 1973 authorized $185 million over three years to states, counties, and other nonprofit agencies to plan, expand, and modernize EMSs (Harvey, 1975). The Act was extended and somewhat expanded in scope twice, in 1976 (P. L. 94–573) and 1979 (P. L. 96–142). The Robert Wood Johnson Foundation played a major role, along with government, in developing the national EMS system (Johnson Foundation).

Three conditions of the basic law are significant. It requires that special consideration be given to rural areas applying for assistance, as well as to applications that will coordinate local systems with statewide EMSs. In addition, the Act provides that the EMS be "organized in a manner that provides persons who reside in the system's service area and who have no professional training or financial interest in the provision of health care with an adequate opportunity to participate in making of policy for the system" (P. L. 93–154). The law also stipulates that emergency services must be provided without prior inquiry as to ability to pay.

Considerable attention has been paid to ambulance design and the qualifications and training of the people who run them (Hoffer). Under the influence of the EMS Act of 1973, the typical ambulance profile has changed from that of the hearse to that of the light van. An essential requirement of modern ambulance design is that it must permit the provision of cardiopulmonary resuscitation (CPR) by an ambulance attendant en route.

The emergency medical technician (EMT) is a new category of health worker spawned by legislation. EMTs are trained to do emergency life-support and injury-management work, primarily out of the hospital. Training has been highly variable, ranging in length from 81 to over 2,000 hours. (The latter figure is impressive in light of the fact that medical school averages about 5,000 hours.) In 1978, a national standard course was established with a length of 185 hours (*National Training Course, Emergency Medical Technician/Paramedic*). As of 1978, there were 262,000 ambulance personnel trained to the EMT-A (81-hour course) level, and 12,000 more with 1,000 or more hours of training, termed "EMT-Paramedics" (*Medical World News*, 1978). As the 1970s came to an end, there was increasing evidence that EMSs were improving the quality of medical care and saving lives (*Medical World News*, 1978; Sherman; Lewis et al.; Hoffer; Montgomery). However, Gibson, a major authority in this area, had his doubts that the evidence in fact reflected reality (1978).

Health Department Services

Ambulatory personal health services are provided by government at the local level in most parts of the United States (see also Chapter 11). Information on these services is limited; they have not been frequently or extensively studied (Miller et al., 1979). The provision of direct personal health service by local health departments has been a subject of controversy since the practice began in the 19th century (Rosen; Winslow, Chapter 17). Private physicians almost always regarded local health departments as competing for their fee-paying patients and therefore threatening their practices, particularly since local health departments—in contrast to local hospital departments—traditionally offered their services free to all persons, regardless of ability to pay. Battles over the role of local health departments were especially fierce during the 1920s. The organizational representatives of American physicians, having successfully reduced medical school enrollments (following implementation of the Flexner Report) and having blocked the passage of any kind of national health insurance program, in which there had been broad national interest during and after World War I (see Chapter 15), struggled to further limit competition and government control over private practice. They were successful in the local health department arena as well, since local health department personal services are generally limited to those areas in which private physicians are either not very interested (routine well-baby examinations) or not especially competent (treatment, case-finding, and contact-investigation of venereal disease and tuberculosis).

In 1975, it was estimated that less than 3% of all ambulatory personal health services were being provided by local health departments, excluding school health services (Roemer, 1975a). The most frequently offered personal health services are tuberculosis control, venereal disease control, well-baby care, crippled children's care, prenatal and family planning services, adult screening programs for chronic disease, mental health diagnostic and follow-up service, and general home public health nursing and homemaker services. These are so-called categorical programs, in which categories of diseases or persons are taken care of. (For a detailed description of the history and problems of maternal and child health programs, see Chapter 4 of Ruth Roemer et al., 1975.) About one-half of local health departments run the school health services in their jurisdictions, the balance being run by boards of education on their own (25%) or in cooperation with the local health department. Very little disease treatment is done in school health programs. Most activity is confined to case-finding to prevent epidemic disease. Screening for vision and hearing difficulties and for inadequate immunization is done by school nurses; referrals are made for diagnosis and treatment.

There have been efforts since World War I to involve local, and sometimes state, health departments in the delivery of general personal health services (Rosen; Winslow, Chapter 17; Myers et al.). These have generally been unsuccessful. Some have expressed optimism that this change in role can be accomplished (Cashman; Romer, 1975a; Miller et al., 1977; Moos and Miller). Given the history of local health departments, their bureaucratic, categorically oriented administrative structure, continuing opposition from the private sector, and their close involvement with politically sensitive, financially pressed local governments (See Chapters 5, 7 of Jonas, 1977), the chances are limited that much headway will be made in this direction.

Group Practice and Health Maintenance Organizations

Group practice, in its simplest sense, means three or more physicians working in the same facility. However, there are a number of different types of group practice, defined by different characteristics—the types of providers included, type of specialties included, mode of association between physicians, patterns of medical practice, mode of physician reimbursement, and mode of patient payment (Terris, 1968).

In terms of types of providers included, some groups can be defined as multidisciplinary, i.e., other health care providers besides physicians are included, in a health care team. Multidisciplinary groups, the most inclusive type, are also the newest in the United States; they are usually found operating in community-based, government-funded neighborhood health centers (see below, p. 151 ff.), although this pattern is now to be seen in some independent prepaid group practices, and also in some hospital ambulatory services.

Physician-only groups may be single-specialty or multispecialty. Single-specialty groups are particularly popular in fields in which out-of-regular-hours calls tend to be fairly frequent. Multispecialty groups usually divide the physicians into two ranks, primary and referral. The primary care rank may consist of internists and pediatricians doing frontline medical practice, or family practitioners, or both. In the referral rank are the medical subspecialists and the surgeons.

The mode of physician association in group practice varies widely. In some groups, physicians may simply share space and perhaps a common billing procedure, but not patients. This sort of arrangement becomes a bit more sophisticated with the addition of a partnership arrangement among the participating physicians. Beyond that some groups are based on a corporation. The AMA defines group practice as "the application of medical services by three or more physicians, formally organized to provide medical care, consultation, diagnosis, and/or treatment through joint use of equipment and personnel, and with the income from medical practice distributed in accordance with methods previously determined by the members of the group" (Goodman et al., p. 2). This definition excludes any combination of physicians that simply shares space, but does not exclude fee-for-service groups.

The pattern of medical practice may be true group or essentially solo. In the latter, each physician has complete responsibility for his own patients with no other physician ever involved, except on formal referral for consultation, or for night or weekend coverage, which is usually shared by group members on a regular rotation basis. In true group practice, physicians share patient-care responsibility.

The mode of physician reimbursement may be fee-for-service (paid either directly by the patient or by the group, even if the patient does not pay the group on a fee-for-service basis); capitation (a flat rate for each individual patient in return for agreeing to provide all needed medical services during a specified time period); or salary. The mode of payment to the group by the patient may be fee-for-service or what is called prepayment, in which the patient or, more usually, the patient's employer or union health fund, pays a premium to cover a set of agreed-to services for a particular time period. Almost every possible combination of the three methods of physician reimbursement and the two methods of patient payment is used somewhere, but the three most common combinations are fee-for-service patient payment with fee-for-service physician reimbursement, patient prepayment with physician reimbursement by capitation, and patient prepayment with physician reimbursement by salary.

The numbers of groups and of doctors working in groups have been rising gradually since the first one was founded by the brothers Mayo in Rochester, Minnesota, in 1887 (Silver; M. I. Roemer et al.). In 1975, the most recent year for which complete figures are available, there were, within the AMA definition, 8,483 groups of all kinds, single specialty, multispecialty, and prepaid, with 66,842 physicians (Goodman et al., Chapter 3). The rate of growth of the institution of group practice is increasing; almost 25% of all active physicians, excluding house staff, are engaged in it. The five most popular specialties for single-specialty grouping (excluding "unspecified") are general/family practice; anesthesiology; radiology; obstetrics and gynecology; and internal medicine (Goodman et al., Chapter 6).

Prepaid group practices. Prepaid Group Practices (PPGP) and their recent incarnation as Health Maintenance Organizations (HMOs) form a special category of group practice. Since the early 1970s, they have received increasing consideration as a possible alternative in the financing and delivery of health services, particularly by those who believe that the U.S. health care delivery system needs significant improvement. PPGPs have been thought by some to be the wave of the future for U.S. health care since the 1920s. The first PPGP was created in 1929 by Dr. Michael A. Shadid in Elk City, Oklahoma (MacColl, pp. 20–24). Basing its recommendations on a 1931 study by Rufus Rorem (1971), the 1932 Final Report of the Committee on the Costs of Medical Care (1970) strongly supported the concept. Axelrod agreed (1956), as did Silver et al. (1957), and Silver again (1963), Falk (1963), MacColl (1966), Weinerman (1968), Saward (1969), the *Harvard Law Review* (1971), Roemer and Shonick (1973), *Consumer Reports* (1974), and M. I. Roemer (1975b).

A good working definition of PPGP is provided by the *Harvard Law Review:*

> Pre-paid group practice may be broadly defined as a medical care delivery system which accepts responsibility for the organization, financing, and delivery of health care services for a defined population. Essentially, it

combines a financing mechanism—prepayment—with a particular mode of delivery—group practice—by means of a managerial-administrative organization responsible for ensuring the availability of health services for a subscriber population. (p. 901)

The use of the term "Prepaid Group Practice" to describe the organization of physicians in groups providing services on a prepaid basis persisted until 1971 when the term "Health Maintenance Organization" was introduced (Ellwood et al.; Center for Health Administration Studies; Myers; USDHEW, 1971). By the late 1970s, the term HMO was being defined by its inventor, Paul Ellwood, as "an organization which offers comprehensive health benefits at a predetermined price to a voluntarily enrolled population which receives its care through a specified set of providers" (Inter Study Health Systems). Voluntary participation by patients in HMOs make them different from other health services provided on a prepaid basis for the military and for institutionalized populations. HMOs have been developed as high-quality, cost-effective, competitive alternatives to fee-for-service forms of practice (Office of Health Maintenance Organizations, 1979a, 1979b; Loebs; Falkson).

The majority of HMOs are multispecialty group practices in which the physicians are either salaried employees of the HMO (staff model) or in an independent group that contracts with the HMO to deliver services (group model). The largest and best known HMOs are group models: Kaiser-Permanente (Kaiser Foundation Medical Care Program; National Advisory Commisson on Health Manpower; Williams; Fleming) and the Health Insurance Plan of Greater New York (Silver et al.; Brindle; Bates). Group Health Association of Washington, D.C., is the oldest and largest of the staff-model plans; it was formed as a consumer cooperative during the 1930s. Another prominent consumer-operated staff model plan is the Group Health Cooperative of Puget Sound (Group Health Cooperative, 1979a, 1979b). While these practices formed the models for the federal legislation promoting HMOs, another alternative is available.

Individual practice associations. The alternative to PPGP that can qualify as an HMO is the Individual Practice Association (IPA), known before that term was developed in the late 1970s as the "Comprehensive Foundation for Medical Care," or FMC (Harrington; Blake and Carnoy; Egdahl; Egdahl et al.; Brian; Newport and Roemer). The IPA combines a prepayment mechanism for patients with fee-for-service solo practice for the physicians. The IPA is an agency that enrolls physicians who agree to a central billing mechanism, peer review of quality, and cost controls. It then contracts, usually with employers and/or union health and welfare funds, to provide a stipulated package of health care benefits to covered persons in return for a per-person payment to the IPA from the contracting entity. Either no fee or a nominal fee changes hands between individual patients and physicians. However, the physicians, working in their own offices, bill the IPA on a fee basis for each item of service provided. There is a maximum amount for which physicians can bill, of course; it is related to the total amount of money paid in by the contractee, and the IPA does monitoring of billing closely. Thus, although physicians charge on a fee-for-service basis, they are actually on a quasi-salary system. IPAs are also concerned with the medical quality of the product that their member physicians are delivering.

HMO—Legislative history. The legislative history of the HMO program is complex (Bauman; Falkson). It began with the introduction by President Nixon in early 1971 of a legislative proposal based on the concepts of Paul Ellwood (Ellwood et al.). In 1972–1973, while specific HMO legislation was being developed, a few organizations received federal money for HMO development under various provisions of the Public Health Service Act and other federal legislation (Center for Health Administration Studies). Congress forced a halt in that kind of activity, however, until specific HMO legislation could be passed. The first HMO Act (P. L. 93–222) was passed in December 1973 (Subcommittee on Health). It authorized $325 million over five years for grants and loans to help HMOs get underway (Starr; Strumpf et al.). To qualify as an HMO, an organization had to provide or contract for the following services: physician care, inpatient and outpatient hospital care, medically necessary emergency health services, short-term evaluative and crisis intervention mental health services, medical treatment and referral services for the abuse of or addiction to alcohol and drugs, diagnostic laboratory and diagnostic and therapeutic radiological services, and preventive health services. Such supplemental services as dental care and prescription drugs could be contracted for as well. But services had to be available and accessible on a 24-hour-a-day, 7-day-a-week basis. The subscriber was to pay nothing, or only a minimal co-payment, at time of service.

The HMO Act of 1973 created an interesting contradiction (Dorsey, 1975). In its attempt to create a model for what comprehensive health care should be, the Act prescribed such a broad range of benefits that many organizations that were interested in sponsoring HMOs declined to do so because the benefit package would carry a very high price tag, in practice making it noncompetitive with existing plans like Blue Cross/Blue Shield, even though the benefits were better. This situation, plus a rather complex set of USDHEW regulations written pursuant to the Act, served to inhibit initiative in HMO development. However, subsequent amendments, in 1976 (P. L. 94–46) and 1978 (P. L. 95–559), created a more workable piece of legislation. The three laws form Title XIII of the Public Health Service Act. The legislation provides grants during a carefully choreographed 3-year planning process and loans during the early years of operations to public or nonprofit private prepaid group practices or individual practice associations. The plan sponsors must agree to and demonstrate that they can meet the stringent federal program requirements mandated by law and regulation. Progress during the planning phase and after commencement of operations is carefully monitored by the Office of Health Maintenance Organizations (OHMO) in Washington and the DHHS regional offices. HMOs meeting the various requirements become "federally qualified." Among other things, this means that employers of 25 or more workers in the HMO's service area that offer health insurance to their employees must offer the HMO service package as an option, the so-called Mandatory Dual Choice System.

The HMO program, entering the 1980s. As of 1979, there were about 210 prepaid health plans, serving approximately 8 million Americans (Office of Health Maintenance Organizations, 1979b, p. 1). Only about half of the HMOs were "federally qualified," but they enrolled about two-thirds of the total HMO membership (Office of Health Maintenance Organizations, 1979a, p. 3). Over 85% of the membership was in prepaid group practices, which accounted for about two-thirds of all plans. HMOs have been shown to be capable of lowering health care costs compared to the cost experienced under conventional health insurance, principally by their ability to substantially lower hospital utilization rates for their enrollees (Luft; Roemer and Shonick; Reidel et al.). Additionally, communities that have HMOs seem to experience lower overall health care costs and hospital utilization than communities without HMOs (Dorsey, 1978). A review of 25 studies of the quality of care provided by HMOs concluded that in 19 of the studies "the general quality of health care, as indicated by the measures applied, was superior to that in fee-for-service or other settings." In the balance of the studies, the quality of care was found to be similar in all settings studied (Williamson et al.).

Building on this base of achievement in maintaining and improving quality while controlling costs, in 1980 the Federal Office of Health Maintenance Organizations embarked on an ambitious "National HMO Development Strategy through 1988 (Office of Health Maintenance Organizations, 1979b). The "Goals for Nationwide HMO Growth" were:

1.   To increase the number of HMOs to improve the public access to comprehensive health sources (pp. 3–4)
2.   To expand enrollment in existing HMOs to increase competition in the health care system (pp. 4–5)
3.   To maximize the cost-savings potential of HMOs (pp. 6–9).

The OHMO hoped to more than double the number of HMOs to 442 by 1988 and increase enrollment to over 19 million (OHMO, Table I). To achieve these goals, OHMO "targeted" about 60 communities for HMO growth, based on various social, economic, demographic, and physical characteristics that indicate a good potential for HMO development and growth (pp. 9–14). Because of their greater potential for cost savings, group practices were favored over IPAs. OHMO stressed that HMOs are "not government-run entities," but rather private corporations, established with federal assistance and guidance (p. 12). OHMO was interested in improving the accessibility of HMOs for the medically underserved and increasing the enrollment of public beneficiaries and federal employees in HMOs (p. 18). It should be pointed out, however, that even with these ambitious plans, the HMO movement still has a long way to go. If the target enrollment figure for 1988 is achieved, HMOs will still be serving less than 10% of the population.

Prepaid group practice and health services.   The medical encounter in the HMO, as in any other medical practice setting, principally involves two persons—the physician and the patient. In 1963, Silver summarized the advantages and disadvantages for physicians of group practice in comparison to solo practice in terms that still apply (1963). The advantages include a regular work schedule, reasonably competitive income, provision of malpractice insurance, the opportunity for collegial medical practice, better access to ancillary personnel and services, and freedom from concern with the business aspects of medical practice. Disadvantages include possible deterioration of the "doctor-patient relationship," limited professional contacts and choice of consultants, limitations on income potential, and a possible rigidity in practice modes and conduct. Advantages for patients include no charge or low charges at time of service; one-stop shopping for 24-hour, 7-day service; continuity of care; and protection against unnecessary surgery. Disadvantages center around the possibility of the development of a clinic atmosphere (Baehr), impersonality, long waits for service, and possible problems of access.

However, the most serious problems of prepaid group practice may be ideological rather than practical. Weinerman, an early, strong advocate of prepaid group practice, reviewed the experience and was disappointed (1968). His observations, although made some time ago, are still pertinent. In essence, he said that PPGP looks great on paper, but the practical results are inconclusive; moreover, the idea really has not caught on to a great extent. He concluded that the mechanical-financial elements of the list of advantages cited above have been implemented, particularly to the benefit of the physicians, but that the ideological aspects of true group

practice have not. Most groups maintain physician elitism. "Group conferences," he said, "medical audits and informal office consultations are, in my
experience, more common in the descriptive literature than in daily practice." He noted (Weinerman, 1968):

> Perhaps most disappointing has been the hesitation on the part of most
> medical groups to effect changes in the "way of life" of the medical team itself.
> This would involve acceptance by the group as a whole of collective responsi-
> bility for the health of its patients or members . . . would mean actively
> reaching out into the community for . . . early detection . . . [and] identifica-
> tion and special protection for those at specific risk of disease . . . [and] would
> imply particular concern for those patients who do not use the service. . . . It
> implies as much concern with rapport as with diagnostic labels, as much with
> education as with prescription. (p. 1429)

Since American medical practice is primarily disease-oriented (Jonas,
1979) and since most physicians bring their "ideological baggage" with
them when they join an HMO staff, the thorough integration of health
promotion and preventive medicine services into the medical and health
services program exists only on paper, if at all, in most HMOs. Weinerman
concluded that only if ideological changes take place, along with organizational and financial ones, will prepaid group practice be successful.

Neighborhood Health Centers

The "Neighborhood Health Center" (NHC) movement of the late 1960s
and early 1970s saw the development of a particular kind of ambulatory
health care facility, based on the concepts of full-time, salaried physician
staffing, multidisciplinary team health care practice, and community involvement in both policy-making and facility operations (Davis and
Schoen; Zwick). The movement was strongly stimulated by the federal
Office of Economic Opportunity (OEO), which was a principal factor in the
so-called War on Poverty conducted by President Lyndon Johnson's administration in the period 1964–1968. The "Neighborhood Health Centers"
discussed here are generally limited to those developed with federal
government support. By the late 1970s, they were being called "Community Health Centers" in federal terminology. Other institutions with similar
features also came into being, sponsored by volunteer groups (Stoeckle et
al.; Schachter and Elliston; Tennant and Day) and other governmental
jurisdictions. However, information available on them is very sketchy, and
by and large their impact was negligible. In any case, the NHCs discussed
herein were prototypical.

The NHC does not represent an entirely new concept in the United
States. The 19th-century dispensary, discussed above, performed some

similar functions, although it was organized differently. Health department ambulatory care programs developed during the last quarter of the 19th century had some elements that would appear later in NHCs, such as districting, but provided primarily categorical services and therefore were not comprehensive. The period 1910–1919 was marked by the development of several health centers in different parts of the country; they truly attempted to offer comprehensive services to designated areas from a freestanding, not hospital-based institution (Rosen). C.-E. A. Winslow noted in 1919: "The most striking and typical development of the public health movement of the present day is the health center" (Rosen). However, he was over-optimistic. Herman Biggs, M. D., then Commissioner of Health of New York State, tried vigorously, but quite unsuccessfully, to get the state and local health departments away from the categorical disease approach and into the business of delivering comprehensive health services during the period 1920–1923 (Winslow, Chapter 17). With the resurgence of political conservatism in the United States following World War I and the concomitant change in policy of the American Medical Association, which came to oppose any health care delivery mode not based on private practice, except for delivery to the very poor, the NHC movement of that period disappeared (Rosen).

The experience with PPGPs in the 1930s, 1940s, and 1950s influenced the development of the NHC movement of the 1960s and 1970s. An ambulatory care service developed at the municipal Gouverneur Hospital on New York City's Lower East Side was significant. Its first director, the late Dr. Howard Brown, came from one of the prototypical PPGPs, the Health Insurance Plan of Greater New York, with many concepts new to municipal health services. A comprehensive ambulatory care program was installed in Gouverneur (Light and Brown). It was very influential in the early development of OEO-NHCs, serving as a model that many persons who were establishing NHCs came to observe.

Another early model OEO-NHC was Montefiore's Neighborhood Medical Care Demonstraton project in the Bronx, New York (Lloyd and Wise; Montefiore "Neighborhood Medical Demonstration"), which became the Martin Luther King Neighborhood Health Center. In a way, this NHC too had its links with the past, since one of the largest and most successful Health Insurance Plan groups in New York City was based at Montefiore. Indeed, the major medical program elements, although not the social, administrative, or political program elements, of the contemporary NHC were proposed in an American Public Health Association policy statement on community health services adopted in 1963 (American Public Health Association).

NHCs appeared in many different shapes and sizes, had a variety of different starting points, various sources of funding, and a variety of programs (Abrams and Snyder; Collins; Davis and Tranquada; C. D. Gibson; Lashof; Schwartz). However, they did share certain common features. NHCs were usually situated in medically underserved, minority-occupied urban areas. They generally attempted—with varying degrees of vigor and success—to institute the concept of multidisciplinary group practice, utilizing nurses, social workers, neighborhood health workers (often people from the area served, specially trained by the NHC, usually with a combination of basic nursing and social service skills), and some-times lawyers, in a health care team to deal with patients and their problems. Latterly, they often added nurse practitioners or physicians' associates to their staffs. Physicians were on salary or paid by the session. Ultimately, the NHCs aimed to institute one-stop shopping for ambulatory care, to provide a comprehensive range of preventive and rehabilitative as well as treatment services that were acceptable, affordable, and of high quality, and to intervene in the cycle of poverty.

Starting an NHC was an expensive proposition. Capital costs were high, staffing to meet multiple health problems was heavy and expensive, and many potential patients had no means of paying for care, either on their own or through a third party. NHCs were funded by a combination of starting-up grants, usually from OEO or HEW, and third-party payments, usually Medicaid and Medicare. NHCs were related in one way or another to a "back-up hospital," which was intended to supply inpatient services, specialist consultation, sophisticated laboratory and X-ray services, and supervision, if not the direct employment, of the medical staff.

The original OEO legislation mandated "maximum feasible participa-tion" in the operation and administration of the NHCs (as well as all other OEO programs) by those persons they served. "Maximum feasible parti-cipation" was never precisely defined. However, its existence as an OEO requirement led to many a conflict between the hospitals and medical schools originally involved to a greater or lesser extent in operating pro-grams and the representatives of the served communities over the ques-tion: "Who's in charge here?" (Geiger; Goldberg et al.; Torrens).

"Community Advisory Boards" were mandated by OEO. Board mem-bers usually came from underserved areas that had often received what little care they did get from the hospital that now had the grant, a hospital that, on the basis of its past performance, was perceived by residents of the service area as being unsympathetic, to say the least. Community boards therefore wanted the final say on major policy questions. The hospitals, on the other hand, had the responsibility for the program, particularly its medical quality, and were reluctant to give up any significant degree of authority. This situation, exacerbated at times by linguistic and cultural barriers, often led to tense and painful experiences for both sides. Later, fiscal responsibility for operation of some NHCs was turned over to non-profit corporations representing the served communities, a long-range requirement of the original OEO program guidelines. These bodies then contracted with the back-up hospitals to provide needed services, retaining primary control for themselves.

Additional problems were created by the OEO view that the provision of job opportunities to residents from the NHC service area was at least as significant a role for the NHCs as was the provision of health care. This created two important areas of conflict. NHCs usually served severely depressed minority-group urban areas where it was most difficult to find persons with requisite health care skills and training, particularly in the professional and semi-professional job categories. Furthermore, control of job positions for which neighborhood residents might be eligible became a plum, for both positive and negative reasons.

Office of Economic Opportunity NHCs and other NHCs were evaluated extensively on a national scale (Davis and Schoen, pp. 177–185). There have been general program evaluations (Orso; Resource Management Corporation); evaluations of quality of care (Morehead; Morehead and Donaldson); and analyses of costs (Sparer and Anderson). By most accounts, in the mid-1970s NHCs seemed to be doing reasonably well in terms of quality. A General Accounting Office report in 1978 noted that there were some problems with overstaffing, with some centers serving the nonpoor while there were many medically underserved areas with no programs at all, and with some failures to collect third-party reimbursement (Comptroller General). The tendency toward expansion of service for the nonpoor in at least some areas may represent an attempt to resolve one of the basic contradictions of the original OEO/NHC program. The health centers' emphasis on the poverty population created a curious dilemma: in attempting to develop an organization to enhance the health of the poor, the NHC was at the same time perpetuating a separate and distinct system of health care for the poor. Ideally, health care for the poor should be integrated into the mainstream of medical care.

At peak development of the original OEO-NHC program in the early 1970s, it was estimated that there were nationally at one time or another about 200 NHCs (*Health PAC Bulletin*). By 1974, that number had fallen to around 150 (M. I. Roemer, 1975a). In the mid-1970s, under the Nixon and Ford administrations, the (renamed) Community Health Center program had its scope more narrowly defined than did the original NHC program. Community Health Centers, or CHCs, which included many of the original NHCs, were to concentrate on the delivery of medical care, deemphasizing other NHC roles of providing employment opportunities and training programs, stimulating social and economic development in their communities, and concerning themselves with environmental as well as personal health problems. In addition, the CHCs were urged to expand their service-availability to the nonpoor (Davis and Schoen, p. 171).

By the end of the 1970s, there were almost 600 CHCs serving over 4.5 million people (Bureau of Community Health Services 1979a), a remarkable resurgence for a program that received little publicity, especially when compared to the HMO program. The program focused on urban and rural medically underserved populations. The CHCs were supported primarily by federal grant funds, plus third-party reimbursements and private fees paid on a sliding scale. Two-year planning grants for new programs were available. The CHCs were to concentrate on the provision of primary-care services.

NHCs and CHCs have been very important in demonstrating the feasibility of new approaches to the provision of health care. However, they require large front-end investments. They operate in areas where most patients simply cannot afford the costs of their own care. If national health insurance comes, a major question will be: Will the private practice sector, which can operate in most lower working-class neighborhoods under a liberal government-financed fee-for-service reimbursement system (Bernstein), allow the NHC movement a new lease on life and a new period of growth and development?

Organized Home Care

One of the oldest and yet most neglected sites of ambulatory care is the home (Brickner). For many persons with chronic diseases in which "cure" is not possible, proper management can make a great deal of difference in their lives. For many who are not acutely ill, but need to spend a great deal of time in bed, the home may be a more comfortable, less isolating, lower-cost alternative to the hospital. (See also Chapter 8.)

The AHA defines home care as the provision of health care to the patient in his or her place of residence (Richter and Gonnerman, 1972). The AHA notes that for some people, care by a family member under the guidance of a doctor is enough, whereas other patients may require care from nurses or occupational and physical therapists. Coordinated home care, according to the USDHEW, is a program "that is centrally administered and, through coordinated planning, evaluation and follow-up procedures, provides for physician-directed nursing, social work, and related services to selected patients at home" (Allen et al.).

Historically, there have been two streams of development in home care (Kasten). A hospital may extend some of its services in the community to provide care in the home under medical direction, or a community agency such as a Visiting Nurse Service or a Public Health Department may build upon an existing program of services in collaboration with one or more hospitals to provide coordinated care (Richter and Gonnerman, 1972, 1974). There are many combinations of service that appear in different home care programs. The prototypical hospital-based program was established at the Montefiore Hospital in the Bronx in the late 1940s (Bluestone). That program provided medical, social, nursing, housekeeping, transportation, medication, occupational therapy, physical therapy, and diagnostic services in the home on a virtually as-needed basis (Cherkasky). The basis of the concept was a "hospital without walls" (Richter and Gonnerman, 1972). Essential to a comprehensive home care program for the chronically ill is guaranteed readmission to the hospital, whether for medical reasons or for "social" reasons, such as "giving the family a rest" in instances when caring for the sick relative is physically or emotionally too demanding.

Lenzer and Donabedian (1967) catalogued the pros and cons of home care. As advantages they cited: the company of one's family; a freer, more cheerful atmosphere; comfort; the support and understanding of a visiting nurse; more personal freedom and dignity than in the hospital. And, of course, the patient who is enjoying these advantages is not occupying a costly hospital bed. In addition, patients treated at home may make more progress in the activities of daily living and experience less deterioration in indices of socioeconomic functioning (Katz). Home care may decrease the number of hospital admissions and nursing home replacements (Nielson et al.) and may also decrease the length of stay for patients treated at home but subsequently admitted to a hospital. The home may be a more effective site for patient learning and motivational activities (Stone et al.), and it may engender a higher level of patient satisfaction than institutionalized care. It may also be less expensive to patient and health care systems (Hurtado et al.). But for home care to be appropriately and effectively utilized, it is essential that physicians be knowledgeable about and in favor of home health services. This is often not the case.

Home care is not without disadvantages. Successful home care requires the deep involvement of family members (House) and may disrupt family functioning at the same time that it permits the family to remain technically intact. The indirect costs may be high, when, for example, cost of family members' time is considered. There may be lack of coordination between physician, home health agency, family, and patient. In addition, we need to know much more about the quality of care delivered in the home before reliable judgments can be made. Nevertheless, if quality can be assured, it can be assumed that home care is an important dimension of a coordinated health care system (Weller).

Primary Care

Primary care is a popular subject in the health care literature (Aiken et al.;
Dorsey, 1970; Hansen; Kirkham; Last and White; Magraw; Mechanic;
Scheffler et al.). Aspects of the subject have already been touched upon in
Chapters 4 and 5. Primary care has been variously defined (Haggerty;
Rogatz; White, 1967, 1973). In fact, when Institute of Medicine staff were
reviewing definitions for their manpower policy study (1978), they found,
and summarized, 33 different ones (Ruby).

Definitions of primary care can be descriptive (what is) or normative
(what ought to be). A working descriptive definition of primary care is:

> The routine, episodic, and ongoing care given to the majority of patients for
> the majority of their ills, the majority of the time.

A working normative definition states that primary care is (Jonas, 1973):

> medical attention to the great majority of ills, provided continuously over a
> significant period of time by the same appropriately trained individual (or
> team), who is sympathetic, understanding, knowledgeable, and equipped,
> who is as capable of keeping people well as he is of returning them to health
> when they fall ill. (p. 177)

Both the descriptive and normative definitions of primary care can be
contrasted with descriptive definitions of secondary and tertiary care.
According to Rogatz (1970);

> Secondary care encompasses most medical and surgical diagnostic and ther-
> apeutic health services such as diagnostic radiology and laboratory studies,
> referrals for consultation, general surgery, most medical and pediatric dis-
> orders requiring hospitalization, and all but the most unusual obstetrical
> problems. Tertiary care is provided at major hospital centers to patients
> requiring diagnostic, therapeutic, or rehabilitative services that transcend
> the capabilities of the average community hospital. (p. 47)

It is quite obvious that there is blurring at the boundaries of these definitions. Certainly some "diagnostic radiology and laboratory studies" are part
of primary care, as is some hospital care. The descriptive definitions of
primary and tertiary care are based in part on exclusion. Whatever the
limitations of the definitions, however, they are generally useful, and make
it quite clear that ambulatory care and primary care are not synonymous,
since there are ambulatory components of both secondary and tertiary
care.

In the late 1960s, a list of functions of an *ideal* primary care *system* was
developed that is still valid (Committee on Medical Schools):

1. Assessment of total [patient] needs before these are categorized by specialty. 2. Elaboration of a plan for meeting those needs in the order of their
importance. 3. Determination of who shall meet the defined needs—physicians, general or specialist; non-physician members of the health team; or
social agencies. 4. Follow-up to see that needs are met. 5. [Provision of such
care] in a continuous, coordinated and comprehensive manner. 6. Attention
at each step . . . to the personal, social and family dimensions of the patient's
problem. 7. [The provision of] health maintenance and disease prevention [at
the same level of importance as the provision of] cure and rehabilitation. (p.
753)

Of course, the ever-increasing specialization and subspecialization of
American medicine in this century has made primary care, particularly
primary care provided by people especially trained in it, increasingly
difficult to find (Freymann, p. 152). Various levels of government have
recognized this fact. Increasingly, government financial aid, particularly to
medical education, has been tied to improving training in primary care.
Several major battles have resulted from this emphasis (Aiken et al.;
Hamerman; Institute of Medicine; Relman 1978, 1979; Scheffler et al.).
One major battle is whether the basic primary care doctor is to be a family
physician or an internist-pediatrician combination (Coordinating Council
on Medical Education; Hudson and Nourse; McWhinney; Perkoff;
Petersdorf). Another is what other specialties, if any, have a legitimate
claim to a piece of the pie (Alpert and Charney, p. 2; Colwill; Rubin et al.).
   One of the possible outcomes of these struggles may be simply a change
of label without touching what is inside the jar (Aiken et al.), a favorite
American solution to problems. Of course, many other categories of health
care provider are necessary to the provision of primary care, but the
centrality of the physician in the American health care delivery system
makes the position of the physicians of central concern. In a medical
education system that trains specialists and biomedical researchers
(Stevens, Chapter 16) and does not focus on the broad needs of the
population at large (Freymann, Chapters 6, 26; Jonas, 1979, Chapters 3,
12), providing for the education of physicians in primary care presents
serious difficulties (Alpert and Charney). As White (1973, p. 362) says:
"One wants to avoid the confusion inherent in the encounter between the
patient who says to the doctor, 'I hope you treat what I've got' and the
physician who says, 'I hope you've got what I treat.' " Simply tinkering with
the curriculum will not do (Jonas, 1979, Chapter 13). As the description of
the *functions* of the primary care physician developed by the Pellegrino
Committee shows, physician primary care is above all not a collection of
services, but a state of mind (Committee on Medical Schools):

[The primary-care physician] must be capable of establishing a profile of the total needs of the patient and his family. This evaluation should include social, economic, and psychologic details as well as the more strictly "medical" aspects. He must know what resources are available for meeting those needs. He should then define a plan of care, deciding which parts are to be carried out by himself and which by others. The plan should have a long-range dimension. It should be understandable to the patient and his family, and it should include a follow-up on whether indicated measures have been undertaken and whether they have been effective. (p. 754)

Which brings us back to ambulatory care.

Although primary care is not limited to ambulatory care, ambulatory care is central to primary care. If primary care is to become a major function for physicians, ambulatory care—service, teaching, and research—will have to become a major function of the institutions that train them.

References

Abrams, H. K., and Snyder, R. A. "Health Center Seeks to Bridge the Gap between Hospital and Neighborhood." *Modern Hospital,* May 1968, p. 96.

Aiken, L. H., et al. "The Contribution of Specialists to the Delivery of Primary Care." *New England Journal of Medicine, 300,* 1363, 1979.

Albin, S. L., et al. "Evaluation of Emergency Room Triage Performed by Nurses." *American Journal of Public Health, 65,* 1063, 1975.

Allen, D., et al. "Agencies' Perceptions of Factors Affecting Home Care Referral." *Medical Care, 12,* 828, 1974.

Alpert, J. J., and Charney, F. *The Education of Physicians for Primary Care.* Washington, D.C.: USDHEW Publication No. (HRA) 74–3113, Autumn 1973.

American College of Surgeons and the American Surgical Association. *Surgery in the United States (SOSSUS).* Baltimore, Maryland, 1975.

American Hospital Association. *Reshaping Ambulatory Care Programs,* Chicago, 1973.

————. *Hospital Statistics. 1979 Edition.* Chicago, 1979.

American Public Health Association. "The Development of Community Health Service Centers—Present and Future: Policy Statement." *American Journal of Public Health, 54,* 140, 1964.

Andrus, L. H. "The Emergency Room Rip-Off." *The Journal of Family Practice, 2,* 147, 1975.

Axelrod, J. "Group Practice of Medicine and Surgery," *Resident Physician, 2,* September 1956.

Baehr, G. "Pre-Paid Group Practice: Its Strengths and Weaknesses, and Its Future." *American Journal of Public Health, 56,* 1898, 1966.

Bates, L. E. "Health Insurance Plan of Greater New York." *Hospitals, J.A.H.A.,* March 16, 1971.

Bauman, P. "The Formulation and Evolution of the Health Maintenance Organization Policy, 1970–73." *Social Science and Medicine, 10,* 129, 1976. (This paper is based on exhaustive primary research.)

Beloff, J. S. "Adapting the Hospital Emergency Service Organization to Patient Needs." *Hospitals, J.A.H.A.,* April 16, 1968.

Bernstein, G. *An Analysis of Private Physician Participation in the New York City Medicaid Program.* New York: Health Services Administration, 1968. Mimeographed.

Blake, E., and Carnoy, J. "The Vanguard of the Rearguard." *Health PAC Bulletin,* February 1973, p. 2.

Block, J. A. "Hospital Innovations in the Community: Ambulatory Care." *Bulletin of the New York Academy of Medicine, 55,* 104, 1979.

Bluestone, E. M. "Home Care: An Extra-Mural Hospital Function." *Survey Midmonthly, 84,* 99, 133, April 1948. Reprinted in: Committee on Medical Care Teaching, of the Association of Teachers of Preventive Medicine, *Readings in Medical Care,* Chapel Hill: University of North Carolina Press, 1958, p. 408.

Brian, E. "Foundation for Medical Care Control of Hospital Utilization: CHAP—A PSRO Prototype." *New England Journal of Medicine, 288,* 878, 1973.

Brickner, P. W. *Home Health Care for the Aged.* New York: Appleton-Century-Crofts, 1978.

Brindle, J. "The Health Insurance Plan of Greater New York Program." Presented at National Forum on Hospital and Health Affairs, May 21, 1971, Duke University, Durham, North Carolina.

Bureau of Community Health Services. *Community Health Centers.* Rockville, Maryland: USDHEW, c. 1979a.

—————. *Hospital-Affiliated Primary Care Centers.* Rockville, Maryland: USDHEW, 1979b.

Cashman, J. *What Thirteen Local Health Departments Are Doing in Medical Care.* Washington, D.C.: Public Health Services, USDHEW, 1967.

Center for Health Administration Studies. *Health Maintenance Organization: A Reconfiguration of the Health Services System.* Proceedings of the Thirteenth Annual Symposium on Hospital Affairs. Graduate School of Business, University of Chicago, 1971.

Cherkasky, M. "The Montefiore Hospital Home Care Program." *American Journal of Public Health, 39,* 29, 1949.

Collins, B. "Denver Builds Citywide Health Network." *Modern Hospital,* May 1968, p. 102.

Colwill, J. M. "Primary-Care Education in Multiple Specialties." *New England Journal of Medicine, 299,* 657, 1978.

Committee on the Costs of Medical Care. *Medical Care for the American People.* Chicago: University of Chicago Press, 1932. Reprinted, USDHEW, 1970.

Committee on Medical Schools and the AAMC in Relation to Training for Family Practice. "Planning for Comprehensive and Continuing Care of Patients through Education." *Journal of Medical Education, 43,* 751, 1968.

Comptroller General. *Are Neighborhood Health Centers Providing Services Effi-*

ciently and to the Most Needy? Washington, D.C.: General Accounting Office, HRD-77-124, June 20, 1978.

Consumer Reports. "HMO's: Are They the Answer to Your Medical Needs?" October 1974, p. 756.

Coordinating Council on Medical Education. "Physician Manpower and Distribution: The Primary Care Physician." *Journal of the American Medical Association, 233,* 880, 1975.

Davis, K., and Schoen, C. *Health and the War on Poverty.* Washington, D.C.: The Brookings Institution, 1978. Chapter 6, "A New Approach to Health Care Delivery," contains a comprehensive review of the program plus an excellent bibliography.

Davis, M. M., and Warner, A. R. *Dispensaries: Their Management and Development.* New York: The Macmillan Company, 1918. Reprinted, New York: Arno Press, 1977.

Davis, M. S., and Tranquada, R. E. "A Sociological Evaluation of the Watts Neighborhood Health Center." *Medical Care, 7,* 105, 1969.

Dorsey, J. L. "Manpower Problems in the Delivery of Primary Medical Care." *New England Journal of Medicine, 282,* 871, 1970.

―――――. "The Health Maintenance Organization Act of 1973 (P. L. 93–222) and Prepaid Group Practice Plans." *Medical Care, 13,* 7, 1975.

―――――. "HMO's and the Cost of Medical Care." *New England Journal of Medicine, 298,* 1360, 1978.

Dutton, D. B. "Patterns of Ambulatory Health Care in Five Different Delivery Systems." *Medical Care, 17,* 221, 1979. (This paper has an extensive bibliography.)

Egdahl, R. H. "Foundations for Medical Care." *New England Journal of Medicine, 288,* 491, 1973.

Egdahl, R. H., et al. "Fee-for-Service Health Maintenance Organizations." *Journal of the American Medical Association, 241,* 588, 1979.

Ellwood, P. M., et al. "Health Maintenance Strategy." *Medical Care, 9,* 291, 1971.

Falk, I. S. "Group Practice Is the Pattern of the Future." *Modern Hospital,* September 1963.

Falkson, J. F. "HMOs: A Look Back, a Look Ahead." *Hospitals,* Aug. 16, 1979, p. 86. (See also Dr. Falkson's book, *HMOs and the Politics of Health System Reform,* Chicago: American Hospital Association, 1979.)

Fleming, S. "Kaiser Foundation—Permanente Program." *Hospitals, J.A.H.A.,* March 16, 1971.

Freymann, J. G. *The American Health Care System: Its Genesis and Trajectory.* New York: Medcom Press, 1974.

Gaffney, J. C., and Glandon, G. L. *Profile of Medical Practice, 1979.* Chicago: Center of Health Services Research and Development, American Medical Association, 1979.

Geiger, H. J. "Community Control—or Community Conflict?" *National Tuberculosis and Respiratory Disease Association Bulletin,* Nov. 1969, p. 4.

Gentile, A. "Physician Visits: Volume and Interval Since Last Visit." Hyattsville,

Maryland: USDHEW. *Vital and Health Statistics.* Series 10, Number 128, 1979.

Gersonde, R. J. "Two Approaches to Providing Physician Coverage in E. R." *Hospital Topics, 49,* 50, February 1971.

Gibson, C. D. "The Neighborhood Health Center: The Primary Unit of Health Care." *American Journal of Public Health, 58,* 1188, 1968.

Gibson, G. "Status of Urban Services." Parts I and II. *Hospitals, J.A.H.A.,* December 1, December 16, 1971.

—————. "Evaluative Criteria for Emergency Ambulance Services." *Social Science and Medicine, 7,* 425, 1973.

—————. "Guidelines for Research and Evaluation of Emergency Medical Services." *Health Services Reports, 89,* 99, 1974.

—————. "How Far Have We Come With Categorization?" *Hospitals, J.A.H.A.,* May 1, 1977a, p. 97.

—————. "Emergency Medical Services." *Proceedings of the Academy of Political Science, 32,* 121, 1977b.

—————. "Emergency Medical Services: Regionalizing Intents and Localizing Effects." In Ginzberg, E., Ed., *Regionalization and Health Care,* Chapter 9. Washington, D.C.: USDHEW, 1978.

Givens, J. D. "Current Estimates from the Health Interview Survey: United States—1978." Hyattsville, Maryland: USDHEW. *Vital and Health Statistics.* Series 10, Number 130, 1979.

Goldberg, G. A., et al. "Issues in the Development of Neighborhood Health Centers." *Inquiry, 6,* 37, 1969.

Goodman, L. J., et al. *Group Medical Practice in the U.S.: 1975.* Chicago: American Medical Association, 1976.

Group Health Cooperative of Puget Sound. *1977 Annual Report,* Seattle, Washington, 1979a.

—————. *Group Health Cooperative's History.* Seattle, Washington, 1979b.

Haggerty, R. J. "The University and Primary Medical Care." *New England Journal of Medicine, 281,* 416, 1969.

Hamerman, D. "Primary Care—Is It Here to Stay?" *Bulletin of the New York Academy of Medicine, 55,* 540, 1979.

Hanlon, John. "Emergency Medical Care as a Comprehensive System." *Health Services Reports, 88,* 579, 1973.

Hannas, R. R. "Emergency Medicine—A Survey." *Southern Medical Bulletin,* December 1971, p. 11.

—————. "Spreading the Specialty Spectrum." *Harvard Medical Alumni Bulletin,* July/August 1975, p. 23.

Hansen, M. F. "An Educational Program for Primary Care." *Journal of Medical Education, 45,* 1001, 1970.

Harrington, D. C. "San Joaquin Foundation for Medical Care." *Hospitals, J.A.H.A.,* March 16, 1971.

Harvard Law Review. "The Role of Prepaid Group Practice in Relieving the Medical Care Crisis." *84,* 887, 1971.

Harvey, J. C. "Categorization of Emergency Capabilities." *Hospitals, J.A.H.A.*, May 16, 1973, p. 69.

————. "The Emergency Medical Services Systems Act of 1973." *New England Journal of Medicine, 292*, 529, 1975.

Health PAC Bulletin. "NENA: Community Control in a Bind." June 1972.

Hoffer, E. P. "Emergency Medical Services, 1979." *The New England Journal of Medicine, 301*, 1118, 1979.

House, M. K. "Home-Style Nursing." *Journal of the American Medical Association, 240*, 2472, 1978. (See also editorial on p. 2471.)

Hudson, J. I., and Nourse, E. S. "Perspectives in Primary Care Education." *Journal of Medical Education, 50*, December 1975, Part 2.

Hurtado, A., et al. "The Utilization and Cost of Home Care and Extended Care Facility Services in a Comprehensive Prepaid Group Practice Program." *Medical Care, 10*, 8, 1972.

Institute of Medicine. *A Manpower Policy for Primary Health Care.* Washington, D.C.: National Academy of Sciences, May 1978.

InterStudy Health Systems. *HMO Growth 1977–78.* Excelsior, Minnesota: Demographic Center, 1979.

Johnson Foundation. *Special Report.* Princeton, New Jersey, 1977.

Jonas, S. "Some Thoughts on Primary Care: Problems in Implementation." *International Journal of Health Services, 3*, 177, 1973.

————. *Quality Control of Ambulatory Care: A Task for Health Departments.* New York: Springer Publishing Co., 1977.

————. *Medical Mystery: The Training of Doctors in the United States.* New York: W. W. Norton, 1979.

Jonas, S., et al. "Monitoring Utilization of a Municipal Hospital Emergency Department." *Hospital Topics, 54*, 43, 1976.

Kaiser Foundation Medical Care Program. *Organized Health Care Delivery Systems: A Historical Perspective.* Oakland, California, 1978.

Kasten, J. "The Case for Standards in Home Care Programs." *The Gerontologist, 3*, 14, 1963.

Katz, S. "Comprehensive Outpatient Care in Rheumatoid Arthritis." *Journal of the American Medical Association, 206*, November 4, 1968.

Kelman, H. R., and Lane, D. S. "Use of the Hospital Emergency Room in Relation to Use of Private Physicians." *American Journal of Public Health, 66*, 1189, 1976.

Kessler, M. S., and Wilson, K. C. "Emergency Department Key Factor in Hospital Admissions." *Hospitals, J.A.H.A.*, December 16, 1978, p. 87.

Kippel, A. P. "Status Categorization Is Dynamic." *Hospitals, J.A.H.A.*, July 16, 1975, p. 151.

Kirkham, F. T. *Issues in Primary Care: The 1976 Annual Health Conference: New York Academy of Medicine. Bulletin of the New York Academy of Medicine 53*, 2nd Series, 5–153, 1977.

Knowles, J. H. "The Role of the Hospital: The Ambulatory Clinic." *Bulletin of the New York Academy of Medicine, 41*, 2nd Series, January 1965, p. 68.

Lane, D. S., and Evans, D. "Study Measures Impact of Emergency Department Ombudsman." *Hospitals, J.A.H.A.*, February 1, 1978, p. 99.

Lashof, J. C. "Chicago Project Provides Health Care and Career Opportunities." *Hospitals, J.A.H.A.*, July 1, 1969, p. 105.

Last, J. M., and White, K. L. "The Content of Medical Care in Primary Practice." *Medical Care, 7,* 41, 1969.

Lenzer, A., and Donabedian, A. "A Needed Research in Home Care." *Nursing Outlook, 18,* October 1967.

Lewis, R. P., et al. "Effectiveness of Advanced Paramedics in a Mobile Coronary Care System." *Journal of the American Medical Association, 241,* 1902, 1979.

Light, H. L., and Brown, H. J. "The Gouverneur Health Services Program: An Historical View." *Milbank Memorial Fund Quarterly, 45,* 375, 1967.

Lloyd, W. B., and Wise, H. B. "The Montefiore Experience." *Bulletin of the New York Academy of Medicine, 44,* 1353, 1968.

Loebs, S. F. "Dramatic Rise in National Growth of HMOs." *Hospitals,* August 16, 1979, p. 96.

Luft, H. S. "How Do Health-Maintenance Organizations Achieve Their 'Savings'?" *New England Journal of Medicine, 298,* 1336, 1978. (This paper has an excellent bibliography.)

MacColl, W. A. *Group Practice and Prepayment of Medical Care.* Washington, D.C.: Public Affairs Press, 1966.

McWhinney, I. R. "Family Medicine in Perspective." *New England Journal of Medicine, 293,* 175, 1975. (Letters in response, *NEJM, 293,* 781, 1975.)

Magraw, R. M. "Trends in Medical Education and Health Services." *New England Journal of Medicine, 285,* 1407, 1971.

Mawardi, B. H. "Satisfactions, Dissatisfactions, and Causes of Stress in Medical Practice." *Journal of the American Medical Association, 241,* 1483, 1979.

Mechanic, D. "General Medical Practice." *Medical Care, 10,* 402, 1972.

Medical World News. "The Crisis in Emergency Care." December 4, 1970.

––––––. "The Emergency Physician." February 1, 1974.

––––––. "ER Use Triggers 'Battle for Bucks.'" September 19, 1977.

––––––. "Emergency Medicine: How Far Has It Come, Where Is It Going?" March 20, 1978, p. 65.

––––––. "Doctors Called Highly Prone to Midlife Crisis." June 25, 1979.

––––––. "Being a Doctor May Be Hazardous to Your Health." August 20, 1979, p. 68.

Mendenhall, R. C. "A National Study of Medical and Surgical Specialties: 3. An Empirical Approach to the Classification of Patient Care." *Journal of the American Medical Association, 241,* 2180, 1979.

Mendenhall, R. C., et al. "A National Study of Medical and Surgical Specialties: 1. Background, Purpose, and Methodology." *Journal of the American Medical Association, 240,* 848, 1978a.

Mendenhall, R. C., et al. "A National Study of Medical and Surgical Specialties: 2. Description of a Survey Instrument." *Journal of the American Medical Association, 240,* 1160, 1978b.

Miller, C. A., et al. "A Survey of Local Public Health Departments and Their Directors." *American Journal of Public Health*, 67, 931, 1977.

Miller, C. A., et al. "A Study of Local Health Departments." *Bulletin of the Association of Public Health Physicians*, 26, No. 1, January 1979.

"Montefiore Neighborhood Medical Demonstration: The Early Experience." A series of articles by several authors. *Milbank Memorial Fund Quarterly*, 45, July 1968.

Montgomery, B. J. "Emergency Medical Services—a New Phase of Development." *Journal of the American Medical Association*, 243, 1017, 1980.

Moos, M.-K., and Miller, C. A. "Outstanding Local Health Departments: Relationships to Other Provider Systems." Presented at American Public Health Association Annual Meeting, New York, New York, November 6, 1979.

Morehead, M. A. "Evaluating Quality of Care in the Neighborhood Health Center Program of OEO." *Medical Care*, 2, 118, 1970.

Morehead, M. A., and Donaldson, R. "Quality of Clinical Management of Disease in Comprehensive Neighborhood Health Centers." *Medical Care*, 12, 301, 1974.

Myers, B. A. "Health Maintenance Organizations: Objectives and Issues." *HSMHA Health Reports*, 86, 585, 1971.

Myers, B. A., et al. "The Medical Care Activities of Local Health Units." *Public Health Reports*, 83, 757, 1968.

National Academy of Sciences, National Research Council. *Accidental Death and Disability: The Neglected Disease of Modern Society*. Washington, D.C., 1966.

National Advisory Commission on Health Manpower. *Report*. Vol. II, Appendix IV: "The Kaiser Foundation Medical Care Program." Washington, D.C.: USGPO, 1967.

National Conference on Cardio-Pulmonary Resuscitation and Emergency Cardiac Care. "Standards for Cardio-Pulmonary Resuscitation (CPR) and Emergency Cardiac Care (ECC)." *Journal of the American Medical Association*, 227 (Suppl.) 837–868, 1974.

National Training Course, Emergency Medical Technician/Paramedic, Course Guide. Washington, D.C.: USGPO, 1978.

Newport J., and Roemer, M. I. "Comparative Prenatal Mortality under Medical Care Foundations and Other Delivery Models." *Inquiry*, 12, 10, 1975.

Nielson, M., et al. "Older Persons after Hospitalization: A Controlled Study of Home Health Aide Service." *American Journal of Public Health*, 62, 1094, 1972.

Office of Health Maintenance Organizations. *Fourth Annual Report to the Congress*. Rockville, Maryland: USDHEW Pub. No. (PHS) 79–13058, 1979a.

——————. *National HMO Development Strategy: Through 1988*. Washington, D.C.: USDHEW, 1979b.

Orso, C. L. "Delivering Ambulatory Health Care." *Medical Care*, 17, 111, 1979.

Perkoff, G. T. "General Internal Medicine, Family Practice or Something Better?" *New England Journal of Medicine*, 299, 654, 1978.

Petersdorf, R. G. "Internal Medicine and Family Practice." *New England Journal of Medicine*, 293, 326, 1975.

P. L. 93–154. Emergency Medical Services Systems Act, 1973.

Reidel, D. C., et al. *Federal Employees Health Benefits Program.* Washington, D.C.: Health Resources Administration, USDHEW, 1975.

Relman, A. S. "The Debate on Primary-Care Manpower." *New England Journal of Medicine*, 299, 1305, 1978. (See associated papers and letters.)

——————. "Generalists and Specialists." *New England Journal of Medicine*, 300, 1386, 1979.

Resource Management Corporation. *Evaluations of the War on Poverty: Health Programs.* Washington, D.C.: General Accounting Office, Contract No. GA–654, 1969.

Richter, L., and Gonnerman, A. "Hospital Administered Home Care Programs." *Hospitals, J.A.H.A.*, May 1, 1972, p. 41.

Richter, L., and Gonnerman, A. "Home Health Services and Hospitals." *Hospitals, J.A.H.A.*, May 16, 1974, p. 113.

Roemer, M. I. "Organized Ambulatory Health Service in International Perspective." *International Journal of Health Services, 1*, 18, 1971.

——————. "From Poor Beginnings, the Growth of Primary Care." *Hospitals, J.A.H.A.*, March 1, 1975a, p. 38.

——————. "A Realistic System: Health Maintenance Organizations in a Regionalized Framework." In Roemer, R., et al., *Planning Urban Health Services.* New York: Springer Publishing Co., 1975b.

Roemer, M. I., and Shonick, W. "HMO Performance: The Recent Evidence." *Health and Society, 51*, 271, 1973.

Roemer, M. I., et al. "The Ecology of Group Medical Practice in the United States." *Medical Care, 12*, 627, 1974.

Roemer, R., et al. *Planning Urban Health Services: From Jungle to System.* New York: Springer Publishing Co., 1975.

Rogatz, P. "The Health Care System: Planning." *Hospitals, J.A.H.A.*, April 16, 1970, p. 47.

Rorem, C. R. *Private Group Clinics.* Publication No. 8, The Committee on the Costs of Medical Care. Chicago: University of Chicago Press, 1931. Reprinted, New York, Milbank Memorial Fund, 1971.

Rosen, G. "The First Neighborhood Health Center Movement—Its Rise and Fall." *American Journal of Public Health, 61*, 1620, 1971.

Rosenberg, C. E. "Social Class and Medical Care in Nineteenth-Century America: The Rise and Fall of the Dispensary." *Journal of the History of Medicine and Allied Sciences, 29*, 32, 1974.

Rubin, A. A., et al. "Effective Primary Care by the Subspecialty Center." *New England Journal of Medicine, 293*, 607, 1975.

Ruby, G., et al. *Definitions of Primary Care.* Washington, D. C.: Institute of Medicine. Staff paper, January 17, 1977.

Satin, D. G., and Duhl, F. J. "Help?: The Hospital Emergency Unit as Community Physician." *Medical Care, 10*, 248, 1972.

Saward, E. W. "The Relevance of Prepaid Group Practice to the Effective Delivery of Health Services." Presented at the 18th Annual Group Health Institute, Sault Ste. Marie, Ontario, Canada, June 18, 1969. Reprinted, USDHEW, n.d.

Schachter, L. P., and Elliston, E. D. "Medical Care in a Free Community Clinic." *Journal of the American Medical Association, 237,* 1848, 1977.

Scheffler, et al. "A Manpower Policy for Primary Health Care." *New England Journal of Medicine, 298,* 1058, 1978.

Schwartz, J. L. "Early Histories of Selected Neighborhood Health Centers." *Inquiry, 7,* 3, 1970.

Sheps, C. G. "Conference Summary and the Road Ahead." *Bulletin of the New York Academy of Medicine,* Vol. 41, No. 1, 2nd Series, January 1965, p. 146.

Sherman, M. A. "Mobile Intensive Care Units: An Evaluation of Effectiveness." *Journal of the American Medical Association, 241,* 1899, 1979.

Shortell, S. M. "Determinants of Physician Referral Rates: An Exchange Theory Approach." *Medical Care, 12,* 13, 1974.

Showstack, J. A., et al. "Fee-for-Service Physician Payment: Analysis of Current Methods and Their Development." *Inquiry, 16,* 230, 1979.

Silver, G. A. "Group Practice—What It Is." *Medical Care, 1,* 94, 1963.

Silver, G. A., et al. "An Experience with Group Practice: The Montefiore Medical Group, 1948–1956." *New England Journal of Medicine, 256,* 785, 1957.

Sparer, G., and Anderson, A. *Cost of Services at Neighborhood Health Centers: A Comparative Analysis.* Washington, D.C.: Program Planning and Evaluation Division Office, Office of Health Affairs, Office of Economic Opportunity, 1975.

Spencer, J. H. *The Hospital Emergency Department.* Springfield, Illinois: Charles C. Thomas, 1972.

Staff, P. "The New Medicine." *The New Republic,* April 19, 1975, p. 15.

Stevens, R. *American Medicine and the Public Interest.* New Haven, Connecticut: Yale University Press, 1971.

Stoeckle, J. D., et al. "The Free Medical Clinics." *Journal of the American Medical Association, 219,* 603, 1972.

Stone, J., et al. "The Effectiveness of Home Care for General Hospital Patients." *Journal of the American Medical Association, 205,* July 19, 1968.

Strumpf, G. B., et al. "Health Maintenance Organizations 1971–1977: Issues and Answers." *Journal of Community Health, 4,* 33, 1978.

Subcommittee on Health. *Health Maintenance Organization Act of 1973, S. 14 (Explanation of Act and Text).* Washington, D.C.: Committee on Labor and Public Welfare, U.S. Senate, USGPO, February, 1974.

Tennant, F. S., Jr., and Day, C. M. "Survival Potential and Quality of Care Among Free Clinics." *Public Health Reports, 89,* 558, 1974.

Terris, M., Conference Chairman. "Group Practice: Problems and Perspectives." The 1968 Health Conference. The New York Academy of Medicine. *Bulletin of the New York Academy of Medicine, 44,* November 1968, pp. 1277, 1434.

——————. "Crisis and Change in America's Health System." *American Journal of Public Health, 63,* 313, 1973.

Torrens, P. "Administrative Problems of Neighborhood Health Centers." *Medical Care*, 9, 487, 1971.

Torrens, P., and Yedvab, D. "Variations among Emergency Room Populations: A Comparison of Four Hospitals in New York City." *Medical Care*, 8, 60, 1970.

USDHEW. *Health Maintenance Organizations: The Concept and Structure*. Washington, D.C.: 1971.

—————. *Health United States, 1979*. Washington, D.C.: USDHEW Pub. No. (PHS) 80–1232, 1979.

Waller, J. A. "A Rural EMS Categorization System." *Hospitals, J.A.H.A.*, October 1, 1974, p. 111.

Warner, J., and Aherne, P. *Profile of Medical Practice. '74*. Chicago: Center for Health Services Research and Development, American Medical Association, 1974.

Webb, S. B., and Lawrence, R. W. "Emergency Services: Physician Staffing and Reimbursement Trends." *Hospitals, J.A.H.A.*, October 1, 1972, p. 69.

Weinerman, E. R. "Problems and Perspectives of Group Practice." *Bulletin of the New York Academy of Medicine*, 2nd Series, 44, 1423, 1968.

Weinerman, E. R., and Edwards, H. R. "Yale Studies in Ambulatory Medical Care I. Changing Patterns in Hospital Emergency Service." *Hospitals, J.A.H.A.*, November 16, 1964.

Weinerman, E. R., et al. "Yale Studies in Ambulatory Medical Care V. Determinants of Use of Hospital Emergency Services." *American Journal of Public Health*, 56, 1037, 1966.

Weller, C. "Home Health Care." *New York State Journal of Medicine*, October 1978, p. 1957.

White, K. L. "Primary Medical Care for Families—Organization and Evaluation." *New England Journal of Medicine*, 277, 847, 1967.

—————. "Organization and Delivery of Personal Health Services—Public Policy Issues." *Milbank Memorial Fund Quarterly*, January 1968. Reprinted, McKinlay, J. B., *Politics and Law in Health Care Policy*. New York: Prodist, 1973.

—————. "Health and Health Care: Personal and Public Issues." The 1974 Michael M. Davis Lecture. The Center for Health Administration Studies, Graduate School of Business, The University of Chicago. 1974.

Williams, G. "Kaiser." *Modern Hospital*, February 1971, p. 67.

Williamson, J. W., et al. *Quality of Health Care in HMOs Compared to Other Settings*. Baltimore, Maryland: Johns Hopkins University, March 1979.

Winslow, C.-E. A. *The Life of Herman M. Biggs*. Philadelphia: Lea and Febiger, 1929.

Wolfe, S., and Badgley, R. F. "The Family Doctor." *The Milbank Memorial Fund Quarterly*, 50, April 1972, Part 2.

Zwick, D. I. "Some Accomplishments and Findings of Neighborhood Health Centers." *Milbank Memorial Fund Quarterly*, October 1972. Reprinted in Zola, I. K., and McKinlay, J. B., Eds., *Organizational Issues in the Delivery of Health Services*, New York: Prodist, 1974, p. 331.

7

Hospitals

Michael Enright and Steven Jonas

Introduction

The hospital is the institutional center of the health care delivery system (Knowles). Because of its complexity, the hospital has been described as a city whose major enterprise is the restoration of its citizens' health. All the major services, resources, and social forces of a city have parallels in a hospital.

Like our cities, the hospital has changed dramatically in character in the past century (Rosenberg). While at the turn of the 20th century a person entering a hospital had less than a 50% chance of leaving it alive, today a patient can expect to benefit from his hospital stay. Typically, 97% of patients admitted can expect to leave the hospital alive. The hospital has evolved from a place of refuge, where a person went to spare his family the anguish of watching him die, to a multiservice institution providing interdisciplinary medical care to ambulatory as well as bed patients. Moreover, the present-day hospital has other functions aside from delivering health and medical services. It is the center of most clinical training, both graduate and undergraduate, and is the principal locus of continuing education, formal and informal, for most physicians. It also trains other health providers and conducts health and medical research. It is the workplace for most United States physicians (in addition to their office practices) and at the present time the only place where they are likely to be subject to peer review of their medical care performance. The hospital also has symbolic importance: being the most visible component of the health care delivery system, it *is* that system in the minds of many laymen. Its increasingly complex and sometimes bewildering structures and methods have come to represent the growing complexity of the delivery system as a whole.

In this chapter we will deal primarily with the most common type of hospital—the short-term, general, acute-care institution under private or nonfederal public ownership. The second-largest category—mental hospitals—is covered in Chapter 9, while federal hospitals are dealt with in

Chapter 11. Certain aspects of rising hospital costs are covered in Chapter 10, while hospital licensing, regulation, and quality control are discussed in Chapters 13 and 14.

Historical Development

The historical development of hospitals has been related to provision of care for poor persons (Stern, Chapters 2, 6; Freymann, pp. 28–29) and to provision of medical care for the acutely ill (Freymann, pp. 21–29, Chapter 4). Hospitals (the word shares a Latin root with "hostel" and "hotel") began in the Middle Ages as places of refuge for the sick, the weary, and the poor. Most were church-sponsored. Beginning in the 17th century, several Western European countries, notably England, began to attempt to deal with the problem of the poor at the local level (de Schweinitz, Chapters 3–5). Under the original Elizabethan Poor Laws (c. 1590), much of the relief provided was given to persons living in their own dwelling-places. However, local governments were also given the authority, and in some cases the responsibility, to build or provide institutions to house the poor. The poor comprised those who were unemployed owing to lack of jobs, skills, or education; orphans or children whose parents could not care for them; the dependent elderly; and the mentally retarded, as well as the ill. These institutions generally were called almshouses or poorhouses. In certain jurisdictions in England and the United States, some or all of these categories of person were housed together, from the first appearance of the poorhouses until well into the 20th century.

In the American colonies, the earliest hospitals were actually infirmaries in poorhouses: at Henricopolis in Virginia (1612); Blockley in Philadelphia (1732); Charity Hospital in New Orleans (1736); and the Public Workhouse and House of Correction in New York City (1736) (Stern, Chapter 6). The first public institution designed solely for the care of the sick was the "pesthouse" built on the same grounds as the New York workhouse. It was not until 1848 that the administrations of the two institutions were formally separated and an independent hospital created (Freymann, pp. 28–29).

Private voluntary hospitals in the United States go back to the 18th century (Freymann, pp. 22–24). These institutions also cared for the poor: since hospitals could do little for their patients, there was no reason for the self-supporting sick to go to them. The first voluntary hospital in the American colonies was the Pennsylvania Hospital in Philadelphia (1751). The New York Hospital was founded in 1769, followed by the Massachusetts General in Boston in 1811 (Freymann, pp. 22–24). However, by 1873, there were only an estimated 178 hospitals in the United States (Stevens, p. 52).

Not until the turn of the 20th century did a patient admitted to a general hospital have a better than even chance of getting out alive. That milestone was achieved largely by the development of general hospital hygiene, asepsis, and surgical anesthesia.

By 1909, there were more than 4,359 hospitals with more than 421,000 beds (Stevens, p. 52). The rapid advance of medical science caused the expansion of the hospital and its evolution as the center of the medical care system (MacEachern, pp. 21–27). Medical care had become too complex for the physician to carry his entire armamentarium in his black bag; special equipment and consultation with other medical specialists became essential.

The types of patients in the hospitals have changed with each medical discovery. In 1923, the discovery of insulin drastically changed the character of diabetes as a hospital disease. Liver extract reduced the incidence of pernicious anemia in 1929. Sulfonamides began to affect the care of pneumonia and some other infectious diseases in 1935, a trend that accelerated with the widespread use of antibiotics beginning in 1943, and the continuing development of immunization techniques. The development of rehabilitation services began to bring more disabled patients to the hospital. The 1950s saw chronic illness becoming progressively more important as a hospital problem. As noted in Chapters 2 and 3, infectious diseases have generally been conquered, leaving hospitals to cope with the pathology of the degenerative and neoplastic diseases, and trauma (Letourneau, 1964, p. 548; Knowles, pp. 100–101; Roemer, 1980; Office of Health Research, pp. 22–26).

In the first half of the 20th century, there was a striking development of specialty hospitals—for example, general surgical, orthopedic, and eye and ear—largely as a result of benefactors' responses to the initiative of individual physicians (Ginzberg, p. 238). Fiscal exigencies, considerations of efficiency, and medical advances have sharply curtailed this development in recent years, and many former specialty hospitals now have closed or admit a full range of patients. Currently, most new specialty hospitals formed are parts of larger medical centers.

Classification of Hospitals

There are two major agencies that count and classify hospitals in the United States—the American Hospital Association (AHA) and the National Center for Health Statistics (NCHS) of the USDHHS. The AHA annually publishes the "Guide Issue" of its journal, *Hospitals*, followed by a companion publication, *Hospital Statistics* (which until 1972 was published as part of the "Guide Issue"). These publications list each AHA-registered hospital, giving its basic characteristics, as well as much summary data. *Hospitals* also includes "Hospital Indicators," compilations of data on trends in hospital use and financing. The NCHS publishes *Health Resources Statis-*

tics on a biennial basis, as well as results of the Hospital Discharge Survey, which appear periodically in *Monthly Vital Statistics Report* and *Health and Vital Statistics*. The Hospital Discharge Survey gathers and analyzes data from a sample of hospitals on demographic characteristics of patients, descriptors of hospitals, morbidity and diagnoses, and surgical operations. Since 1976, a congressionally mandated annual report to the President entitled *Health: United States* has appeared. It includes some data on hospitals, as well as health and financial data. (All of these publications are discussed in Chapter 3 and Appendix I.) This chapter uses AHA definitions and data, except as specifically noted.

The American Hospital Association classifies hospitals and reports comparative data principally by the variables listed below.

Hospital size. Hospital size is determined by the number of adult and pediatric beds regularly available, excluding bassinets (American Hospital Association, 1979a, p. xxviii).

Hospital type. The four types of hospital are mental, tuberculosis, other special, and general. "Other special" hospitals include narcotics addiction; maternity; eye, ear, nose, and throat; rehabilitation; orthopedic; chronic disease; mental retardation; and alcoholism—or some combination of the above, such as children's psychiatric (American Hospital Association, 1979c p. A–2). "General hospital," that is, all nonspecial, is the category that includes the majority of hospitals in the United States. The AHA has an all-inclusive descriptor for the bulk of U.S. hospitals: "community hospital" (Georgeopoulos, 1962). It is defined as "all non-federal, short-term general or other special hospitals—excluding hospital units of institutions [such as prisons and universities]—whose facilities and services are available to the public" (American Hospital Association, 1979b, p. xvi).

Mode of ownership. There are two principal modes of ownership: private and public. Private hospitals are categorized by the use to which they put their surplus income. They may be investor-owned for-profit (proprietary) or not-for-profit (voluntary). Public hospitals are categorized by the level of government jurisdiction that owns and operates them: federal, state, or local.

Length of stay. Length-of-stay categories are "long" and "short"; in the former, the average length of stay is 30 days or more, whereas in the latter the average length of stay is less than 30 days.

Types of Hospitals: Data

Table 7.1 provides some statistics on the various types of hospitals, showing number of hospitals, beds, average daily census, and occupancy rate by type, ownership, and length of stay. The voluntary general short-term hospital is the most common type, followed by the local government general short-term hospital. The other principal groups are the federal short-term hospitals, the state mental hospitals, and the proprietary short-term hospitals. In terms of beds, the two major groups are the short-term hospitals (average size, 169 beds), and the long-term (average size, 511 beds). Altogether in 1978, there were almost 1.4 million beds in 7,015 hospitals, with an average daily census of 1.04 million patients and an overall occupancy rate of 75.5% (American Hospital Association, 1979b, Tables 1, 2A, and 2B).

Table 7.2 shows selected characteristics of community hospitals for 1964, 1973, and 1978. Between 1964 and 1973 the number of hospitals increased by 1.33%, while between 1973 and 1978 the number increased by 1.06%. The peak number of community hospitals in the U.S., 5,881, was reached in 1977. Between 1964 and 1978 the number of beds increased from 721,000 to 975,000, or 35%. At the same time the average number of beds per hospital increased by 32%, reflecting the decline in the number of small hospitals (American Hospital Association, 1979b, pp. vii–viii). For example, between 1968 and 1970, the percentage of total beds in community hospitals of less than 100 beds decreased from 20.1% to 15.1%, while the proportion of hospitals with more than 400 beds increased from 27.5% to 33.3%. Therefore, while the number of community hospitals changed little in the period 1968–1978 (+0.5%), the average size grew substantially from 138 beds to 166 beds (20%). The wide variation in the size of community hospitals is related to a variety of factors: community size, availability of manpower, number of hospitals serving a given community, and availability of funds for construction and operation.

In the period 1968–1978, total admissions to community hospitals increased by 26.5%, while the average daily census increased by 14% (American Hospital Association, 1979b, p. vii). During the same time, the total U.S. population increased by slightly more than 9% (Bureau of the Census, Table 2), so increased admissions and average daily census reflect a real increase in hospital utilization. Average length of stay has been less stable than would appear from the figures in Table 7.2, because they do not show the peak of 8.4 days in 1968, when the upward pressure of Medicare on length of stay reached its peak, before financial controls were introduced.

Teaching Hospitals

The term "teaching hospital" generally refers to hospitals in which undergraduate and/or graduate teaching of medical students and/or house staff (interns, residents, and specialty fellows) takes place. The term is not applied to hospitals with teaching programs for nurses, technicians, therapists, and other allied health workers who are not physicians. The AHA publishes information on hospitals affiliated with medical schools, which account for most teaching hospitals (American Hospital Association, 1979b, Table 8). In 1978, there were 794 teaching hospitals (13.5% of all hospitals,

Table 7.1

Short- and Long-Term Hospitals Registered with the American Hospital Association, 1978

Type and Category	Short-Term				Long-Term			
	No.	Beds (× 1,000)	Average daily census (× 1,000)	Occupancy rate	No.	Beds (× 1,000)	Average daily census (× 1,000)	Occupancy rate
General								
Nongovernmental not-for-profit	3278	676	515	76.2	3	0.3	0.2	86
Investor-owned (for profit)	698	79	51	64	1	0.1	0.08	81
Local government	1685	182	124	68	4	0.9	0.8	86
State government	137	29	21	71	4	0.8	0.7	83
Federal government	329	87	66	76	12	9.3	7.7	83
Total	6127	1054	777	74	24	11.5	9.5	82
Psychiatric								
Nongovernmental not-for-profit	47	3.5	2.8	81	47	6.3	5.9	94
Investor-owned (for profit)	85	5	3.4	66	54	5.2	3.9	76
Local government	10	1	0.8	80	6	3.4	2.8	83
State government	33	11	9.0	80	244	199.2	161.3	81
Federal government	0	0	0	0	24	23.0	19.9	86
Total	175	20.8	16.0	77	375	237.2	193.8	82

TB and other respiratory diseases

Nongovernmental not-for-profit	1	0.07	0.04	51	1	0.1	0.04	40
Local government	1	0.63	0.08	76	1	0.2	0.08	67
State government	0	0.00	0.00	0	11	2.4	1.46	60
Total	2	0.14	0.09	62	13	2.6	1.58	60
Other special								
Nongovernmental not-for-profit	82	7.9	5	69	73	10	8.7	86
Investor-owned (for profit)	34	1.7	0.8	52	9	1	0.8	81
Local government	8	1.8	1.5	80	34	13	11.8	87
State government	13	1.6	1.1	71	41	14	11.7	80
Federal government	2	1.0	0.7	74	3	1	1.0	65
Total	139	14.	9.7	69	160	41	34.0	83
Total	6443	1089	803	74	572	292	239	82

Source: American Hospital Association, *Hospital Statistics*, Chicago, 1979, Tables 2A and 2B. (See Appendix I, A10.)

Table 7.2

**Selected Characteristics of Community Hospitals Registered
with the American Hospital Association, 1964, 1973, 1978**

	1964	1973	1978
Number of hospitals	5,712	5,789	5,851
Number of beds (thousands)	721	898	975
Average number of beds per hospital	126	155	167
Total admissions	26,000	32,000	34,506
Average daily census (thousands)	550	680	718
Average length of stay (days.)	7.7	7.8	7.6
Occupancy, percent	76.3	75.7	73.6
Outpatient visits (millions)	91	173	202

Source: American Hospital Association, *Hospital Statistics,* 1975, pp. vii–xvi, and *Hospital Statistics 1979*, p. vii. (See Appendix I, A10.)

a 50% increase since 1974), with 349,000 beds (36% of all beds). Their average size, excluding mental hospitals, was around 440 beds, while the average size for all short-term hospitals was around 170 beds. They provided 12.1 million admissions (35% of the total), and, on the average day, cared for 38% of all hospitalized patients. They provided one-third of all outpatient visits. Their occupancy rate was 79.2% and the average length of stay was 8.3 days. Thus, teaching hospitals have an importance in the hospital system quite out of proportion to their number.

Hospital Utilization

There are several measures of hospital utilization, which are for the most part self-explanatory: admissions; average daily census (average number of patients in the hospital); occupancy rate (percentage of beds occupied); average length of stay; total patient days (the product of average daily census by number of days in time period considered); and discharges. These data can be modified and compared in various cross-tabulations: by geography (region, state); by hospital characteristics (bed-size, type, category of ownership); and by patient age, sex, and demographic modifiers. Analyses of hospital utilization data are vast; we will cover only a small portion of them.*

---

*As mentioned elsewhere, hospital utilization data are available from several recurrent sources. The AHA's "Guide Issue" and "Hospital Indicators," as well as *Hospital Statistics*, are very useful in giving provider-perspective information. Provider-perspective information for short-term hospitals is also collected in the Hospital Discharge Survey (see Chapter 3).

In 1978, there were 37.2 million admissions to hospitals in the United States (American Hospital Association, 1979b, Table 1). Of the admissions, 93% were to community hospitals, although only two-thirds of the patient-days of care were in such hospitals (American Hospital Association, 1979b, Table 2); 71% of these admissions were to voluntary general hospitals, 21% to local government hospitals. Although only 1.6% of admissions were to nonfederal short- and long-term psychiatric hospitals, these accounted for 18% of the total average daily census.

There are many determinants of hospital admission. Being separated or divorced, having comprehensive insurance, and having a long traveling time to a regular source of medical care all increase an individual's chance of being hospitalized (Andersen et al., p. 13). The length of stay in a hospital is most closely associated with degree of anxiety about health, but is also related to a person's age, family structure, beliefs about health care, and availability of hospital services (Andersen et al., p. 13).

Women are more likely to be hospitalized than men (National Center for Health Statistics, 1979b, p. 2). Women use about 25% more days of care per 1,000 population than do males. When obstetrical admissions are eliminated, the average length of all admissions is about the same for males and females. Length of stay in a hospital decreases with patients' level of education and with higher income, and increases with age (Phelps, p. 112).

The use of community hospitals varies among age groups of the population. Persons age 65 years and over are discharged from the hospital at more than twice the rate of persons aged 15–44 and at more than 5 times the rate of those under 15 years of age (National Center for Health Statistics, 1978, p. 303). Diagnosis-specific length of stay has been declining with medical progress. In 1947, pneumonia patients stayed 16 days in hospital; in 1977, they stayed 8.4 days. An appendectomy once resulted in an average of 14 days of hospitalization; by 1977, it resulted in an average of 4.9 days. The average maternity stay in 1947 was 10 days; by 1972, it was · down to 3.4 days (Commission on Professional and Hospital Activities).

In 1977, the leading discharge diagnoses from nonfederal short-stay hospitals were: diseases of the circulatory system, 4.8 million discharges; diseases of the digestive system, 4.3 million discharges; normal delivery and complications of pregnancy, 4.3 million discharges; accidents, poisonings, and violence, 3.8 million discharges; diseases of the genitourinary system, 3.6 million discharges; and diseases of the respiratory system, 3.5 million discharges (National Center for Health Statistics, 1979b). Among the most common specific discharge diagnoses were: malignant neoplasm, 1.7 million; fractures, 1.2 million; pneumonia, 820,000; and diabetes mellitus 574,000.

The ten most common surgical procedures were: diagnostic dilation and curettage of uterus, 995,000; hysterectomy, 705,000; tonsillectomy, 617,000; sterilization of females, 585,000; hernia repair, 533,000; ovariectomy, 458,000; Caesarean section, 455,000; gall bladder removal, 446,000; operations of muscles and related tissues, 371,000; and setting of fracture, 351,000. Note that 5 of the first 7 most common surgical procedures are for females only.

The average length of stay (ALOS) in community hospitals in 1978 was 7.6 days (American Hospital Association, 1979b, p. vii). It had remained essentially unchanged for three years. There is wide variation in length of stay by age ("Hospital Indicators," March 16, 1979). In 1979, patients aged 65 and over stayed an average of about 10.6 days, while those 65 and under stayed about 6.0 days per admission ("Hospital Indicators," May 1, 1980). There is variation in the ALOS by region and hospital bed-size. For example, the ALOS in community hospitals ranged from 5.2 in Utah and Wyoming to 8.9 in Minnesota and 9.7 in New York (American Hospital Association, 1979b, Table 6). Variation in length of stay by as much as 5 days may also be found in hospitals of less than 50 beds when compared to hospitals of more than 500 beds. Variation in ALOS by hospital size may be explained in part by variation in severity of disease, but regional differences are difficult to explain on medical bases alone (Goran, pp. 4–7). By type of short-term hospital, the ALOS is 6.6 days in the investory-owned hospitals, 7.8 days in the not-for-profit, with local government hospitals averaging 7.4 days (American Hospital Association, 1979b, Table 1).

Distribution and Relative Bed Supply

In 1948, there were approximately 3.4 nonfederal general medical and surgical hospital beds per 1,000 civilian resident population, with a geographical range from a low of 2 beds per 1,000 population in the South to a high of 6 beds per 1,000 population in the industrial North and far West. By 1976, the general medical and surgical hospital bed-population ratio was 5.0 beds per 1,000. There was some variation around the mean, ranging from 3.6 per 1,000 in Utah to 7.2 per 1,000 in North Dakota, among the contiguous states, and from 3.3 per 1,000 in Hawaii to 9.8 in the District of Columbia (National Center for Health Statistics, 1979a, Table 213). The ratio in a majority of states lies within ± 0.6 beds per 1,000 of the mean. Nevertheless, there are no known variations in health status, positive or negative, which can explain the variations that do exist.

Although improvements in bed distribution and increase in bed supply since World War II have been regarded as an achievement in providing access to hospitals for people in rural areas, the overall number of hospital beds in the United States has come to be regarded as excessive. This is difficult to quantify because a generally accepted definition of an excess bed cannot be found (Sattler and Bennett, p. 30). The number of beds required for a given geographic region is a function of the number of patient-days of hospital care required by the population (expressed as average daily census) and the occupancy level deemed appropriate for the hospitals of a given area (Sattler and Bennett, p. 30). However, beds have not been built in accordance with such a rational formula, but rather because of medical need, local wealth, civic pride, and competition.

Once built, the availability of hospital beds promotes their use (Klarman, p. 139). The popular formulation of this relationship is known as Roemer's Law (Roemer, 1961), abbreviated as "a built bed is a filled bed." Thus, adding beds can cost the system money even if the beds are all used, because they may be filled with patients who do not need hospital care.

A relatively high proportion of hospital costs are either fixed, or varied with difficulty in the face of short-term changes in utilization. Personnel costs accounted for 57% of community hospital costs in 1979 ("Hospital Indicators," Oct. 16, 1979, Table 1). Of the balance, capital costs for plant already purchased do not vary and utility costs can be reduced only slightly. Only expenditures for food and consumable supplies do not have to be made when a bed is empty. For these reasons, it can be estimated that on a short-term basis an empty bed costs about 70% as much to maintain as does a filled one (Blue Cross/Blue Shield). High occupancy provides a stimulus to shorten length of stay and pressure for maximum use of diagnostic and therapeutic facilities. However, increased occupancy raises hospital costs only modestly, while raising hospital income dramatically, assuming that the patient has a payment source. Thus, the incentive for hospitals is to admit patients. The only way to really save money in the hospital sector is to close beds and eliminate those high fixed costs. Simply holding down admissions will not solve the problem. It saves insurance dollars in the short run, but does not reduce total health expenditures effectively in the long run.

Overbedding

A great deal of controversy has been generated in recent years over the related, but different, questions of overbedding and overutilization of beds. Overbedding means an excessive bed supply, resulting in unused beds. In the mid-1970s, researchers at the University of Michigan's Program and Bureau of Hospital Administration determined that a general hospital of 300 beds or more could easily operate in the 85%–95% occupancy range (Sattler and Bennett, pp. 36–39). In 1975, the national community hospital adult bed occupancy rate for hospitals of all sizes was around 75% ("Hospital Indicators," April 16, 1976, Table 1). By the end of the decade, it was down to about 74%. Although in 1974 the president of the AHA said, "We've already got more beds than we need" (*Medical World News*, Nov. 8, 1974, p. 114), in 1975 the AHA officially took the position that the 75% occupancy figure does not necessarily mean that there are too many beds and stated that the ideal bed/population ratio has not been determined, flexibility is needed to meet emergency situations, and that there are variations in occupancy rate by region and medical service that are not reflected in national figures (American Hospital Association, 1975b). In 1976, as part of an effort to control hospital costs, the American Hospital Association took an official position against building new hospitals or expanding existing ones, but did not argue against replacing dilapidated ones or recommend closing existing ones (American Hospital Association, 1975c; *Medical World News,* November 8, 1974).

In the study cited above, Sattler and Bennett concluded that for 1975 the estimated national community hospital bed excess was about 70,000 (pp. 40–42). They assumed that although larger hospitals could safely operate with a 90% occupancy rate, smaller ones could not: enough beds to allow for emergencies must be provided. They suggested that a weighted national average occupancy rate of 81% for hospitals of all sizes would be optimal. Estimating the average cost of carrying an excess bed to be $18,250, the authors found that the 81% rule would produce an annual savings of over $1 billion (p. 46).

The Comptroller General of the Unites States (p. 98) pointed out that excess beds are accompanied by sophisticated equipment, often purchased with little assurance of use sufficient to justify cost. Because of this "over-equipping," an estimated 25% of the population receives hospital care in facilities with expensive equipment that inflates costs, but that is not necessary for patient care. This is a point that was being made with increasing frequency by the end of the decade (Westerman; *Consumer Health Perspectives*).

In 1975, the Health Research Group (HRG) of Public Citizen, the Ralph Nader organization, and the AHA had a sharp exchange on the issue of overbedding (Ensminger; American Hospital Association, 1975d; Health Research Group). The HRG concluded from its examination of the data that the excess bed figure was 100,000. The AHA did not agree. However, in 1976, the Institute of Medicine issued what is considered to be an authoritative report, recommending a reduction in nonfederal short-term general hospital bed-to-population ratio from the then 4.4 per 1,000 to 4.0 per 1,000 by 1981. That would have required a reduction of about 70,000 beds from the 1976 total of about 950,000.

In 1974, before the AHA had adopted its end-to-expansion-in-certain-circumstances policy in 1976, Rogatz, among others, had recommended an almost complete moratorium on additional hospital bed construction (1974a, 1974b). Further, the devising of legally acceptable means of closing beds down was recommended, while the necessity of finding a way to support geographically essential but underutilized hospitals was recognized. For the rest of the 1970s, however, the industry was going the other way. By 1979, the total number of beds in the community hospital category was 988,000, about 13% more than the 4/1,000 figure recommended by the Institute of Medicine study and in fact set as a goal in the national health planning guidelines (*Federal Register*, p. 13,045).

In 1980, the Carter administration proposed a set of strict controls on federal support of hospital capital expenditures (*Hospital Week*, June 13, 1980). The American Hospital Association did not like the idea. However, the voluntary approach to hospital bed expansion, which the AHA had been advocating since the mid-1970s, was not working. The hospitals were not heeding warnings that if they did not mind their own business, the government would (Enright and Jonas, p. 176). Nevertheless, the AHA was, at the time at least, very powerful in Congress. It remained to be seen what would come of the idea.

At the end of the 1970s, although not reflected in national figures, in certain regions control on the number of beds had begun to occur, primarily in an unplanned way as a result of financial pressures, and secondarily as a result of the Certificate of Need process (see Chapter 13). Some hospitals closed due to bankruptcy. Robert Cunningham, a long-time observer of the industry, believes that in the 1980s, bankruptcy will be the principal method of hospital bed reduction (1980a). The number of hospital corporate entities has been reduced by mergers and consolidations. Financial resources to provide support for geographically necessary but underutilized hospitals, especially in rural areas, brought about special consideration of their problems by the American Hospital Association. Survival of such hospitals presents special problems and requires special solutions (Munroe and Schuman).

Overutilization

Overutilization means that a significant proportion of hospital admissions are unnecessary. If the unnecessary admissions were not made, the occupancy rates would be even lower than they already are, and the excess bed figure would be even higher. There is significant evidence to support this position.*

*See: Roemer and Shonick, pp. 281–291; Reidel et al; Ensminger, pp. 26–28; Gaus et al.; Luft; and other papers cited in the Health Maintenance Organization section in Chapter 6 (pp. 144 ff.). The geographic variation in average length of stay and occupancy rate without evidence of variations in health or illness levels (American Hospital Association, 1979b, Tables 5B and 5C); surgical procedure rates (Gittelsohn and Wennberg pp. 101–104); and Medicare hospital discharge and multiple-stay rates (Gornick) are also impressive.

The analysis of possible overutilization of hospitals has focused particularly closely on surgery. John Bunker, comparing the frequency of surgery in England and Wales with that in the United States, said: "There are twice as many surgeons in proportion to the population in the United States as in England and Wales, and they perform twice as many operations. . . . Indications for surgery are not sufficiently precise to allow determination of whether American surgeons operate too often or the British too infrequently . . ." (p. 135). It appeared from this study that there might be a Roemer's Law for surgeons too: when surgeons are present, they will operate.

The controversy flared into the national press in 1975 when Congressional hearings were held by Representative John Moss. The Congressmen examined a New York City study in which second opinions were required before surgery could be authorized; the study concluded that 17.6% of operations are unnecessary (McCarthy and Widmer). They also reviewed evidence that the surgery rate for Medicaid recipients in the U.S. is almost 2½ times that for the general population ("Getting Ready for National Health Insurance," July 18). Ensminger, citing the McCarthy-Widmer study, as well as a study by Lewis and a book by a pseudonymous Dr. Williams (1971), estimated that the national excess surgery rate is 20% (pp. 17–19). He estimated the dollar cost of that surgery at $3 billion. (Added to the $2 billion for excess beds and an estimated $3 billion for overlong hospital stays, Ensminger arrived at his $8 billion overrun total.) Ensminger also raised the issue of unnecessary death as the ultimate side-effect of unnecessary surgery. He estimated that if there are 3 million unnecessary surgical operations each year, there must be about 15,000 unnecessary deaths (assuming normal surgical and anesthetic mortality) resulting from the unnecessary operations (p. 18). This dispute blossomed further when in early 1976 *The New York Times* projected McCarthy and Widmer's figures nationally. Their estimates were somewhat lower than Ensminger's, but still substantial: 2.4 million unnecessary operations and almost 12,000 needless deaths (*New York Times*, January 27, 1976).

The response of organized medicine to these charges was as sharp as the AHA's response to the overbedding instigations. Dr. Francis D. Moore, chief of surgery at the Peter Bent Brigham Hospital in Boston, said: "Fraudulent operations are extremely rare and it's irresponsible to suggest otherwise. . . . The person who wrote that story in *The New York Times* ought to be horsewhipped" (*Medical World News*, May 3, 1976, p. 50). *The American Medical News*, the AMA newspaper, criticized *The Times* "for exaggeration, for distortion of admittedly true facts, for extrapolating sound data beyond reasonable limits" (*American Medical News*, p. 4). A former AMA President, Malcolm Todd, said: "These figures are outrageously exaggerated" (*American Medical News*, p. 15).

The issue does have a long history. *Medical World News* compiled a lengthy bibliography with citations going back to 1946 (1976, p. 66). The second half of the 1970s saw increasing attention paid to the issue of unnecessary surgery. In 1976 and again in 1978, the Subcommittee on Oversight and Investigations of the House Commerce Committee issued reports claiming that there was a good deal of unnecessary surgery with resulting avoidable deaths (Subcommittee on Oversight, 1976, 1978). A study by the American College of Surgeons and the American Surgical Association examined, among other things, the supply of surgeons, their training and qualifications, and the amount of surgery (American College of Surgeons). The study on supply expanded on the classic work of Hughes and his colleagues (1972). The so-called SOSSUS (Study on Surgical Services in the United States) report was so controversial that readers of it and participants in its creation could not even agree upon what it actually said (Blackstone; Colton; Hughes et al., 1977; Moore), much less agree on the value of its recommendations. John Bunker and many colleagues carried out an exhaustive cost-benefit analysis of surgery and concluded, among other things, that more research was needed (Bunker et al.). An analysis of a mandatory surgical second-opinion program in Massachusetts Medicaid concluded that "only" 7.7% of procedures were unnecessary (Gertman et al.). A lay perspective on the problem was provided by Stroman. However, Annas thought that the debate obscured more important issues. Pauly was not even sure that unnecessary surgery occurred; his was certainly not the majority view. The likelihood is that, as with overbedding, the question is not whether unnecessary surgery and overutilization occur, but to what extent they prevail and what should be done about them. It is up to the hospital industry and the medical profession to determine the true state of affairs and then to take action to save dollars and lives.

Hospital Structure

The Operating Divisions of a Hospital*

The principal hospital operating divisions are medical, nursing, other diagnostic and therapeutic support, financial, personnel, hotel, and community relations. Most hospitals provide services both to inpatients, who are admitted to the hospital and assigned a bed, and to outpatients, who come to an emergency department, an outpatient clinic, or a diagnostic or therapeutic service for a procedure not requiring admission.

---

*We are here considering primarily community hospitals, as defined above. Although some of the broad generalizations and principles apply to other kinds of hospitals, many of the details do not. For more specific information on state mental hospitals see Chapter 9 and for more information on federal hospitals, see Chapter 11.

Medical division. The medical division is generally organized along the lines of the medical specialties. The larger the hospital and the more specialized the medical services, the more medical departments are found, particularly in teaching hospitals. There is no universal logic to the way in which medical departments are categorized. Some are separated from the others by type of skill involved, some by the age or sex of their main patient group, and some by the organ or organ system that is their primary purview.

The principal departments are:

- *Internal medicine*—diagnosis and therapy for adults, in general with problems involving one or more internal organs or the skin, in which the principal tools do not involve a physical alteration of the patient's body by the physician;
- *Surgery*—diagnosis and therapy in which the principal tools involve a physical alteration of the patient's body by the physician;
- *Pediatrics*—diagnosis and therapy for children, primarily but not entirely with nonsurgical techniques;
- *Obstetrics/gynecology*—diagnosis and therapy relating to the sexual/reproductive system of women, which uses both surgical and nonsurgical techniques;
- *Psychiatry*—diagnosis and therapy for people of all ages with mental and emotional problems, using primarily nonsurgical techniques.

A sixth important medical department in many hospitals is general–family medicine—diagnosis and therapy for people of all ages with all conditions, using nonsurgical and surgical techniques, although the practice of the latter in general–family medicine has been declining in recent years.

Other medical departments, when they exist, tend to be organized around organs and organ systems: ophthalmology (eye); otolaryngology (ear, nose, and throat); urology (male sexual/reproductive system, and the renal system for both males and females); orthopedics (bones and joints); and so on. Radiology, the use of X-ray and other radiation sources, is a medical department with a primarily diagnostic function, although radiotherapy is also important. With the development of certain non-X-ray scans and the separation of therapeutic nuclear medicine in some institutions, some radiology departments are now called departments of "Diagnostic Imaging." Pathology, in medical practice, serves only a diagnostic function, both before and after treatment. Anesthesiology is principally concerned with preparing patients so that they may be surgically operated upon with no pain or discomfort during the procedure.

Other health services. The functional divisions of the nursing service follow the pattern discussed in Chapter 5. The diagnostic and therapeutic services, which may or may not be attached to one of the medical departments, include: laboratory (usually under the direction of the department of pathology); electrocardiography (usually a part of internal medicine); electroencephalography (part of neurology); radiography (part of radiology); pharmacy; clinical psychology; social service; inhalation therapy (often part of anesthesiology or pulmonary medicine); nutrition as therapy; physical, occupational, and speech therapy (often attached to the department of rehabilitation medicine, if there is one); home care; and medical records (American Hospital Association, 1979c, p. A–2).

Administrative functions. Financial, personnel, and hotel service are the major operating functions of the hospital administration. The hotel services include maintenance of plant and equipment, housekeeping, laundry, and dietary (cooking and delivery of meals). Other primarily administrative functions include community/public relations, organizing volunteer services, operating the medical library, and long-range planning.

Administration

Health administration encompasses planning, organizing, directing, controlling, and coordinating the resources and procedures by which needs and demands for health and medical care and a healthful environment are fulfilled, by provision of specific services to individual clients, organizations, and communities (Austin, p. 139). The hospital's chief administrator is the direct representative of the board of trustees or other governing authority in the management of the hospital, and is responsible to the governing authority alone for the performance of his or her duties. The administrator is responsible for seeing that all policies approved by the board, including medical staff by-laws, are implemented.

Hospital management is primarily concerned with efficiency, in terms of controlling expenditures, and effectiveness, in terms of assuring benefits (Georgeopoulos, 1971). The hospital has a major incentive to contain costs in order to increase its ability to provide a broader range of services to as many of the sick as possible. Opportunities to contain hospital costs exist in five areas: planning of facilities, planning of services, scheduling of patients and patient services, medical control of facilities utilization and quality of service, and administrative control of manpower and expenditures (Phillips).

Financial aspects of administration are complemented by other administrative skills such as planning the evolution of the hospital role; defining and redefining corporate objectives; and developing policies with appropriate strategies to assure their implementation. Areas in which these skills are utilized are medical staff and board of trustees relations; maintenance of the physical plant and equipment; maintaining awareness and responsiveness to the legal environment; and fostering educational programs, medical and health care delivery research, and cooperation with other hospitals and health agencies (Davis and Henshaw, pp. 5–7).

Community relationships in administration. Hospital administrators, in addition to dealing with professional medical concerns, have a special role in filling community demands for health care (Rogatz, 1980). Some hospitals are regarded as detached from their communities, and demands are being made that they change their institution-centric (Freymann, Section V) mode of functioning and share control of decision-making processes with community groups. Social roles in which hospitals that choose to can become involved include eliminating unemployment and underemployment in their communities, improving inadequate educational services, and combating personal and institutional racism (Dornblaser). While this type of community involvement was popular with some progressive hospitals in the late 1960s and early 1970s, it has never become a significant activity, except for some urban hospitals in communities where social problems were so intertwined with the delivery of health care that they were impossible to ignore.

Currently, community activities of hospitals focus on efforts to combine health promotion and health information in programs for the community (Adamson et al.; Carpenter; Green; Jonas, 1979b; Lane; Vickery). Typical programs are health education centers; wellness centers; home visit programs; hospital orientation programs for children; disease-specific programs; cardiopulmonary resuscitation courses for community groups; and life-style programs on nutrition, exercise, and aging (Longe). The AHA is lending active support to these efforts with its Center for Health Promotion (Behrens). Within the institution, services to patients have been improved by the presence of patient advocates, who serve as hospital ombudsmen. In 1979, there were nearly 1,000 of them working in the nation's larger hospitals (Lane and Evans; Sun).

In developing its role in relation to its community, the hospital must also consider other health agencies and community health programs. In some communities, it may be quite logical to have health services centralized in the hospital, while in others it may be appropriate to decentralize some services to a neighborhood health center or other agency, which may be either independent of the hospital or contractually related (see Chapter 6).

Providing outpatient care, which is either preventive or treats a problem that might otherwise have necessitated hospital admission, could lower the cost of medical care, but may also increase demand for inpatient services by referrals for admission to the hospital from the clinic. At any rate, it will probably increase the average cost per admission because of the higher proportion of more seriously ill patients admitted when minor illness is no longer a cause of hospital admission. In a time of increasingly scarce resources, it is not clear whether hospitals will expand or contract their community role. The relationship between consumer expectations and hospital financial problems will continue to force hospitals to make difficult choices.

*Sharing strategies.** Some administrators make efforts to see that the services that their hospitals do provide are accessible to the community and appropriate to its health needs. To achieve this end, the range of services must be broad enough to leave no critical needs unmet, but not so broad as to require wasteful investment of community resources in high-cost, low-utility technology if it can be made available to the community through cooperation with some other agency. In the past few years, there has been an increasing recognition of the need to deal with wasteful practices. Administrators also attempt to see that the services provided are continuous rather than episodic and that hospital services interface through appropriate referral mechanisms with other health services in the community or, through sharing services, with other agencies.

Some institutions have historical relationships with a geographically, ethnically, or religiously discrete patient population, and are reluctant for political and social reasons to appear to be reducing services. A sharing strategy among hospitals is sometimes used to reduce the burden of a given service. For example, one hospital may be responsible for emergency medical care, and back-up services can be provided by one or several others.

The sharing strategy is also being implemented by administrators on a larger scale in the consolidation of hospitals through various forms of mergers (Brown and Money; Connors; Hepner, Part 7). Further, management of some hospitals is being provided under contract by other hospitals or management firms. The result is the development of multiple hospital chains under centralized management that can afford expensive management expertise. In at least one instance, ten multihospital systems have joined together to form an even larger chain to benefit from certain shared services (Parker and Wardell). Many of these chains are investor-owned operations, which will be subject to the pressures of public expectations that a wide range of services be provided (Brown and Money). Using this strategy, not-for-profit institutions are establishing consulting offices; this enables them to expand their services and influence without new capital

*See also Hepner, parts 4 and 6.

and to acquire and use the range of talent essential in modern hospital operations.

As the pace of growth and variety of institutional arrangements expand to include more pervasive types of hospital consolidation along a continuum of management to partnership to ownership, interaction among multihospital systems is beginning to develop. More cooperation and economic consolidation with concomitant increases in power are anticipated. However, several antagonists to such expansion exist, including antitrust and tax laws, reimbursement regulations, and organizational barriers. Growth will change the nature of hospital-clinician relationships and the production and distribution of clinical and administrative manpower (Zuckerman).

The proportion of hospital expenses that are accounted for by personnel costs varies according to the intensity of the technology used in treating patients. In high-technology cancer treatment centers, personnel costs may be only 40%; in community hospitals, the range is between 46% and 60%; in psychiatric hospitals, personnel costs may consume more than 80% of the operating budget. The number of personnel required to provide patient care in acute-care hospitals is increasing constantly. In 1950, there were 1.31 full-time equivalent employees per patient bed in nonfederal short-term general hospitals. In 1973, the number had increased to 3.15 (American Hospital Association, 1975a, p. xii). By 1978, the number had decreased to 2.72, largely due to cost pressures on hospitals (American Hospital Association, 1979b, derived from Table I, p. 5).

New medical technology, which is being developed continuously, has a direct effect on hospital personnel costs. For every new piece of high-technology equipment purchased for the hospital, additional staff, who may require extensive training, and often licensing or certification, are hired to perform tasks required by the new technology. Further, as medical care becomes more complex, many duties formerly carried out by physicians or nurses are delegated to other persons who are specifically trained to provide a broad range of related services.

Personnel costs contribute to hospital inflation not only because there are more employees, but also because they now earn proportionately more than in the past. Increases in the minimum wage, the infusion of funds that followed the implementation of Medicare, unionization, and the greater skills demanded of those who work with complex medical technology have all resulted in increased wages (Raske, 1974, p. 68).

Hospital employees are now covered under the Federal Wage and Hour Standards Act. The right of collective bargaining through hospital unions is protected by law and may be enforced by state labor agencies. Unionization, collective bargaining, and the occasional strike are being seen more frequently, although the vast majority of health workers are not unionized

(Bognanno and Champlin; Metzger; Wolfe). Three factors have influenced the impact of unionization on hospital wages: (1) the percent of hospital employees covered; (2) laws requiring nonprofit hospitals to recognize collective bargaining agents; and (3) spreading union coverage for workers in general (Sloan, p. 36). It has been argued that these measures serve the public interest because the state should assure decent wages for all persons working in its jurisdiction, while hospitals must be able to maintain a qualified and stable labor force, which must be sought in the competitive labor market (Shain and Roemer).

Hospital Governance in the Private Sector

The majority of hospitals in 1980 were voluntary. The voluntary principle is historically associated with charity, emphasis on good quality of care, concern for the public interest, and involvement in education and training. These elements are found also to various degrees in all types of hospitals, often deriving from the example of the private not-for-profit hospital. Many not-for-profit hospitals still want to continue their charity role, providing care without charge to patients who have no source of payment, as both a moral and social commitment. Federal law now requires hospitals that have received federal funds under the Hill-Burton program to provide a proportion of free care to medically indigent patients (Raske, 1980; Wing, pp. 154–156). However, this care costs money. Its provision has caused problems for certain hospitals with little or no endowment income and little or no charitable income.

Investor-owned and not-for-profit hospitals differ in that economic criteria are most important in decision-making in for-profit hospitals, whereas a wider variety of criteria influence decision-making in nonprofit hospitals (Rushing). These differences influence the way that the hospital operates. Specifically, not-for-profit hospitals have a higher ratio of personnel to patients than do for-profit hospitals with the same occupancy levels. Also, average daily charges of for-profit hospitals are positively associated with community wealth; for nonprofit hospitals, there is no evidence of such a relationship (Rushing, pp. 474, 477).

Trustees

The typical private community hospital is organized according to a constitution and by-laws, investing in a board of trustees the responsibility for all aspects of the operation of the hospital, including ultimate responsibility for the medical care delivered in that institution (Cunningham, 1980b; Umbdenstock, 1979, 1980). That responsibility is then delegated to a medical staff, which has its own set of by-laws, approved by the board of trustees (Letourneau, 1964, p. 92; Roemer and Friedman, 1979, p. 281).

Hospitals receive authority to operate from the government of the state in which they are located. The agency with hospital licensing powers varies from state to state. Boards of voluntary hospitals are given the legal authority to operate the hospital, set policy, and make all major decisions. Day-to-day decisions are made by the administrative and professional personnel who manage the hospital. New York State law, for example, specifies that the board shall appoint the hospital administrator, shall appoint members of the medical staff, and shall approve the by-laws and regulations of the medical staff (Somers, p. 108). Boards of trustees for voluntary hospitals were formed originally out of a sense of obligation felt by the upper class in the United States to provide for the welfare of the sick poor in the cities. This was done by financing the building and operation of hospitals. Hospital trusteeship has since become legally formalized in all states.

Making and soliciting philanthropic contributions has not been a major activity of hospital trustees for quite some time (Stephenson, p. 38). Although the amount of dollars contributed to hospitals has remained relatively constant, the increases in national medical care expenditures have made such contributions relatively less significant. In 1974, philanthropic contributions amounted to $3.9 billion, covering around 10% of total hospital expenditures (American Hospital Association, 1976). In 1977, 8% of the $68 billion total of hospital expenditures, $5.25 billion, was covered by charitable contributions. The appropriateness of funding with financial gifts projects that have not been approved by planning agencies has been subject to federal scrutiny. Further, proposed changes in the federal tax structure may remove charitable incentives to the extent they are associated with tax relief (Cunningham, 1978).

Before the 1940s and 1950s, when hospital administration had not yet emerged as a career, hospitals actually needed trustees to deal with the administrative problems that most senior administrators were not trained to handle (Cunningham, 1980b). As hospitals moved from caring for the sick and poor to caring for the community at large, medical matters became more important to trustees. Their role changed from providing minimal charity services to guaranteeing that each patient is maximally safe when he enters the hospital (Stephenson, p. 40).

The board of trustees is the body legally responsible for the operation of the hospital. It acts as an organ of review, appraisal, and appeal in a judicial manner. It assures the physical integrity of the hospital. It must be cognizant of the appointments and privileges granted to each physician and be assured that all services provided in the hospital are of adequate professional caliber and it must review the medical staff constitution and by-laws (Stephenson, pp. 40–41). It must intelligently manage the relationship between the hospital and its paid staff on the one hand, and the private medical staff, which admits the patients and has primary responsibility for their care, on the other (Thompson). Most importantly, it has the responsibility for establishing the goals and objectives of the hospital and evaluating the hospital's performance in pursuit of those goals and objectives.

Some characteristics of hospital trustees in the mid-1970s were identified in a survey conducted by the American Hospital Association Bureau of Research Services (Kessler, pp. 21–26). It reported that 39% of the respondents had annual incomes of more than $40,000. More than one-half of the trustees surveyed indicated no limit on the number of years they could serve without interruption. In general, boards of trustees cannot be considered to be broadly representative of the communities their hospitals serve. In Detroit in 1971, 76% of board members were business or professional people (*Health Perspectives*, Table II (a)). In 1973, among the memberships of the boards of trustees of hospitals with 300 or more beds in Manhattan, New York City, 87% were male, 67% were business people or non-health professionals, and another 3% were health professionals (*Health Perspectives*, Table II (b)).*

Studies in the late 1970s showed that upper- and middle-class representation on boards of trustees still excluded lower income and minority groups from most hospital boards. One study considered the characteristics of trustees and their impact on the hospital by analyzing the flow of information between the administration and the board. Results indicated that larger boards were associated with higher costs. But there was little support for the proposition that representation from specific occupational groups was associated with more or less efficient operation of the hospital. A recommendation was made that boards be used to link hospitals to community resources. Another was that trustees should pay more attention to the kind of information that administrators and physicians have, rather than worry about obtaining the information themselves (Kaufman et al.).

Some observers believe that changes are imminent in the membership of hospital boards. A professional trustee may develop in the future, with expertise in a specific area and with experience on boards of several hospitals. Ex officio members who represent other agencies will be given seats on hospital boards; in exchange for their information, they will acquire an informal base for political action outside the traditional structures (Mott and Chalk; Umbdenstock, 1979, 1980).

*Given that trustees are often business people and that they substantially influence hospital expenditures, conflicts of interest can arise when hospitals do business with firms with which their trustees are associated (*New York Times*, Dec. 26, 1975, April 18, 1976; *Newsday*, February 27, March 15, 1976).

Broader representation of the users of hospital services may be in the offing. Those who argue for it say that the wishes and value systems of the vast majority of persons in the community are represented only to the extent that upper- and middle-class board members understand those wishes and value systems and choose to pay attention to them (Mott and Chalk).

The wealthy are no longer providing the level of financial support that originally brought about their appointment. It is possible that broadening the makeup of the governing board will bring improvements, or at least a system that the majority of people want. If members of the community are recruited, the board's broadened power base might yield greater community support; the likelihood of relevant decision-making would increase; and a legitimate testing ground for new ideas would be provided.

Trustees of all powerful community institutions are being made aware of public scrutiny of the power they hold, the influence they wield, and the responsibility they must demonstrate. The AHA has taken an active role in trustee development (American Hospital Association, 1979a). Hospital trustees are developing a new awareness of their responsibilities in response to the public feeling that "the health care system is out of control and needs to be changed." Trustees are expected to represent hospitals to the community and vice versa. They are expected to become partners with the government in developing responsible laws, and they are being called upon by some hospitals for specific expertise (Umbdenstock, 1979). Further changes in the composition and activities of boards of trustees can be expected as the necessity for community cooperation, interagency sharing, and trustee expertise becomes apparent to even the most traditional boards (Cunningham, 1980b; Mott and Chalk).

Public Hospitals

Governance

There are a variety of governance forms for public hospitals. At the federal level, the Department of Defense, the Veterans' Administration, and the Public Health Service operate their hospitals without boards of trustees or their equivalent. The hospital directors are directly accountable to their administrative superiors, and indirectly to the President and the Congress. (See Chapter 11 for additional information on federal government hospitals.) State hospitals are also run directly by government departments, usually Mental Health or Hygiene for psychiatric facilities, and Health for the remaining tuberculosis sanatoria and the few state general or other special hospitals. These hospitals usually do not have boards of trustees, although the government department may be in part responsible to a Board of Mental Hygiene, or Health, which may exert some board-of-trustee-like influence on individual hospitals. As at the federal level, state hospital directors are mainly accountable to their administrative superiors, and indirectly to the Governor and the state legislature. (See Chapter 9 for additional information on state mental hospitals.)

The governance of local public general hospitals, with which the balance of this section is primarily concerned, is a more complex matter. For example, until 1969 in New York City, the 18 municipally owned hospitals were operated by a Department of Hospitals (by 1979, there were 17). Hospital directors were directly accountable to the commissioner, who was accountable to the mayor and the City Council. (A similar situation currently prevails in Los Angeles, San Francisco, and Boston.) Hospital boards, where they existed, were mere window-dressing.

In 1969, New York City adopted the public corporation approach. A semi-independent Health and Hospitals Corporation was established. Public officials sit on the board but do not have a majority of its seats. All appointments are made by elected officials. The chief operating officer is the corporation's president, elected by the board, usually on recommendation from the mayor. The president is under the mayor's control through the latter's control of part of the corporation finances and the fact that the mayor directly or indirectly appoints 10 of the 15 board members. However, there is no formal administrative line from the corporation president to the mayor. The hospital directors report directly to the corporation president, and the corporation board functions like the board of trustees of a voluntary hospital. There are "community advisory boards" for each municipal hospital, but their powers are limited.

County hospitals in semiurban, suburban, and rural areas may be run directly by a department of the county government or may have a board of managers, as is the case in Nassau County, New York. These boards are usually appointed by the chief executive officer of the county and/or the county legislative body. The purse-strings are usually controlled by the county government, but in certain jurisdictions, county hospital boards are independent authorities with the power to levy their own taxes and sell their own bonds for capital construction, as in Houston, Texas.

Public General Hospitals

The public general hospital is defined by the Commission on Public General Hospitals of the American Hospital Association as "short-term general and certain special hospitals—excluding federal, psychiatric, and tuberculosis hospitals—that are owned by state and local governments" (Commission on Public-General Hospitals, p. v). As of 1978, there were 1,693 local government general and other special hospitals and 150 state government general and other special hospitals with a total of 215,000 beds (American Hospital Association, 1979b, Table 2A). Together, these 1,843 hospitals (31% of all community hospitals) provided 22% of the beds, 21% of the inpatient admissions, and 27% of the outpatient visits for all community hospitals (American Hospital Association, 1979b, derived from Table 1).

Public general hospitals usually provided care for poor persons, including an estimated 5 million undocumented aliens (Friedman, May 1, 1980). They often are the only institutions that will provide care for persons with special social problems: the "shopping bag lady," the poor prostitute, the poor drug addict or alcoholic, the disruptive psychiatric patient, the destitute aged person, and the prisoner. In certain areas, they are the only source of care for the patients with special medical problems: the badly burned, the distressed neonate, the high-risk mother, and the victim of accidental or criminal life-threatening trauma (Friedman, 1980a). In many areas they are also an important locus for health sciences education and for local employment.

Problems of public general hospitals. Public hospitals have many problems (Shonick). They may have poor management, which can be due to a cumbersome civil service or patronage job system. They are saddled with the "pauper stigma," which has a long history and is deeply ingrained in the national psyche. Staffing by medical school specialty physicians, where it occurs, often impedes the development of comprehensive care. The location of hospitals in declining and poor areas of the city results in more poverty clients and more difficulty in recruiting staff. Declining occupancy figures, and the closing of county hospitals in California (Blake and Bodenheimer) and municipal hospitals in New York, Philadelphia, and St. Louis are regarded by some as a harbinger of similar events in other states. They point out that Medicare and Medicaid give the patient free choice of physician and hospital, and the private sector is increasingly being chosen. In California, 30% of all patients requiring hospitalization switched from the public to the private sector between 1966 and 1974.

Where municipal hospitals are principal teaching institutions of medical schools—New York's Bellevue, Boston City, New Orleans Charity, Chicago's Cook County, and Los Angeles General—the technical medical quality is probably superior to that of the average community hospital. However, in general surroundings, amenities, overall staffing, buildings, equipment, and budgeting, many local government hospitals are distinctly inferior.

There are periodic scandals involving New York City hospitals that go back over decades, usually as a result of journalistic or political exposés. The findings are always the same: staff shortages, antiquated buildings, broken equipment, dirt, insects, poor food, unattended patients, and so on. Outpatients in particular have suffered a great deal from long waits, hard benches, understaffing, poor recordkeeping, and inefficient organization. The results of the investigation usually were negligible. To its credit, New York City embarked on a major hospital construction program after a major exposé in the mid-1960s, replacing some of its most antiquated buildings. Ironically, the new buildings came on line in the mid-1970s, just at a time when the city was facing its worst financial squeeze. The Health and Hospitals Corporation was then forced to close some of its facilities, including one new building, stop its construction program, and curtail services at all of its institutions. The care in a new building with staff shortages cannot be much better than that in an old building with staff shortages, and could be worse (New York Times, July 30, 1976). By the end of the decade, newspaper articles were still being written that had in them the sound of the 1960s—and, indeed, the 1930s (New York Times, May 21, November 26, December 24, 1978, September 19, December 18, 1979).

The future of the public general hospital. The Commission on Public-General Hospitals identified three major issues on which the future of these institutions rests (Applebaum):

● Whether the governmental jurisdictions that own [them] continue to perceive health care delivery roles for themselves in the future, and, if so, whether they choose to carry out these roles by delivering care directly or by divesting themselves of operating responsibility by such means as establishing an independent operating authority, or purchasing care in the private sector.
● Whether the federal and state governments assume greater responsibility for financing the care of the poor.
● Whether the public-general hospitals are able to adapt their roles and governance to planning and regulatory pressures to become more efficient while improving the quality of services and to provide adequate health service capacity while eliminating duplication. (p. 96)

The Commission on Public-General Hospitals concluded (pp. 1–4) that public general hospitals should be maintained since they are a major, established health service, they provide services frequently not provided elsewhere, they are "an indispensable resource" for health sciences education and training, they offer few barriers to care, and they are designed to respond to government-mandated policies and programs. According to the Commission, their future depends upon: (1) their "ability to become broad-based community resources" operating within "rationally planned and organized community health care delivery systems"; (2) the establishment of "governance and management capabilities that enable them to identify and assume viable services roles, reconcile public accountability and management flexibility, and work with the community, with other providers, and with planners and regulators"; and (3) the solution of the "financial problems that threaten [their] ability . . . to serve their communities. . . ."

Would that it were so simple. If all local governments saw their hospitals as an opportunity to provide service rather than an increasingly heavy financial burden that they would sooner be rid of, it might be. However, there are local governments, critics say, in St. Louis and Philadelphia that have followed the latter course (Wilkins). On the other hand, the New Jersey state government took special steps to keep open the Jersey City Medical Center (Malloy), and New York City, while shrinking its system, is trying to provide alternative and substitute services while obtaining direct federal aid for local hospitals, one of the first local governments to do so (*The New York Times*, June 20, 1980).

New York City has found through a 10-year experience that establishing an independent hospital authority does not make the problems go away. Although management is simpler outside local government rules and regulations, the mayor's authority is diluted while the city's financial responsibilities have remained sizable. Chicago gave up a 10-year experiment with a semi-independent authority operating Cook County Hospital, and in April 1980 turned management of the institution over to a private company, Hyatt Medical Management Services, Inc. (Friedman, 1980b). The Hyatt team's first present from the Cook County Board of Commissioners was a 33% daily rate increase (*Hospital Week*, April 25, 1980). One wonders what wonders the old Governing Commission would have been able to achieve with the additional money.

With some kind of universal financial entitlement to health services for all Americans still a possibility (see Chapter 15), the question of what to do with local government hospitals becomes pressing (Haughton). Should they be improved and strengthened? Should advantage be taken of universal coverage to put them on a sound financial basis, since it should be possible for them to exist almost entirely on third-party reimbursement for services rendered? Should they be upgraded so that they could attract private patients, as some already are? Or should it be assumed that the Poor-Law heritage and the pauper stigma, civil service rules, detrimental local political influence and ever-increasing financial problems have injured them beyond repair? The public receives little benefit from having poor-quality hospitals. Maintaining local government hospitals in an era of universal financial entitlement might well perpetuate the two-class system. Moreover, voluntary hospitals that were significantly accountable to public authorities might actually be more attuned to the communities than public hospitals have been in the past. Nevertheless, for the time being it is apparent that many people, for whom the local public general hospital is the sole source of care, will suffer if it is closed.

Medical Staff

The physician is traditionally described as a guest in the hospital and as its primary customer. Except when a physician chooses to run a hospital for profit, he has no personal responsibility to see that the hospital is available to provide care for his patients. The physician uses the hospital as his workshop, as noted above. In exchange for this privilege, he is obligated to participate in governance of the medical staff and hospital. Further, he is obligated to participate in care given in areas of the hospital for which the medical staff accepts collective responsibility, such as the emergency room or outpatient clinic (Letourneau, 1964, pp. 20–26). In fact, the demands of private practice on physicians have made it difficult for them to honor these obligations. Many emergency rooms and ambulatory care departments are now staffed with full-time paid physicians (see Chapter 6).

When a physician admits a patient to the hospital, in many instances he is free to order whatever tests or treatments he deems necessary. Thus, he basically determines the amount of services used and consequent costs of the individual patient's care. He also influences the growth and expansion of the institution. Physicians have every reason to want the best possible institutional setting in which to practice medicine, especially when it is provided at no personal cost to them.

Although the doctor is technically a guest in the hospital, the hospital is responsible for the care its staff renders his patients on the physician's orders. Until relatively recently, hospitals could not be held liable for the wrongful conduct of a physician, but this principle has been significantly changed by a series of judicial decisions (Health Law Center, pp. 31–34). Changing legal doctrines of negligence and corporate liability of hospitals have established that hospitals are legally responsible and, to the extent that they cause a tort (a civil wrong involving negligence) to a patient, financially responsible for the care provided by their entire professional staff, including physicians (Johnson; Somers, pp. 32–36). There is a wide variety of medical staff patterns of organization, which have been analyzed in great detail by Roemer and Friedman (1971).

The medical staff by-laws specify procedures for election of medical staff officers by the membership. The officers are given authority under the by-laws to enforce rules and regulations. The officers delineate privileges and recommend disciplinary action when necessary through the committee structure. They enforce the by-laws and must oversee the committee structure and submit reports of medical staff activities to the board of trustees.

There are numerous medical staff committees. The executive committee coordinates all activity, sets general policies for the medical staff, and accepts and acts upon recommendations from the other medical staff committees. The joint conference committee acts as liaison between the medical staff and the governing board in deliberations over matters involving both medical and nonmedical considerations. The credentials committee reviews applications by physicians to join the medical staff and considers the qualifications of education, experience, and interests before making recommendations to the executive committee, which will then make recommendations for appointment to the board of trustees. In some hospitals the conference committee is also involved in this process.

The infections control committee is responsible for preventing infections in the hospital through routine preventive surveillance, tracking down of outbreaks of infection, and education of hospital personnel. The pharmacy and therapeutics committee reviews pharmacologic agents for inclusion in the list of drugs approved for use in the hospital. The tissue committee is responsible for insuring quality control of surgery, principally by examining and evaluating bodily tissues removed during operations.

The medical records committee is responsible for certifying complete and clinically accurate documentation of the care given to patients. The committee also acts as a judge of clinical care based on the written record.

The utilization review committee evaluates the appropriateness of admissions and length of stay in the hospital and may review use of services and facilities for patients whose hospital care is being paid for by Medicare. Utilization review never worked very well, for reasons that are not entirely clear. In the mid-1970s, it was allied with the Professional Standards Review Organization (PSRO) system (see Chapter 14).

The tissue, medical audit, and utilization review committees and the PSRO provide for review of physician's professional work by other physicians. (See Chapter 14 for a description of the 1980 Joint Commission on Accreditation of Hospitals [JCAH] requirements for quality assurance and utilization review.) As the hospital has become more complicated and more critical of medical practice, the medical staff has been subjected to more scrutiny. In the hospital, the medical chain of authority exists side by side with an administrative chain. There are many areas of confused jurisdiction and overlapping or conflicting powers. Hospital-physician cooperative efforts attempt to integrate these hierarchies. Thus physicians have become more involved in hospital governing boards; boards of trustees review the methods used to appoint physicians to hospital staffs; and more full-time salaried physicians have been hired, resulting in direct physician-hospital reporting lines (Jacobs; Wilson). There has developed an erosion of the traditional power of the physician as increasing regulation has made the medical staff more accountable to the board and administration (Petersen et al.). One result has been the evolution of the medical staff from one of collegiality to one of collective accountability and liability (Johnson).

Because of the vested interests of various medical departments in a hospital, and latent or open conflict with trustees or administration, the method of selecting a full-time or part-time chief of the medical staff or of medical departments is potentially explosive. To avoid controversy, in some hospitals appointments are made for a specified period of time rather than for indefinite or lifetime periods of tenure. As full-time chiefs of service become more common, many functions now handled by volunteer committees—such as quality-of-care review, medical records, and continuing medical education—may gradually be taken over by full-time paid employees (McGill; K. Williams).

Many hospitals are now hiring salaried medical care directors and quality-of-care review teams. As hospitals are made more accountable for alleged misconduct of attending physicians, much attention has been focused on the concept of due process. If a physician is to be deprived of his medical staff privileges, the process by which the decision was made must be capable of standing the scrutiny of the courts (Southwick). Further, hospitals may now require physicians to have malpractice insurance as a condition of staff membership (Hollowell).

As more salaried physicians are being hired by hospitals, private physicians are beginning to fear their impact. The American Medical Association reports that the number of hospital salaried physicians other than house staff increased from 10,000 in 1963 to 38,000 in 1977, almost quadruple. Salaried physicians are employed in the hospital to supervise medical care in intensive care units, outpatient departments, and medical education. Nonsalaried physicians could fear competition for patients, the possibility of a closed medical staff, additional supervision of their medical care, a change in traditional patient care orientation to more emphasis on teaching and research, and reduced availability of beds (*Medical World News*, October, 1974).

The Economics of Hospital Operations

The hospital is the largest user of the health care dollar (see Chapter 10). The rate of increase of hospital costs is a serious problem (Congressional Budget Office, Chapter I; Council on Wage and Price Stability; see also Chapter 10 for a discussion of rising health care costs). The flow of resources into the hospital industry is subject to several constraints and is likely to be altered considerably in the future under any national health insurance program, and by increased regulation. Currently, funds come from commercial and government insurance, philanthropy, private payment from a small number of patients, and various other sources of grant and contract funding for demonstrations and experiments.

Hospital costs are defined as the expenses that hospitals incur in the treatment of patients. They are usually expressed in terms of U.S. average cost per patient-day. Unfortunately, patient-days are not a unit of output, only a time frame in which hospital services are provided. When hospital expenses are expressed in terms of a patient-day, the result is average cost per day. Comparing the cost per patient-day in 1967 ($53.14) and in 1972 ($96.70), we find an apparent increase of 82.1%. By 1978, this figure had increased to $194.34. However, real hospital costs rose by about only one-half of that figure. The rest was due to inflation. The real increase results from the fact that a patient-day in 1972 and in 1978 involved more tests, more personnel, more education, and more diagnostic and therapeutic services than in 1967 (Abernethy and Pearson, Section I; Raske, 1974).

The USDHEW, after analyzing the rise in hospital unit costs over the 20-year period from 1952 to 1972, concluded that approximately half of the average annual increase in hospital unit cost was attributable to hospitals increasing the number and the quality of their labor and nonlabor inputs (Raske, 1974). In a slightly more recent study of the period 1950–1973, Worthington (1975) similarly concluded that the most important factor in rising hospital costs is technological change, as reflected in increased real inputs. Inflation is only one problematic aspect of advances in technology. Others are adoption of technology without knowledge of risks, inappropriate use of technology, lack of a method to equitably allocate resources among patients due to the high costs of technology, and the lack of a sound technology-acquisition decision model (Arnstein; Office of Technology Assessment). By the end of the decade, with double-digit inflation, the AHA was claiming that inflation, rather than changes in the hospitals' product, had become the major cause of hospital cost increases (*Hospital Week*, April 25, 1980). It is likely that the absolute contribution of technological change to hospital cost increases has not changed; it is smaller relative to general inflation because the latter rate has increased so much.

Hospitals experience financial difficulties as a result of one or a combination of the following: (1) a decrease in volume of services sold; (2) an inability to increase charges because of constraints imposed by third-party payors; (3) poor financial planning; (4) bad management planning and control; (5) lack of coordination and cooperation between medical and administrative staffs; (6) the notion that quality is a function of cost; (7) too tight control by the board of directors, who lack adequate training or experience over the operation of the institution (Berman and Weeks; Sattler and Bennett, p. 59).

If there are too many beds in a community, it is obviously impossible to have high occupancy and controlled use of hospital resources. Strategies to maximize revenues, payrolls, or prestige run counter to a general movement toward cost containment. More careful cost budgeting, consistent occupancy goals, better reporting of exceptional expenditures, and cost-benefit justification are all necessary for adequate financial control (Griffith et al.).

Voluntary hospitals have traditionally acknowledged that part of their responsibility is to provide care to the medically indigent. Funds for this purpose were generated by pricing certain hospital services higher than the cost of providing them, to those who could afford to pay, so that a number of medically indigent patients could receive those services for free. Traditionally, laboratory and radiology services have been used to generate this excess revenue. Now, with 88% of patients having their hospital bills paid by a third party, which is not willing to pay more than the actual costs of services received, this source of revenue is rapidly disappearing. Although Medicare and Medicaid programs have reduced to some extent the number of persons seeking free care, in many states large numbers of the poor still have no source of payment. Medicaid eligibility levels are changed periodically by state governments, and the future of the program is problematic (see Chapters 10 and 15). Thus the sources of funds used by hospitals to care for the poor are not constant. Few hospitals have endowments sufficient to finance this care; few can generate excess revenue and, for those which can, there are many other competing uses for it. However, the discretionary aspect of free care has been removed from the hospitals' control. As noted above, in 1978, a federal regulation was promulgated that required hospitals that had received Hill-Burton construction funds to provide a reasonable volume of services to persons who are unable to pay (Raske, 1980). As of 1980, legal challenges to the regulation were still being adjudicated. Ironically, the infusion of federal funds under the Medicare and Medicaid programs, which were once stimuli to inflation in health care costs by providing guaranteed payments for medically indigent patients, are now causing downward cost pressure on hospitals as the government reduces the scope of its programs.

Another regulation, promulgated in 1979, challenges the basis of average costs upon which third-party reimbursement is universally based. Based upon a review of malpractice experience of hospitals, the Health Care Financing Administration concluded that Medicare beneficiaries have fewer and less serious malpractice claims than other hospital patients. HCFA proposes to pay for malpractice insurance only 5% of the average hospital per diem cost. This is a reversal from previous Medicare policy whereby reimbursement to hospitals was based on overall average costs rather than specific costs allocated to each patient. For hospitals with contracts with private insurance companies, which will pay only average costs, malpractice costs would be lowered for patients having such coverage as well since their costs would no longer be overall average costs. This would mean that the entire balance of the burden of malpractice insurance costs would fall upon the relatively small portion of patients who are self-paying or who have private insurance that pays on an other-than-average cost basis. The legality of the 1979 regulation was also undergoing court challenge in 1980.

Lowering Hospital Costs

In hospitals, there are many incentives to reduce costs. Ironically, many efforts to reduce the cost of medical care to the community increase the cost of providing medical care in the hospital, as we have pointed out earlier. Providing care on an ambulatory basis, when possible, to avoid hospitalization, or making efforts to shorten the length of stay for hospitalized patients, may increase the cost of a day of hospital care, for several reasons. Patients who do occupy hospital beds may be sicker and require more services per day. A reduction in occupancy means less expenditure by the third-party payors, which reimburse hospitals on an item-of-service basis, but it also means less revenue for the hospitals, which still have their relatively high fixed expenses. Shortening length of stay also lowers third-party expenditures, but it increases cost per patient-day because more technical services have to be provided each day, on the average. As pointed out above, the only long-term way to lower costs is to reduce the capital investment and operating expenses by not building additional beds or adding new equipment and by closing existing beds. Reimbursing hospitals for providing days of hospital care rewards them for admitting patients, not for providing a spectrum of health services that might, or might not, include hospitalization for any particular patient.

This is a complex social problem that could be partially solved by altering the financial structure used to pay for care. Decisions made would have to take into account the effect of the procedure on the patient, the cost, the patient's ability to pay, and the recommendation of his physicians. The appropriate use of high-cost technology is a central issue in providing hospital services. The number of hospitals offering special, expensive services has increased over the past two decades. Facilities for open-heart surgery, radioisotope diagnosis and therapy, cobalt therapy, renal dialysis, electronic fetal monitoring, and computerized axial tomography have proliferated (Office of Technology Assessment). Regional planning for the distribution of specialized, expensive hospital services has been a subject of much talk, but little action.

The Health Planning and Resources Development Act of 1974 (see Chapter 13), which could restrict payment by federal third-party payors for services rendered in nonapproved facilities and programs, to some degree in some areas has discouraged implementation of technological advances that have not been proven necessary or effective. It may encourage regional planning among hospitals for the distribution of new equipment, procedures, and services on a rational basis, rather than the present all-too-common competitive approach. PSRO admission certification and appropriateness review may have a similar effect.

However, in the past, such controls have been relatively ineffective. If a hospital could justify sufficient use of such equipment to make it pay for itself, or even generate a profit, it was possible to justify it to planning agencies on the basis of adequate demand. The extent to which this demand was manufactured by the novelty of the diagnostic effort was not considered. Another approach that may have some effect is the refusal of certain private third-party payors to reimburse hospitals for the performance of expensive specialized services like open-heart surgery, if their volume of service does not meet minimum levels. This should encourage the closing of marginal, underutilized services with high fixed costs.

In some cases new technology does not lead to increased costs. The hospital laboratory and the accounting and materials management functions can reduce the numbers of people required to carry out work, because the materials with which the new equipment comes in contact are not living patients, but specimens or information. However, while there has been extensive automation in laboratories since 1965, the absolute number of personnel has not declined: costs per test are dropping, but the total number of tests performed is increasing. Thus, the cost benefits of few productivity increases are being passed on to consumers, while the health benefits of many of them remain to be evaluated.

"Cost-containment" and the "voluntary effort." "Cost-containment" for hospitals was a by-word of the Carter Administration. The Administration's approach, introduced as H. R. 2626 in 1979, was to put an artificial "cap" on allowable hospital revenue and expenditure increases by setting a fixed permitted percentage for them (Congressional Budget Office, pp. 23–29). The hospital industry did not like this idea at all. It offered a two-prong response. One prong was the "voluntary effort" (VE); the other was a large, intense, and well-orchestrated lobbying effort in Congress led by the AHA, joined by the AMA, the AAMC and the Federation of American Hospitals (the investor-owned hospitals' organization), to defeat the Administration's proposal. The latter was effective (Washington Report). After a lengthy and sometimes stormy debate, the House of Representatives rejected the bill.

The "voluntary effort" began in 1978 (American Hospital Association, 1978). It was based primarily on exhortation to the hospitals and their medical staffs to hold down expenditure increases to a target percentage. The goal percentage was set between the Administration's goal and an estimate of what expenditure increases would have been without the VE. Both by the AHA's own estimation (*Hospital Week*, March 23, 1979; "Hospital Indicators," February 16, 1980; American Hospital Association, 1980b) and by that of the Congressional Budget Office (pp. 13–16), the program was a success. The Carter Administration remained unconvinced (*Hospital Week*, January 25, 1980). It remained to be seen if the Congressional Budget Office's suspicion would be borne out: that the key to the success of the VE was the real threat of federal legislation and that removal of the threat would sap the strength of the VE. In 1980, the AHA was doing its best to make sure that that would not be the case (American Hospital Association, 1980b).

There are other approaches to cost-containment for hospitals. State rate review ("Rate Regulation") has met with some success in some states according to some observers (Fielding and Weiner; McDaniel) but not others (American Hospital Association, 1979d). In 1980, New Jersey began an experiment to reimburse some hospitals with a lump sum per case, the amount to be determined by the patient's admitting diagnosis (Simler). This is the so-called diagnostically related groupings (DRG) approach, designed to replace the customary daily rate cost-plus reimbursement mechanism. Also in 1980, Blue Cross/Blue Shield announced an experimental plan to reimburse selected hospitals by a capitation method (*Hospital Week*, May 2, 1980). After two years of planning, the experiment was to run for three years from 1982.

Any approach to cost-containment, however, will have to deal with what David Kinzer, President of the Massachusetts Hospital Association, calls the ten "exposed nerves" of the hospital system (p. 92). We have identified some of these "exposed nerves" elsewhere in this chapter and others, but it is useful to list them together here:

1. The system rewards those who do more.
2. Spending more money is the only way to get more money.
3. Hospitals compete for customers who don't care about the price.
4. Services will be used up to the limits of their availability.
5. Open access to medical services is a basic "right."
6. Hospitals now have the capacity to spend more money on health services than society can afford.
7. Hospitals have no effective control of their main salesmen and users, the physicians.
8. The more government depends on health care, the more it will control those who get the money.

9. Hospitals have not been able to relate inputs or outcomes to price.
10. Hospitals assume that nothing the government can do to them will make them better off than they now are, so they must assume that any government action will only make things worse.

Capital costs.   Capital expenditures are limited by the reimbursement formulas of Blue Cross, Medicare, and Medicaid. Capital projects must, therefore, be funded by such external sources as private and government grants and long-term commercial borrowing. Of the total expenditure for hospital construction in 1973, $820 million came from government grants, philanthropy, and internal operations, while $1.25 billion came from borrowing, a ratio of 2 to 3 (Sattler and Bennett, p. 51). In 1969, debt financing constituted one-fifth of the total funds for construction; by 1978, almost two-thirds came from that source (Mullner et al.). All other sources of revenue, government, philanthropy, and hospital reserves, had declined in relative importance. All community hospitals show a similar pattern except state and local government hospitals, which required less than 40% debt financing.

The price of capital for hospitals seemingly has been increasing faster than prices of capital for other industries. Yet payment of depreciation and interest costs by third parties may enable a hospital to cover the cost of expansion whether it is justified or not. Therefore, it is essential that planning agencies continue to attempt to exercise controls, including approval of capital expenditures. Although in the past, being subject to political pressure from health care providers, they have not been able to fulfill this responsibility (Lave and Lave, p. 63), Health Systems Agencies are becoming increasingly effective in requiring rationality in hospitals' capital expenditures (see Chapter 13). Nevertheless, Medicare and Medicaid did facilitate access to capital markets for hospitals by replacing revenue from private patients with a more reliable revenue source (Lightle). According to an official in the New York State Health Department, real control over capital formation in the hospital industry is the single most important step in cost control (Fleck).

In June 1980, in the wake of its defeat over mandatory hospital expenditure controls, the Carter Administration launched a campaign to sharply curtail hospital capital construction, through a variety of measures, as noted above (*Hospital Week,* June 13, 1980). It remained to be seen if this effort would be any more successful than the previous one. Some observers fear that if nothing is done to control hospital costs, in the future hospital services could become so expensive that they will be unavailable except in absolutely life-threatening situations.

Conclusion: Problems of Hospitals

If the first problem hospitals face is costliness, the second is the imbalance in the hospital sector between acute and long-term care. The major problem of the cost of hospital care is exacerbated by the inadequate supply of long-term care beds for patients who have recovered from the acute phase of their illness but are still plagued by the chronic diseases of old age. Although the patients should be placed in facilities that are less costly than hospitals, the supply of these beds is inadequate. Beyond that, there is a pressing need for appropriate housing with social and support services for the elderly who cannot live entirely on their own in ordinary housing, but nevertheless do not need institutionalization of any kind (Rogatz, 1980). Recent proposals to convert surplus hospital beds to long-term care beds have foundered on the necessity to fund depreciation of modern facilities at hospital construction cost rates.

The imbalance that does exist, however, by no means developed accidentally, as Freymann noted:

The mold from which today's health care system was cast took its shape around 1850. There were still relatively few general hospitals or health facilities of any type in Britain [our most important medical *organizational* forebear] and the fledgling United States, but the institutional organization of health care was already firmly established. Separate administration and staffing of the curative services—for acute, chronic, and psychiatric illnesses—became such a strong precedent that it continues even when all three components have a common source of support, as they do now in Britain. . . . As the four disparate fragments of our system for delivering care developed [acute, long-term, psychiatric, and preventive services], the voluntary hospital component was the only one whose primary institutional objective was *always* treatment of disease. Voluntary hospitals were able to cater to patients selected for certain illnesses, generally acute ones, because donors were entitled to prescribe the scope of their charity, and because a medical staff that contributed its time without remuneration could reasonably dictate the nature of its worth. Both the philanthropic trustees and the medical staffs agreed on leaving to the state the prevention of disease and the intractable problems of mental illness and chronic infirmity. . . .

The contrast between the history of voluntary hospitals and that of the other three fragments of the health care system is striking. A common thread runs through the chronicle of the last three—entanglement with overwhelming numbers of people and with complex social, economic, and political problems. . . . Voluntary hospitals have been able to limit their involvement for almost 200 years, while the other three components sequestered the problems which were destined to become the main health concerns of the late 20th century. (pp. 47–48)

The third major problem concerns the mode by which most physicians taking care of patients in hospitals are paid, and the influence that physicians have over hospital operations. The physician makes most of the decisions regarding the commitment and use of hospital resources. Yet, as noted above, because he is usually paid directly by the patient or his insurer, he has no direct financial relationship to the hospital, nor any responsibility for its financial status. It is as if modern school boards provided everything necessary for education except payment of the teachers, who would proceed to collect fees directly from the students, as indeed they did before the educational reforms of the mid-19th century.

Fourth, hospitals have problems with vertically organized administrative structures that are not well integrated horizontally at the service levels. In many hospitals the operating divisions to which we referred earlier fall roughly into three separate vertical organizational groupings: medical staff, nursing, and support/hotel services. Within each of these structures there can be further fragmentation; e.g., the different medical services, internal medicine, surgery, pediatrics, etc., may function quite separately from each other. The vertical lines of authority may meet in the office of the director; sometimes they never meet. This kind of separation can make it very difficult to provide integrated programs of patient care in which unitary direction is needed at the functional level in order to best meet patient needs. For example, in outpatient services, it is very difficult to provide comprehensive patient-centered care when there is no coordinated leadership at the functional level of service for the medical, nursing, social work, and clerical personnel who are all essential to providing that care (Jonas, 1973).

A fifth problem is the isolation of many hospitals from the real health and medical needs of their communities. This does not apply solely to short-term general hospitals. In health terms, Freymann describes the present era as the Age of Darwin and Freud, since "most of our woes now stem from two causes: either our genetic heritage or the buffeting of our environment or both" (p. 74). However, he says many health care institutions, not just short-term hospitals, are still armed primarily to fight the wars of the era immediately past, the Age of Pasteur, when "infection was the main foe of medicine" (p. 13). This orientation, of course, arises not only from institutional rigidity but also from the character of medical practice, which is still largely stuck in the Age of Pasteur as well.

In most hospitals, outpatient services have a distinctly second-class status, preventive medicine is practiced to a minimal extent, home care and rehabilitation services are treated as luxuries. Community-based chronic disease control programs are not undertaken. Mental hospitals have little to do with community mental health. Proprietary nursing homes have not the least interest in dealing with the complications of aging in a positive way, since they want patients *in*, not *out*. Hospitals and other health care institutions, with certain impressive and encouraging exceptions, to be sure, resolutely turn inwards, wishing that everyone would just go away and leave them to do their job as they see it: taking care of sick people in bed.

Solutions

Complex problems do not have simple solutions, and we do not pretend to offer panaceas. But in the context of a program of universal financial entitlement to health services, an approach to hospital reform is available. We turn once again to Freymann, who has developed the concept of the "mission-oriented hospital" (Chapter 18).

The mission-oriented hospital has two principal attributes: (1) Each hospital has a mission defined and continuously modified by the specific needs of the community it services; (2) individuality and flexibility are secured by ongoing use of a rational planning process (p. 248).

The concept is based on four "theorems":

1. The need for medical *cure* that dominated men's minds from the dawn of time to the end of the Age of Pasteur will wane, but the need for total health *care* will remain.
2. Health care must be a continuum because a healthy life is a continuum from conception to death—not a vacuum punctuated by episodes of illness.
3. Since the needs of each individual vary widely, an organization meeting these needs cannot be frozen into classification by organ, by diagnosis, or by medical specialty.
4. Since the mission of the health care system is to maintain health, the system should interfere as little as possible with the functional capacity of those it serves. Ambulatory or home care are ideals; confinement to an institution must be dictated only by biologic necessity. (pp. 247–248)

Freymann recognizes that "the word 'hospital' itself presents a problem, for today it connotes a building that houses patients. I think 'hospital' could be used in a different sense—to signify a dynamic complex of facilities and skilled personnel organized to provide all types of health services" (p. 247). He points out that:

> . . . while general hospitals were originally intended only for the acutely sick, history has dictated that they become the centers about which the American health care system revolves. To consider creating new centers for the care of the well and limiting 6,000 general hospitals to their 18th-century function is

to fly in the face of reality. But [to meet their new functions] they must be designed [physically and programmatically] not as enclaves but as open accessible places where the scattered fragments of the health care system can at least be brought together. (p. 212)

To accomplish this goal, we must end the "tyranny of the bed" (Freymann, pp. 197–223, 249). In this "tyranny," as we have seen in this chapter, the principal measures of what a hospital is, and does, are related to beds—that is, admissions, length of stay, occupancy, average daily census, and bed-days of care—rather than to any measures of illness or health.

The mission-oriented approach would in fact make the hospital into a health center rather than an illness center. The hospital would relate to the needs of its community in a rational, planned, dynamic manner. By definition, the acute-chronic-preventive distinctions would become things of the past. Cost problems would be dealt with directly because we already know from group practice experience that in reasonably comprehensive ambulatory care, even without special prevention programs, and where there is no special incentive for physicians to hospitalize patients, hospitalization rates are significantly lowered.

The present-day administrative problems would not be automatically resolved by a mission-oriented approach. Rather, they would have to be solved in order to accomplish mission orientation. It demands an administrative structure that is functionally decentralized to operate integrated programs requiring staff teams at the patient-care level, not one which has vertically organized reporting lines separating health care providers into independent hierarchies.

Some movement in this direction is already occurring. As we noted above, hospitals are becoming increasingly involved in health promotion and outreach programs. Sharing strategies are becoming more frequently adopted. The planning process of the Health Systems Agencies system (see Chapter 13) is becoming more of a way of life for more hospitals, whether they participate in it willingly or unwillingly. Conversions of acute-care beds to long-term care beds, either permanently or on a "swing-bed" basis, are becoming more common, despite the difficulties associated with the changes. Peter Rogatz (1980), a respected observer of the hospital scene, has predicted that the following changes will take place during the 1980s:

- The supply of hospital beds will decrease, the average hospital will increase in size, and hospitals increasingly will offer complex services;
- Regulation will become more, not less, a part of hospital life;

- Ambulatory surgery will become increasingly common;
- Home care services will expand;
- Long-term care facilities will increase and special housing for the elderly will become more commonplace;
- Hospitals will become increasingly interested in and attached to health maintenance organizations;
- The hospice movement (see Chapter 8) will expand.

Many of these changes are in the direction of creating the mission-oriented hospital. However, a major challenge in implementing mission-orientation lies in finding the personnel who can do it. To change hospitals to mission orientation will require "mission-oriented" physicians and other staff who can understand health and illness in populations as well as in individuals, and can see patients in their socioeconomic context. But the bulk of health sciences training takes place in our present-day, inward-directed hospitals. How to break out of this vicious circle requires a separate discussion (Jonas, 1979b). Solutions and resources are available to do so. We will need to summon the will and deal with many very complex political realities.

References

Abernethy, D. S., and Pearson, D. A. *Regulating Hospital Costs*. Ann Arbor, Michigan: AUPHA Press, 1979.

Adamson, G. J., et al. "Hospital's Role Expanded with Wellness Effort." *Hospitals, J.A.H.A.*, October 1, 1979, p. 121.

American College of Surgeons and American Surgical Association. *Surgery in the United States*. (No city), 1975.

American Hospital Association. *Hospital Statistics, 1975*. Chicago, 1975a.

————."Are There Too Many Hospital Beds?" *Hospitals, J.A.H.A.*, April 1, 1975b, p. 17.

————*Annual Report*. May 1975c.

————*A Critique of the Public Citizen Health Research Group Report $8 Billion Hospital Bed Overrun*. Chicago: Bureau of Research Services, July 1975d.

————"Health Philanthropy Registers a 2.6 Percent Gain in 1974." *Hospitals, J.A.H.A.*, March 16, 1976, p. 29.

————Voluntary Effort: A New Spirit of Cooperation." *Hospitals, J.A.H.A.*, July 1, 1978, p. 55.

————*Trustee Development Program*. Chicago, 1979a.

————*Hospital Statistics, 1979*. Chicago, 1979b.

————*Guide to the Health Care Field, 1979*. Chicago, 1979c.

————"Hospitals Headlines. New York State Blamed for 80 Percent of Hospitals Incurring Losses During 1977." *Hospitals, J.A.H.A.*, February 16, 1979d, p. 17.

──────"Cost Watch: Many Little Efforts Bring Large Success to Voluntary Effort." *Hospitals, J.A.H.A.*, June 1, 1980a, p. 49.

──────"Hospitals Headlines. Voluntary Effort Seeks Cut in 1980 Inpatient Expenses." *Hospitals, J.A.H.A.*, January 16, 1980b, p. 17.

American Medical News. "Unnecessary Surgery." February 9, 1976.

Andersen, R., et al. *Equity in Health Services: Empirical Analyses in Social Policy.* Cambridge, Massachusetts: Ballinger, 1975.

Annas, G. J. "The Extravagant, Wasteful, and Superfluous Debate About Unnecessary Surgery." *Hastings Center Report*, April 1979, p. 13.

Applebaum, A. L. "Commission Report Addresses Future of Public General Hospitals." *Hospitals, J.A.H.A.*, May 16, 1978, p. 95.

Arnstein, S. R. "The Uses and Abuses of Assessing Health Technology." Presented to the American Public Health Association Annual Meeting, Los Angeles, California, October 1978.

Austin, C. J. "Emerging Roles and Responsibilities in Health Administration." In *Education for Health Administration*, Vol. 1, pp. 137–151. Ann Arbor, Michigan: Health Administration Press, 1975.

Behrens, R. "AHA Center for Health Promotion." *Physician's Patient Education Newsletter*, Vol. 3, No. 3, June, 1980, p. 8.

Berman, H. J., and Weeks, L. E. *The Financial Management of Hospitals.* Ann Arbor: Hospital Administration Press, 1979.

Blackstone, E. A. "The Condition of Surgery." *Health and Society*, 55, 429, 1977. See also p. 485.

Blake, E., and Bodenheimer, T. *Closing the Doors on the Poor: The Dismantling of California's County Hospitals.* San Francisco: Health/PAC, 1975.

Blue Cross/Blue Shield of Greater New York. "Just How Much Hospital Does This City Need?" *New York Times*, August 24, 1976.

Bognanno, M. F., and Champlin, F. "Collective Bargaining in the Health Care Industry" in Misek, G. I., Ed., *Socioeconomic Issues of Health: 1979*, Chicago: American Medical Association, 1979.

Brown, M., and Money, W. "The Promise of Multihospital Management." *Hospital Progress*, August/September 1975, p. 36.

Bunker, J. P. "Surgical Manpower." *New England Journal of Medicine*, 282, 135, 1970.

Bunker, J. P., et al., Eds., *Costs, Risks, and Benefits of Surgery.* New York: Oxford University Press, 1977. The combined bibliography is comprehensive.

Bureau of the Census. *Statistical Abstract of the United States, 1979.* Washington, D.C.: U.S. Dept. of Commerce, USGPO, 1979.

Carpenter, D.C. "Hospitals Should Be Fitness Centers." *Hospitals.* February 16, 1980, p. 148.

Colton, T. "Quality of Care and Unnecessary Operations." *Health and Society*, 55, 461, 1967.

Commission on Professional and Hospital Activities. *Length of Stay in PAS Hospitals U.S., 1977.* Ann Arbor, Michigan, 1978.

Commission on Public-General Hospitals. *The Future of the Public-General Hospital.* Chicago: Hospital Research and Educational Trust, 1978.

Comptroller General of the United States. *Study of Health Facilities Construction Costs*. Washington, D.C.: USPGO, 1972.

Congressional Budget Office. *Controlling Rising Hospital Costs*. Washington, D.C.: USGPO, 1979.

Connors, E. J. "Multihospital Systems Are Changing the Health Care Landscape." *Trustee*, July 1979, p. 24.

Consumer Health Perspectives. "Conferences on Medical Technology." Vol. V, Nos. 5 and 6, 1978; Vol. V, No. 8, 1979; Vol. VI, No. 1, 1979.

Council on Wage and Price Stability. *The Rapid Rise of Hospital Costs*. Washington, D.C.: USGPO, 1977.

Cunningham, R. M. "Philanthropy Thrives Despite Adversity. *Hospitals*, *J.A.H.A.*, June 16, 1978, p. 143.

————. "Whither Hospitals and Associations?" *Hospitals*, *J.A.H.A.*, January 1, 1980a, p. 81.

————. "The Way We Were—and Are." *Hospitals*, *J.A.H.A.*, February 1, 1980b, p. 54.

Davis, S., and Henshaw, S. *Decision Analysis in Hospital Administration*. Washington, D.C.: Association of University Programs in Health Administration, 1974.

de Schweinitz, K. *England's Road to Social Security*. New York: 1943. Reprinted, A. S. Barnes and Co. Perpetual Edition, 1961.

Dornblaser, B. M. "The Social Responsibility of General Hospitals." *Hospital Administration*, Spring 1970, p. 6.

Enright, M., and Jonas, S. "Hospitals." In Jonas, S., Ed., *Health Care Delivery in the United States*, Chapter 7. New York: Springer, 1977.

Ensminger, B. *The $8 Billion Hospital Bed Overrun*. Washington, D.C.: Public Citizen's Health Research Group, 1975.

Federal Register. "Health Planning: National Guidelines." March 28, 1978, Part IV.

Fielding, J. E., and Weiner, S. "Controlling Hospital Costs in Massachusetts." *New England Journal of Medicine*, 299, 1249, 1978.

Fleck, A. Personal communication. March 7, 1975.

Freymann, J. G. *The American Health Care System: Its Genesis and Trajectory*. New York: Medcom Press, 1974.

Friedman, E. "Public Hospitals: Is 'Relevance' in the Eye of the Beholder?" *Hospitals*, May 1, 1980a, p. 83.

————. "Hyatt Management Team." *Hospitals*, June 1, 1980b, p. 21.

Gaus, C. R., et al. "Contrasts in HMO and Fee-for-Service Performance." *Social Security Bulletin*, May 1976, p. 3.

Georgeopoulos, B. *The Community General Hospital*. New York: Macmillan, 1962.

Georgeopoulos, B., Ed. *Organization Research on Health Institutions*. Ann Arbor: Michigan: University of Michigan Press, 1971.

Gertman, P. M., et al. "Second Opinions for Elective Surgery." *New England Journal of Medicine*, 302, 1169, 1980.

"Getting Ready for National Health Insurance: Unnecessary Surgery." Hearings before the Subcommittee on Oversight and Investigations of the Committee on Interstate and Foreign Commerce, House of Representatives. Washington, D.C.: July 15, 17, 18 and September 3, 1975.

Ginzberg, E. *A Pattern for Hospital Care*. New York: Columbia University Press, 1949.

Gittelsohn, A. M., and Wennberg, J. E. "On the Incidence of Tonsillectomy and Other Common Surgical Procedures." In Bunker, J. P., et al., Eds., *Costs, Risks, and Benefits of Surgery*. Chapter 7. New York: Oxford University Press, 1977.

Goran, M. J. "The Evolution of the PSRO Hospital Review System." *Medical Care*, 17, No. 5, Supp., May 1979.

Gornick, M. "Medicare Patients: Geographic Differences in Hospital Discharge Rates and Multiple Stays." *Social Security Bulletin*, June 1977, p. 22.

Green. L. W. "How to Evaluate Health Promotion." *Hospitals, J.A.H.A.*, October 1, 1979, p. 106.

Griffith, J., et al. "Practical Ways to Contain Hospital Costs." *Hospital Financial Management*, January 1975, p. 46.

Haughton, J. C. "Role of the Public General Hospital in Community Health." *American Journal of Public Health*, 65, 21, 1975.

Health Law Center. *Problems in Hospital Law*. Rockville, Maryland: Aspen Systems Corporation, 1974.

Health Perspectives. "Profile of Governing Bodies of New York City Voluntary Hospitals." November 1973–January 1974

Health Research Group–Public Citizen. *Consumer Health Action Network*. January 1976, p. 7.

Hepner, J. O., Ed. *Health Planning for Emerging Multihospital Systems*. St. Louis, Missouri: The C. V. Mosby Co., 1978.

Hollowell, E., J. D. "No Insurance—No Privileges." *Legal Aspects of Medical Practice*, April 1978.

"Hospital Indicators." *Hospitals, J.A.H.A.*, April 16, 1976, p. 45.

——————. *Hospitals, J.A.H.A.*, March 16, 1979, p. 67.

——————. *Hospitals, J.A.H.A.*, October 16, 1979, p. 56.

——————. *Hospitals*, February 16, 1980, p. 66.

——————. *Hospitals, J.A.H.A.*, May 1, 1980, p. 57.

Hospital Week. "$1.48 Billion Saved in First Year, VE Report Shows." March 23, 1979.

——————. "Carter Repeats Need for Hospital Cost Cap Bill." January 25, 1980.

——————. "Hyatt to Run Cook County Hospital." April 25, 1980.

——————. "Blue Cross to Test Fixed Payments to Hospitals." May 2, 1980.

——————. "Carter Proposes Capital Financing Cut for Hospitals." June 13, 1980.

Hughes, E. F. Y., et al. "Surgical Workloads in a Community Practice." *Surgery*, 71, 315, 1972.

——————. "The Study on Surgical Services in the United States." *Health and Society*, 55, 465, 1977.

Institute of Medicine. *Controlling the Supply of Hospital Beds*. Washington, D.C.: National Academy of Sciences, 1976.

Jacobs, M. "Administrators, Boards, and Physicians Must Help Change Health System." *Hospitals, J.A.H.A.*, August 1, 1978.

Johnson, E. "Medical Staff Liability for Individual Acts of Physicians." *Health Care Management Review*. Fall 1978.

Jonas, S. "Some Thoughts on Primary Care: Problems in Implementation." *International Journal of Health Services*, 3, 177, 1973.

──────. *Medical Mystery: The Training of Doctors in the United States*. New York: W. W. Norton, 1979a.

──────. "Hospitals Adopt New Role." *Hospitals, J.A.H.A.*, October 1, 1979b, p. 84.

Kaufman, K., et al. "The Effects of Board Composition and Structure on Hospital Performance." *Hospital and Health Services Administration*, Winter 1979.

Kessler, R. "A Profile of the Hospital Trustee." *Trustee*, January 1975, p. 21.

Kinzer, D. M. "Cost Reductions Remain Goal of Federal Regs." *Hospitals*, January 1, 1980, p. 91.

Klarman, H. E. *The Economics of Health*. New York: Columbia University Press, 1965.

Knowles, J. "The Hospital." In Williams, S. J., Ed. *Issues in Health Services*. New York: Wiley, 1980, Chapter 8.

Lane, D. S. "Patient Education in the Community Hospital." *The Journal of Biocommunications*, 5, 6, 1978.

Lane, D. S., and Evans, D. "Study Measures Impact of Emergency Department Ombudsman." *Hospitals, J.A.H.A.*, February 1, 1978, p. 99.

Lave, R., and Lave, L. *The Hospital Construction Act*. Washington, D.C.: American Enterprise Institute for Public Policy Research, 1974.

Letourneau, C. U. "A History of Hospitals." *Journal of the International College of Surgeons*, 35, 527, 1961.

──────. *The Hospital Medical Staff*. Chicago: Starling Publications, 1964.

Lewis, C. E. "Variations in the Incidence of Surgery." *New England Journal of Medicine*, 281, 880, 1969.

Lightle, M. A. "'70s See New Approaches to Capital Financing for Hospitals." *Hospitals, J.A.H.A.*, June 16, 1978, p. 135.

Longe, M. "What's Going on in the Community?" *Hospitals, J.A.H.A.*, September 16, 1979, p. 171.

Luft, H. S. "How Do Health-Maintenance Organizations Achieve Their 'Savings'?" *New England Journal of Medicine*, 298, 1336, 1978.

McCarthy, E. G., and Widmer, G. W. "Effects of Screening by Consultants on Recommended Elective Surgical Procedures." *New England Journal of Medicine*, 291, 1331, 1974.

MacEachern, M. T. *Hospital Organization and Management*. Berwyn, Illinois: Physician's Record Co., 1962.

McDaniel, J. P. "We Have Seen Rate Review and It Works." *Hospitals, J.A.H.A.*, April 16, 1978, p. 71.

McGill, C. S. "A Look into the Hospital of the Future." *Trustee*, December 1974, p. 14.

Malloy, J. "Public Hospitals Must Survive." *The New York Times*, August 5, 1979.

Medical World News. "Full-Time Physicians in Hospitals." October 4, 1974, p. 41.
――――. "'More Beds than We Need,' AHA Admits." November 8, 1974, p. 114.
――――. "How Much Unnecessary Surgery?" May 3, 1976, p. 50.
Metzger, N. "Hospital Labor Scene Marked by Union Issues." *Hospitals*, April 1, 1980, p. 105.
Moore, F. D. "Board Requirements for Economists Who Write on Medical Subjects?" *Health and Society*, 55, 455, 1977.
Mott, A., and Chalk, A. "The Board Structure Has to Change." *Trustee*, January 1975, p. 28.
Mullner, R., et al. "Hospital Trends in Construction Financing, Costs." *Hospitals*, June 1, 1980, p. 59.
Munroe, S. A., and Schuman, J. "Small/Rural Hospitals Must Innovate in 80's." *Hospitals*, January 1, 1980, p. 99.
National Center for Health Statistics. *Health, United States, 1978*. USDHEW Pub. No. (PHS) 78–1232, USGPO, 1978.
――――. *Health Resources Statistics: 1976–77 Edition*, Washington, D. C.: DHEW Pub. No. (PHS) 79–1509, USGPO, 1979a.
――――. "Utilization of Short-Stay Hospitals." *Vital and Health Statistics*, Series 13, No. 41, March 1979b.
Newsday. "Poll Shows LI Hospital Conflicts." February 27, 1976.
――――. "60 Doing Business as Hospital Trustees." March 15, 1976.
New York Times. "Hospitals Lay on Conflict of Interest Data." December 26, 1975.
――――. "Incompetent Surgery Is Not Found Isolated." January 27, 1976.
――――. "Hospitals Resist a Trustee Conflict-of-Interest Bill." April 18, 1976.
――――. "Care at Lincoln Hospital Scored." July 30, 1976.
――――. "New York Municipal Hospitals Found 'Plagued' by Nurse Shortage." May 21, 1978.
――――. "Lincoln Hospital's Chaos Traced to 'Battle' Conditions in Bronx." November 26, 1978.
――――. "A Symposium on Hospitals: 'That Patient Is Dying.'" December 24, 1978.
――――. "A Hospital on the Edge: Metropolitan and the Business of Survival." September 19, 1975.
――――. "A Grim Midnight Tour at a City Hospital." December 18, 1979.
――――. "2 City Hospitals in Harlem Saved by a 3-Way Pact." June 20, 1980.
Office of Health Research, Statistics, and Technology. *Health, United States, 1978*. Hyattsville, Maryland: USDHEW Pub. No. (PHS) 80–1232, USGPO, 1980.
Office of Technology Assessment. *Assessing the Efficacy and Safety of Medical Technologies*. Washington, D.C.: USGPO, 1978.
Parker, S. S., and Wardell, K. S. "Multihospital Systems Form a Cooperative for Sharing Services." *Hospitals*, June 16, 1980, p. 79.
Pauly, M. V. "What Is Unnecessary Surgery?" *Health and Society*, 57, 95, 1979.
Petersen, L. P., et al. "Medical Staff: Physicians Seek New Responses to Mounting Pressures." *Hospitals, J.A.H.A.*, April 1, 1979.
Phelps, Charles E. "Effects of Insurance on Demand for Medical Care." In

Anderson, R., Kravits, J., and Anderson, O., Eds., *Equity in Health Services*. Cambridge, Massachusetts: Ballinger Publishing Co., 1975.

Phillips, D. F. "American Hospitals: A Look Ahead." *Hospitals, J.A.H.A.*, January 1, 1976, p. 73.

————. "Utilization Review in the United States: Results of the 1976–77 National Survey." *Medical Care Supplement*, August 1979.

Raske, K. E. "The Components of Inflation." *Hospitals, J.A.H.A.*, July 1, 1974, p. 34.

————. "Of Rates, Reimbursement, and Regulation." *Hospitals*, April 1, 1980, p. 69.

"Rate Regulation." *Topics in Health Care Financing*, 6, Fall 1979.

Reidel, D. C., et al. *Federal Employees Health Benefits Program Utilization Study*. USDHEW Pub. No. (HRA) 75–3125. Washington, D.C.: USPGO, 1975.

Roemer, M. "Bed Supply and Hospital Utilization: A Natural Experiment." *Hospitals, J.A.H.A.*, November 1961.

————. "Health/Disease Trends to Shape Hospital Role." *Hospitals, J.A.H.A.*, January 1, 1980.

Roemer, M. I., and Friedman, J. W. *Doctors in Hospitals*. Baltimore, Maryland: The Johns Hopkins Press, 1971.

————. "Medical Staff Organization." In Kovner, A., and Neuhauser, D., Eds., *Health Services Management*. Ann Arbor, Michigan: Hospital Administration Press, 1979.

Roemer, M., and Shonick, R. "HMO Performance: The Recent Evidence." *Health and Society*, 51, 271, 1973.

Rogatz, P. M. "Excessive Hospitalization Can Be Cut Back." *Journal of the American Hospital Association*, August 1, 1974a, p. 51.

————. "Let's Get Rid of Those Surplus Hospital Beds." *Prism*, October 1974b, p. 13.

Rogatz, P. "Directions of Health System for the New Decade." *Hospitals*, January 1, 1980, p. 67.

Rosenberg, C. E. "The Origins of the American Hospital System." *Bulletin of the New York Academy of Medicine*, 55, 10, 1979.

Rushing, W. "Difference in Profit and Nonprofit Organizations: A Study in Effectiveness and Efficiency in General Short-Stay Hospitals." *Administrative Science Quarterly*, 19, 474, 1974.

Sattler, F. L., and Bennett, M. D. *A Statistical Profile of Short-Term Hospitals in the United States as of 1973*. Minneapolis: Interstudy, 1975.

Shain, M., and Roemer, M. I. "Hospitals and the Public Interest." *Public Health Reports*, 76, 401, 1961.

Shonick, W. "The Public Hospital and Its Plight." *International Journal of Health Services*, 9, No. 3, 1979.

Simler, S. L. "New Jersey Testing New DRG-Based Rate Setting." *Modern Health Care*, April 1979, p. 56.

Sloan, F. A. *Determinants of Hospital Wage Inflation*. Washington, D. C.: National Center for Health Services Research, 1974.

Somers, A. *Hospital Regulation: The Dilemma of Public Policy*. Princeton, N. J.: Princeton University Press, 1969.

Southwick. A. "Due Process: The Physician's Right to Due Process and Equal Protection." *Hospital Medical Staff*, June 1978.

Stephenson, H. R. "Hospital Trusteeship." *Hospitals, J.A.H.A.*, December 16, 1963, p. 38.

Stern, B. J. *Medical Services by Government*. New York: The Commonwealth Fund, 1946.

Stevens, R. *American Medicine and the Public Interest*. New Haven, Connecticut: Yale University Press, 1971.

Stroman, D. F. *The Quick Knife: Unnecessary Surgery U.S.A.* Port Washington, N.Y.: Kennikat Press Corporation, 1979.

Subcommittee on Oversight. *Cost and Quality of Health Care: Unnecessary Surgery*. Washington, D.C.: House of Representatives, January 1976.

———. *Surgical Performance: Necessity and Quality*. Washington, D.C.: House of Representatives, December 1978.

Sun, M. "Patient Reps Burgeoning in Nation's Hospitals." *Medical News Report*, November 17, 1979, p. 8.

Thompson, R. E. *Helping Hospital Trustees Understand Physicians*. Chicago: American Hospital Association, 1979.

Umbdenstock, R. J. "Governance: Trustees Are Closing the Gap Between Hospitals and Communities." *Hospitals, J.A.H.A.*, April 1, 1979, p. 111.

———. "Hospital Governance Comes of Age." *Hospitals*, April 1, 1980, p. 85.

Vickery, D. "Is It a Change for the Better?" *Hospitals, J.A.H.A.*, October 1, 1979, p. 87.

Washington Report. "House Defeats Administration Cost Control Legislation." *Hospitals, J.A.H.A.*, December 1, 1979, p. 23.

Westerman, J. H. "Technology: Lauded and Rapped in '79." *Hospitals*, April 1, 1980, p. 167.

Wilkins, R. "Loss of Hospitals in Central Cities Said to Cause Array of Problems." *The New York Times*, September 17, 1979.

Williams, K. "The Role of the Medical Director." *Hospital Progress*, June 1978.

Williams, L. *How to Avoid Unnecessary Surgery*. Nash Publishing, 1971.

Wilson, R. N. "The Physician's Changing Hospital Roles." *Human Organization*, Winter, 1959–60, p. 179.

Wing, K. R. *The Law and the Public's Health*. St Louis, Missouri: C. V. Mosby, 1976.

Wolfe, S. *Organization of Health Workers and Labor Conflict*. Farmingdale, N.Y.: 1978.

Worthington, N. L. "Expenditures for Hospital Care and Physicians' Services: Factors Affecting Annual Changes." *Social Security Bulletin*, November 1975, p. 3

Zuckerman, H. "Multi-Institutional Systems: Promise and Performance." *Inquiry*, Winter 1979, p. 297.

8

Long-Term Care

David A. Pearson and Terrie T. Wetle

Introduction

The goal of long-term care is not to cure the patient, but rather to improve or maintain the individual's ability to function. Currently, there is no single generally accepted definition of long-term care. Various definitions have been used over the years, reflecting the biases of professional groups as well as changes in the field. Early definitions emphasized inpatient medical care of 30 days or more. For example, the 1956 report of the Commission on Chronic Illness used a definition developed by Public Health Service personnel (Perrott et al.), stating that long-term care patients were:

> Persons suffering from chronic disease or impairments who require a pro-
> longed period of care, that is, who are likely to need or who have received
> care for a continuous period of at least 30 days in a general hospital, or care for
> a continuous period of more than 3 months in another institution or at home,
> such care to include medical supervision and/or assistance in achieving a
> higher level of self-care and independence. (p. 7)

Definitions of long-term care patients have also recognized that long-term care services involve millions of Americans with such conditions as chronic disabilities, injuries due to accidents, mental retardation and illness, congenital disabling diseases, and other defects. For example, the U.S. Department of Health, Education and Welfare (1963) states that:

> A long-term patient is an individual who, because of physical or mental
> illness, deterioration or disability, requires medical, nursing, or supportive
> health care for a prolonged period of time. Also included in this category is
> the individual who, because of severity of acute illness or injury, or resulting
> complications, requires an extended period of convalescence or treatment.
> (p. 8)

One problem with such definitions is the implication that all persons with chronic disease, disabilities, or impairments need long-term care services. Weissert (1978, p. 92) explains that various definitions "stress that [the] mere presence of such conditions may not be as valid an indicator of the need for long-term care as the effect they have on ability to function." In this respect, function includes activities that are basic to daily living such as feeding, dressing, and toileting, as well as a person's ability to perform his or her role as a homemaker or salaried employee. Brody (1977, p. 14) states: "Long-term care refers to one or more services provided on a sustained basis to enable individuals whose functional capacities are chronically impaired to be maintained at their maximum level of health and well-being."

Recent definitions also recognize that long-term care involves a broad array of services and not those limited solely to health and medical care (e.g., finance, human, and social services plus physical, mental, legal, and technological services). According to Sherwood (1976, p. 8): "Someone is a long-term care person who has reached, either suddenly or gradually, a state of collapse or deterioration in human behavioral functioning which requires—for survival, slowing down the rate of deterioration, maintenance, or rehabilitation—the services of at least one other human being."

Pollak (1979, p. 2) concisely states the more commonly held definition of long-term care: "Long-term care refers to health and social services provided within or outside institutions over extended periods to chronically ill, functionally impaired persons, most of whom are elderly."

The Public Health Service definition is similar in focus (Weissert, 1978):

> Long-term care consists of those services designed to provide diagnostic, preventative, therapeutic, rehabilitative, supportive, and maintenance services for individuals of all age groups who have chronic physical and/or mental impairments, in a variety of institutional and noninstitutional health care settings, including the home, with the goal of promoting optimum levels of physical, social, and psychological functioning. (p. 93)

The Need for Long-Term Care

Estimates of the proportion of the population that needs long-term care are difficult to make and vary depending on the nature or type of services included. A review of changes in demographic trends and in our social values, however, provides some insight into the need for care.

Demographic trends. Chronic illness, functional impairment, and advancing age are directly related to the need for long-term care. Demographic trends in the 65 and over age group are of particular importance, because members of this age group are five times more likely than the general population to be functionally disabled (Congressional Budget

Office). In 1940, only 9 million people were aged 65 and over. By 1975, this number increased to over 22 million, or 10% of the United States' population; by the year 2030, aged persons will number about 52 million, or 1 out of every 4 individuals (Kovar). More relevant to the potential demand for long-term care services are the increasing numbers and proportion of persons in the "old-old," or over 75 age group. The proportion of those 65 and over who are "old-old" was 38% in 1970, and is expected to be 44% by the year 2000 (Kovar).

The increase in the aged population is important in determining long-term care need, because the prevalence of chronic disease and impairment increases with age. For example, 15% of all physician visits in 1978 were made by persons aged 65 and over, and it is estimated that this will increase to 18% by the year 2003; 43% of all hospital-care days in 2003 will be rendered to aged persons, compared to 37% in 1978; and there will be a dramatic increase in the number of nursing home residents—from the current 1.3 million to a projected 2.8 million in the year 2003 (Wylie).

The increase in the proportion of the "old-old" is reflected in projected nursing home statistics. Of all nursing home residents in 1978, 35% were aged 85 or over, compared to a projected 52% in 2003 (Wylie). Increasingly, nursing homes will be taking care of older and older patients, who in turn require higher levels of service.

Changing social values and patterns.   The simple effects of the demographic changes listed above are exacerbated by a series of changes in social values and patterns. The social change most often associated with increased long-term institutionalization is the historical shift from extended to nuclear families. There has been a clear and steady decrease in the proportion of older persons living with adult children (Soldo). Exercising an option to live with adult children, however, is a viable means of postponing institutionalization; this is evidenced by higher ages and more serious impairments of persons entering nursing homes from relatives' houses as opposed to those who lived alone prior to admission (Townsend).

There are multiple causes for the shift from family care to institutional care: children moving to different cities to attend schools, seek employment, and set up households; children seeking advice and support from professional counselors rather than from parents; and, as the divorce rate increases, a diluting of the strength and quality of the parent-child relationship (Soldo). Increased resources through retirement benefits and Social Security facilitate independent living for the elderly, a majority of whom prefer an independent arrangement (Shanas et al.; Lopata; Field). This prevents an early transition into an extended family relationship, while reciprocation of services is still possible, and makes a later transition into a family setting less likely.

This pattern is not equally prevalent among major subcultures in the

United States. For both blacks and Spanish Americans, forms of the extended family are common in both urban and rural settings (Shimkin and Frate), which explains, in part, the underrepresentation of blacks and Spanish Americans in nursing home populations.

Another important social change is the increased participation of women in the labor force, thereby reducing the number of "at home" caretakers of the chronically impaired. By the end of the 1980s, it is estimated that two-thirds of all married women under age 55 will be working, as compared to 20% in 1947, making institutionalization more likely for those elderly with adult children. In the longer run, the shift in infertility patterns to smaller families will probably decrease the availability of adult children to provide home care (Soldo). Divorce, in addition to weakening parent-child ties, increases the number of older persons living alone. Glick estimates that the number of divorced older persons will almost double during the last quarter of the century, from 12% of those over 65 in 1975 to 22% of the older population in the year 2000. In addition, new technologies, better treatments, and prevention of disease result in increased survival rates for the chronically impaired of all ages, and increase the likelihood that healthy individuals will survive long enough to incur chronic disease.

In summary, by studying changing demographic trends, social values, and fertility patterns, we can begin to predict the need for long-term care. A conservative estimate is that 10 or 11 million elderly will need some form of long-term care in 1990. In the aggregate, upwards of 20 million people of *all* ages will require long-term care by the end of this century.

Historical Development

In the pre-Christian era, impaired and aged people depended on their families for care or they died. The lack of specialized facilities was due mainly to the marginal position these persons held in society. Because they were considered to be a drain on society's resources, their usual treatment during the Greco-Roman eras was abandonment (Moroney and Kurtz). The first community hospital was built in 369 A.D. by Justinian at Caesarea; it provided services to aged people and orphans as well as the ill; therefore it is considered the precursor to long-term care (Litman, 1974).

During the middle ages, Christianity brought about a change in attitudes toward the sick and "Houses of God" *(Hôtels de Dieu)* were established to provide shelter, food, and medical care (Sigerist). Religious and economic reformations of the 16th century, however, returned to the sick and needy the burden of "moral" responsibility for their own problems. The English Poor Law Act of 1601 held families responsible for the care of the aged and disabled and, if no relatives were available, aged and disabled persons were placed in miserable almshouses (Pumphrey and Pumphrey; Friedlander; Stewart). The almshouse approach and philosophy were transferred to the United States and continued throughout the 19th century, as evidenced by the Poor Law Commission Report of 1834. The destitute, aged, and impaired were not only considered responsible for their plight, but also were "put on display in workhouses as horrible examples" (Gold and Kaufman).

The Charitable Organization Society, with a philosophy of voluntary rather than public almshouse care for the aged and impaired, created a system of private homes and "out-door" (non-facility-based) relief in the early 1900s (Miles). During the 1920s and 1930s, the acceptance of hospital-based medical practice by physicians, as well as the introduction of voluntary health insurance, accelerated the centralization of medical care. At the same time industrialization, urbanization, and increased family mobility led to a greater demand for residential alternatives for older persons. Boarding homes filled this need. At first they offered only food and shelter, but, as their residents became older and sicker, they offered nursing services and eventually evolved into convalescent homes (Moroney and Kurtz).

The passage of the Social Security Act in 1935 legislated support to the elderly through Old Age Survivors Insurance (OASI) and Old Age Assistance (OAA), which provided monthly payments to eligible persons aged 65 and over—through insurance in the case of OASI, and welfare assistance for the needy in the case of OAA. The impact for long-term care came through guaranteed monthly incomes, which allowed the elderly to purchase boarding home care or nursing home care; payments could not be made to persons in public institutions such as almshouses or county farms (Friedlander).

Public Law 89–97, which included Medicare and Medicaid, was passed in 1965, making public monies available for the purchase of institutional and selected community health services for the long-term care patient (See Chapters 10 and 15).

Organization and Delivery of Long-Term Care Services

Increasingly, health care systems are viewed in relation to their availability, accessibility, and comprehensiveness. This section, therefore, will explore a variety of services available to long-term care patients in institutions as well as those services organized, provided, or coordinated through community organizations and in special delivery systems.

Institutional Services

Long-term care institutions are those that offer services to persons with an average length stay of 30 days or more, e.g., nursing homes; homes for the aged; psychiatric institutions; and facilities for children, mentally handicapped people, physically handicapped people; plus other institutions such as chronic disease hospitals and the extended care facilities of short-term hospitals (American Hospital Association). In 1976, the United States had over 23,600 long-term care facilities of all types (U.S. Department of Commerce). The overwhelming majority of these (77%) were nursing homes. Facilities for the mentally handicapped and psychiatric institutions each represented about 7%; almost 6% were associated specifically with long-term care services for children; facilities for the physically handicapped represented about 2%; and chronic disease hospitals and other facilities were only 1.5% of the total (U.S. Department of Commerce).

Most long-term care facilities (79.5%) in 1976 were relatively small, having less than 100 beds. Significantly fewer (19.3%) were medium-sized (100–399 beds), and still fewer (1%) were large (400 beds or more). About 53% of the 23,600-plus long-term care facilities were proprietary (operated for profit); about 39% were run by private, nonprofit organizations (churches, nonprofit corporations); and only 8% were operated by government (local, state, federal). Occupancy rates vary significantly among long-term care facilities. Overall, about 90% had an occupancy rate of more than 75%. However, only 40% of facilities for the physically handicapped, 46% of institutions for children, and 75% of chronic disease hospitals had 75% or more of their beds occupied in 1976 (U.S. Department of Commerce).

According to the U.S. Department of Health, Education and Welfare (1979a), a facility is a nursing home if nursing care is its primary and predominant function and it meets the following criteria: it employs one or more registered nurses or licensed practical nurses; and 50% or more of the residents are receiving nursing care, that is, one or more of the following: nasal feeding, catheterization, irrigation, oxygen therapy, full bed bath, enema, hypodermic injection, intravenous injection, temperature-pulse-respiration check, blood pressure reading, application of dressings and bandages, and bowel and bladder training.

In general, nursing homes tend to be classified according to their certification status as providers of care under the Medicare and Medicaid programs. In general, there are three types of certification: skilled nursing facility (19.2% of all nursing homes), which refers to a facility being certified as such under Medicare and/or Medicaid; intermediate care facility, which refers to certification only under Medicaid (31.6%); and those 24.2% of all nursing homes that are certified as both skilled nursing and intermediate care facilities; 25% of all nursing homes are not certified (U.S. Department of Health Education and Welfare, 1979a).

The number of skilled nursing homes, the number of beds in such facilities, and the average bed size all have increased, especially since the introduction of Medicaid and Medicare in 1965. Two years before Medicaid and Medicare, there were just over 8,100 homes and 319,000 beds. Four years after these programs were introduced, the number of homes had increased by 41% to over 11,400; the number of beds had increased by 121% to over 704,000; and the average bed size was 61. Today, there are over 18,300 homes, with over 1,380,000 beds, and the average number of beds is about 90.

In 1976, there were almost 453 million resident days in all types of nursing homes, and the median length of stay was 75 days. There were about 1,367,000 admissions (98 per 100 beds) that year, and about 1,117,500 discharges (59 live discharges per 100 beds, 21 dead discharges per 100 beds). The occupancy rate for all nursing homes in 1976 was 89% (U.S. Department of Health, Education and Welfare, 1979a, p. 9).

The age distribution of the current nursing home population is as follows: less than 65 years old, 14% of total nursing home population: 65–74 years old, 16%; 75–84 years old, 36%; 85–94 years old, 31%; and older than 95 years, 3% (U.S. Department of Health, Education and Welfare, 1979a, Table 19, page 29).

Of all persons aged 65 and over, only 4.8% are in nursing homes, but the percentage of aged persons in nursing homes increases with age; 10% of all persons 75 and over and 22% of those 85 and over are in nursing homes (U.S. Department of Health, Education, and Welfare, 1980). The average age of a nursing home resident is 81. Most residents (71%) are women, reflecting, in part, the greater life expectancy of women (77 years as compared to 69 years for men.)

As reported by Litman (1979), almost 50% of all nursing home residents have no visible relationships with a close relative. Over half (55%) are mentally impaired. Concerning activities of daily living, less than half can walk unassisted, over half (55%) require assistance in bathing, almost half (47%) require help in dressing, 11% need help in eating, and about one-third are incontinent. Over half (55%) were admitted to a nursing home from their own or a relative's home, 22% came from hospitals, and about 13% came from other living arrangements, including other long-term care facilities.

Expenditures for all types of long-term care are difficult to identify; however, the federal government reports data on nursing homes. In 1965, the year Medicare and Medicaid began, about $1.9 billion was spent for nursing home care, or about 5% of all expenditures for health and medical care. Since then, both the amount and the percent of the total have increased significantly. By 1975, the amount was almost $9.9 billion or 7.5% of the total. As of 1978, $15.8 billion was spent for nursing home care; this represented over 8% of all national health expenditures. Of the $15.8 billion, about 46% came from direct payments, that is, directly from the patient or the patient's family. Third parties (government, philanthropies, insurance companies) cover the remaining 54%, the lion's share of which was paid by the government (52%). Concerning only public (governmental) expenditures for nursing home care, Medicare represented only 5%, whereas Medicaid pays for 87%; the Veterans Administration plus other federal and state agencies made up the remaining 8% (Gibson, 1979).

Litman (1979) summarizes the 1974 report of the Subcommittee on Long-Term Care of the U.S. Senate's Special Committee on Aging, which identified a number of problems associated with care of the long-term patient. First, there is a lack of coordinated policies on goals and methods. Many citizens go without needed care; others are located in inappropriate facilities. Regardless of the sizable and ever-growing amount of funds spent on nursing home care, the federal government has not issued forthright standards directed at providing minimum protection for patients, and there is no direct enforcement of federal standards.

The summary by Litman of the subcommittee's report also points out a variety of nursing home problems. Patient abuse in nursing homes has been well documented: cruelty, lack of human dignity, dangers from fire and food poisoning, negligence (Moss and Halamandaris; Temporary State Commission on Living Costs and the Economy; Thomas). Similarly, there is concern about the high cost of drugs for nursing home patients, and that the flow of drugs in nursing homes is largely without controls. Physicians are said to have generally shunned responsibility for the care and treatment of nursing home patients, and many medical schools lack a seriousness of purpose about teaching geriatrics and long-term care topics. Further, nursing home personnel generally are unlicensed and untrained, are frequently overworked, and are paid at or near the minimum wage; the annual turnover rate among such workers is about 75%. The subcommittee also reported fraud, illegal kickbacks, bribes, haphazard enforcement of regulation, and collusion plus conflict of interest among legislators and public officials.

On the other hand, nursing homes are convenient scapegoats for the overriding problems of long-term care and there are a large number of facilities providing good quality care. Nursing home administrators point to problems of overwhelming paperwork and inadequate and confusing reimbursement strategies plus the shared problem of rapidly rising costs (Brody; Vladeck).

Community-Based Services

The lion's share of public monies is expended for facility-based institutional services; for example, state and federal Medicaid expenditures in 1977 totaled only $241 million for home health care benefits, while institutional care expenditures were $5.8 *billion* (Comptroller General of the United States, 1977a). Although the institutionalized group may be more impaired, many of them could receive adequate care in a noninstitutional setting, and possibly at lower cost. A description of noninstitutional services follows.

In-home services. (See also Chapter 6.)   Scanlon et al. explain that home health care is generally considered to include the provision of skilled nursing services (medical services furnished or directed by a licensed nurse); rehabilitation services (improving function in activities of daily living through physical, occupational, and speech therapies); and personal care services (assistance in activities of daily living, e.g., bathing, toileting, eating, and ambulation). Home health services are provided by both nonprofit organizations, e.g., Visiting Nurses Associations, and proprietary organizations and private parties, with fragmented funding available from a variety of sources including Medicaid, Medicare, Title XX of the Social Security Act, Title III of the Older Americans Act, and the Veterans Administration. It should be noted, however, that the Congressional Budget Office estimates that less than 10% of federal health reimbursements are allocated to noninstitutional settings.

Hospice   is a set of services intended to improve the quality of life for terminally ill patients (Cohen; Osterweis and Champagne). While some hospice care is provided in institutions, the emphasis is on home care, with intentional inclusion of family in both settings (Hackley; Plant). There is a strong emphasis on an interdisciplinary care team and the use of a "polypharmacy" approach to pain management (Leigner). The overall goal of hospice care is to avoid suffering and "heroic" interventions as much as possible, while offering support to the patient and family during the process of dying.

Homemaker and chore services   are the general housekeeping services needed to keep someone in his or her home (e.g. house cleaning, shopping, meal preparation, minor repairs, financial management, laundry, and errands). Wide variation exists in both the types and quality of services provided, and the amount of public funding is rather limited. The major resource is Title XX of the Social Security Act; about 19% of all Title XX expenditures goes for homemaker and chore services (Scanlon et al.). The effectiveness of homemaker and chore services in reducing the use of nursing homes has yet to be demonstrated, but levels of contentment, social function, and mental functioning are definitely sustained or improved when patients remain at home (Weissert et al.).

Home-delivered meals   are an important resource for persons who are unable to shop, cannot prepare meals, or who have special dietary requirements they are unable to adequately address. The major source of funding for these services has been the Older Americans Act, which provided funding for two programs: congregate meals for the elderly, and home delivered lunches, "Meals on Wheels." Both of these national programs receive a major part of their support through community volunteers and church and civic organizations; it is estimated that there are between 300 to 500 home-delivered meal programs across the country (U.S. Senate).

Monitoring services are intended to supervise, or keep in touch with, chronically impaired or frail persons living alone. They include organized, active services such as telephone networks and friendly visiting as well as more "passive" services such as alert apartment managers, friendly neighbors, and alarm systems. Elderly impaired persons are often particularly isolated, living in single-room occupancy hotels and rooming houses. Monitoring often occurs as a by-product of other services such as home delivered meals, but receives little formal financial support as an independent service.

There also are informal services for long-term patients. Among this population, successful problem-solvers obtain help first from informal sources such as family, friends, and neighbors, followed as needed by additional aid from more formal agencies and organizations (Lebowitz). Those elderly without informal networks of family and friends tend to show a higher use of formal services (Kammeyer and Bolton); report lower personal well-being (Tannenbaum); have more difficult adjustments to crises (Lopata); have a lower mental health status (Lowenthal and Haven); and have an increased likelihood of institutionalization (O'Brien and Wagner; Wagner). The range of services offered by informal helpers is as broad as those delivered by formal organizations; providers can render services as simple as bringing in mail and as complex as complete, total care. The role of the formal service system, therefore, is to supplement and enhance these informal services, rather than to replace them at often greater cost and with a loss of social contact and life satisfaction.

Community Facility Services

Older persons have an average of 6.6 physician contacts per year, more than do persons aged 45–64, who have 5.6 visits per year. These visits are more likely to be for chronic conditions and tend to be with general practitioners and internists. While the overall utilization rate for physician care has not changed since the enactment of Medicare and Medicaid, there has been increased utilization among the elderly poor and a corresponding decrease in utilization by the nonpoor (U.S. Department of Health, Education and Welfare, 1977; National Council on the Aging).

Acute-care hospital utilization increased during the same period (1965–1975), particularly among the elderly poor. Not only is the average length of stay for older persons longer than it is for the general population (11.6 days for older persons and 7.7 days for the general population, but hospital discharge rates, a common measure of utilization, are twice as high for those over 65 and three times as high for those over 75 (Scanlon et al.). Much of this acute hospital care is considered unnecessary. Studies in

Monroe County, New York (Williams and Hill), and in Massachusetts (Tolkoff-Rubin et al.) demonstrate that as many as 18% of the elderly are misplaced in acute-care hospitals, often waiting for placement in long-term care facilities such as nursing homes.

Adult day care, while relatively new in the United States, is used extensively in Europe (Farndale; Brocklehurst). In the United States, Weissert (1976, 1977) has identified two types of day care programs. The first, the "day hospital" program, typically has rehabilitation as its goal and is affiliated with a health care institution. The second type, a "multi-purpose program," focuses more on social programs and activities, and is more likely to be affiliated with a community service agency. Day care programs have been initiated as a cost-saving alternative to institutionalization, but when the costs of food and rent incurred at home are included in cost comparisons between day care and institutional patients, the savings drop considerably (Weissert, 1978).

Congregate meals, supported in great part by funding under the Older Americans Act plus a large voluntary effort, serve hot meals to an estimated 2.85 million elderly (U.S. Senate). They are considered to be important not only for providing the elderly with one-third of the daily nutritional requirement five times a week, but also because they provide the opportunity for social contact and recreation. The meal program sites are also used to conduct health screening, education, and outreach programs (Wetle).

Community mental health clinics are intended to provide ambulatory care and other services to the mentally disabled. Epidemiological data indicate that about 5% of the elderly population have severe psychiatric disorders, and approximately 15% of older people are in need of mental health treatment (U.S. Department of Health, Education and Welfare, 1979b). The elderly are considered to be underserved by community mental health programs, in part because of their reluctance to seek counseling and therapy and in part because of negative attitudes toward the elderly on the part of the mental health workers.

Given the broad array of programs to serve the chronically impaired, it should not be surprising that the long-term care field is marked by fragmentation, confusion, and inappropriate placement of clients. Federal, state, and local officials admit that services to the chronically impaired are not effectively coordinated (Comptroller General, 1977a). Title III of the Older Americans Act created Area Agencies on Aging (AAA) across the country to coordinate services for older persons, provide access assistance to agencies and, in some cases, fill gaps in service. The effectiveness of the AAAs and other coordinative efforts have been limited by lack of both funding and authority (O'Brien and Wetle).

Problems with individual services within the system occur in part because of features common to many service programs. Services tend to be organized around a single problem in professional specialization, whereas the chronically impaired have a variety of problems. Many services tend to be facility-based, making access difficult for persons with mobility problems. Formal services often do not take into account the clients' informal support system, and many fail to recognize the impact of their service on the total individual (e.g., a person served a home-delivered meal may lose the social contact of the neighbor who previously brought groceries). What are needed, therefore, are person-centered coordinated delivery systems (Wetle and Whitelaw).

A few special projects have tested models of coordinated services. One project, TRIAGE, provided evaluation, access, and monitoring services to more than 2,000 older persons in central Connecticut. Supported by funding from the Administration on Aging, the National Center for Health Services Research, and the Connecticut State Department on Aging, this project provides "a single entry mechanism to coordinate delivery of institutional, ambulatory, and in-home services on behalf of the elderly" (Shealy et al., p. 1–2). This was accomplished in part through comprehensive Medicare waivers, which authorized payments for many ancillary and supportive goods and services not traditionally covered by Medicare, such as pharmaceuticals, dental care, mental health services, homemakers, eyeglasses, and hearing aids.

A recent evaluation of this project compared a subsample of TRIAGE patients with a similar group of individuals in another geographic area. Findings indicate that expenditures for hospital care and physician's services were lower for the TRIAGE group, but social, home health, and homemaker costs were higher. Overall, TRIAGE was able to provide a comprehensive array of health and social services for a cost comparable to that spent for health services alone for the comparison group. Equally important, a higher proportion of the TRIAGE group maintained or improved their ADL (activities of daily living) abilities during the study period (Shealy et al.).

A joint effort between the Administration on Aging and the Health Care Financing Administration will fund special demonstration and research "channeling" projects to investigate similar programs. This is an effort to create a full continuum of care for the chronically impaired so that appropriate, efficient, and effective service placements can be made.

Policy Issues

The importance of long-term care is reflected in the Department of Health, Education and Welfare's response to a Government Accounting Office report entitled *Entering a Nursing Home—Costly Implications for Medicaid and the Elderly:* " . . . Dependence on nursing home care is a social and economic problem that far transcends health concerns alone. . . . No issue is of greater interest and concern to HEW's Health Care Financing Administration . . . at this time" (Comptroller General of the United States, 1979, p. 165). Thorny problems make difficult the translation of this interest into feasible, efficient, long-term care policy and programs.

A history of long-term care and a projection of increased demand and spiraling costs of long-term care have been presented in this chapter. Efforts to limit federal expenditures come into direct conflict with public demand for increased home-health and community-based services, plus national concern and outrage over the deplorable conditions documented in some facilities. The question, therefore, becomes whether good quality care at an appropriate level is the right of every chronically impaired person. Regardless of the answer to that question, how are the admittedly limited resources to be distributed?

An issue closely related to expenditures is regulation. Who should regulate long-term care and for what purposes? Does enforcement of regulations necessarily lead to good quality of care? Exactly what constitutes "good quality care" is hotly disputed. Additionally, the problems of assessing quality, even if there were agreement as to its components, have led to confusing, ineffective, and sometimes counterproductive regulation.

A third issue is the development of a comprehensive continuum of care for the chronically impaired. As was demonstrated earlier, the major proportion of federal long-term care expenditures goes for institutionally based care. However, pressure has grown for the initiation and support of community-based services, which enable the chronically impaired to remain in or return to their own homes in the community setting (O'Brien and Whitelaw). While the cost-effectiveness of these programs in comparison to institutional care is still in question, the quality-of-life benefits for many chronically impaired persons have been clearly demonstrated. Will major support be available for these services, and which clients will qualify? Should those most in need be given priority, or should services be provided to those who will most successfully benefit?

Finally, the current dominant philosophy of long-term care, the medical model, should be reexamined. Thinking of the chronically impaired simply in terms of health needs disregards the broad impact of functional problems on the total person. A multidisciplinary team approach to both assessment and service delivery must be taken not only to ensure survival but, of equal importance, to maximize quality of life for each individual.

References

American Hospital Association. *Guide to the Health Care Field*. Chicago: 1979, p. A13.
Brocklehurst, J. C. "Geriatric Services and the Day Hospital." In Brocklehurst, J.

C., Ed., *Textbook of Geriatric Medicine and Gerontology*, pp. 673–691. Edinburgh: Churchill-Livingstone, 1973.

Brody, E. *Long-Term Care of Older People: A Practical Guide*. New York: Human Sciences Press, 1977.

Cohen, K. P. *Hospice: Prescription for Terminal Care*. Germantown, Maryland: Aspen Systems Corp., 1979.

Comptroller General of the United States. *Home Health—The Need for a National Policy to Better Provide for the Elderly*. A Report to the Congress, HRD 78–19, Washington, D.C. : USGPO, December 30, 1977a.

————. *The Well-Being of Older People in Cleveland, Ohio*. A Report to Congress, HRD 77–70. Washington, D.C.: USGPO, April 19, 1977b.

————. *Entering a Nursing Home—Costly Implications for Medicaid and the Elderly*. A Report to the Congress. Washington, D.C.: PAD 80–12. Washington, D.C.: USGPO, November 26, 1979.

Congressional Budget Office. *Long Term Care for the Elderly and Disabled*. Washington, D.C.: USGPO, February 1977.

Farndale, J. *The Day Hospital Movement in Great Britain*. New York: Pergamon Press, 1961.

Field, M. *The Aged, the Family and the Community*. New York: Columbia University Press, 1972.

Friedlander, W. *Introduction to Social Welfare*. Englewood Cliffs, New Jersey: Prentice-Hall, 1961.

Gibson, R. M. "National Health Expenditures, 1978." *Health Care Financing Review*, *1*, 1, Summer 1979.

Glick, P. G. "The Future of the American Family"—A Statement Prepared for Joint Hearings of the House Select Committees on Population and Aging. U.S. House of Representatives: Washington, D.C., pp. 287–306, May 23, 1978.

Gold, J., and Kaufman, S. "Development of Care of the Elderly." Presented at the Gerontological Society Meeting, Denver, Colorado, 1968.

Hackley, J. A. "Full Service Hospital Offers Home, Day and Inpatient Care." *Hospitals*, *51*, 21, 84–87, November 1, 1977.

Kammeyer, K., and Bolton, D. "Community and Family Factors Related to the Use of a Family Service Agency." *Journal of Marriage and the Family*, *30*, 488, 1968.

Kovar, M. G. "Health of the Elderly and Use of Health Services." *Public Health Reports*, *92*, 9, January–February 1977.

Lebowitz, B. "Statement on Research into Crimes Against the Elderly." Testimony before the Subcommittee on Domestic and International Scientific Planning, Analysis and Cooperation of the Committee on Science and Technology, U.S. House of Representatives, 95th Congress, Washington, D.C.: January 31, 1978.

Liegner, L. M. "St. Christopher's Hospice, 1974." *Journal of the American Medical Association*, December 8, 1977, *234*, 10, 1047.

Litman, T. J. *Syllabus on Long Term Care*. Washington, D.C.: Association of University Programs in Health Administration, 1974.

Litman, T. J. *Health and Health Care in the United States: Some Facts, Figures and*

Observations. Minneapolis: Department of Sociology, University of Minnesota, 1979. (Mimeographed.)

Lopata, H. F. *Widowhood in an American City.* Cambridge, Massachusetts: Schenkman, 1973.

Lowenthal, M., and Haven, C. "Interaction and Adaptation: Intimacy as a Critical Variable." *American Sociological Review, 33,* 20, 1968.

Miles, A. *Public Welfare,* Boston: D.C. Heath & Co. 1949.

Moroney, R. M., and Kurtz, H. R. "The Evolution of Long Term Care Institutions." In Sherwood, S., Ed., *Long Term Care: A Handbook for Researchers, Planners and Providers,* pp. 81–121. New York: Spectrum Publications, 1975.

Moss, F. E., and Halamandaris, V. J. *Too Old, Too Sick, Too Bad: Nursing Homes in America.* Germantown, Maryland: Aspen Systems Corp., 1977.

National Council on the Aging. *Fact Book on Aging: A Profile of America's Older Population.* Washington, D.C.: National Council on the Aging, 1978.

O'Brien, J. E., and Wagner, D. L. "Primary Associations: A Conceptual Framework for Analyzing Behavior." Unpublished manuscript available from the Institute on Aging, Portland State University, Portland, Oregon, 1979.

O'Brien, J. E., and Wetle, T. *Analysis of Conflict in Coordination of Aging Services.* A Report to Administration on Aging. Institute on Aging, Portland State University: Portland, Oregon, 1975. (Mimeographed.)

O'Brien, J. E. and Whitelaw, N. *Analysis of Community Based Alternatives to Institutional Care for the Aged.* Final Report to Oregon State Program on Aging and Administration on Aging. Institute on Aging, Portland State University: Portland, Oregon, 1973. (Mimeographed.)

Osterweis, M., and Champagne, D. S. "The U.S. Hospice Movement: Issues in Development." *American Journal of Public Health, 69,* 492, 1979.

Perrott, G. St. J., et al. *Care of the Long-Term Patient: Source Book on Size and Characteristics of the Problem.* PHS Pub. No. 344, Washington, D.C.: USGPO, 1954.

Plant, J. "Finding a Home for Hospice Care in the United States." *Hospitals, 51,* pp. 53–62, July 1, 1977.

Pollak, W. *Expanding Health Benefits for the Elderly, Volume 1: Long-Term Care.* Washington: The Urban Institute, 1979.

Pumphrey, R., and Pumphrey, M. W. *The History of American Social Work.* New York: Columbia University Press, 1961.

Scanlon, W., et al. "A Framework for Analysis of the Long Term Care System." pp. 49–123. In Urban Institute, *Long Term Care: Current Experience and a Framework for Analysis.* Washington, D.C.: The Urban Institute, 1979.

Shanas, E., et al. *Old People in Three Industrialized Societies.* New York: Atherton Press, 1968.

Shealy, M. H., et al. *TRIAGE: Coordinated Delivery of Services to the Elderly.* Final Report to National Center for Health Services Research, DHEW, Plainville, Connecticut: Triage, 1979.

Sherwood, S., Ed. *Long-Term Care: A Handbook for Researchers, Planners, and Providers.* New York: Spectrum Publications, 1976.

Shimkin, D. B., and Frate, D. A., Eds. *The Extended Family in Black Societies.* The Hague: Mouton, 1975.

Sigerist, H. E. "The Social History of Medicine." In Katz, A. H., and Felton, J. S., Eds., *Health and Community*, pp. 3–11. New York: The Free Press, 1965.

Simmons, L. "Aging in Pre-Industrial Societies." In Tibbets, C., Ed., *Handbook of Social Gerontology*, pp. 62–69. Chicago: University of Chicago Press, 1960.

Soldo, B. S. "The Living Arrangements of the Elderly in the Near Future." An unpublished paper prepared for the Conference, "The Elderly of the Future," sponsored by the Committee on Aging of the National Research Council's Assembly of Behavioral and Social Sciences, National Academy of Sciences, Annapolis, Maryland, May 1979.

Stewart, E. M. "The Cost of American Almshouses." *U.S. Bureau of Labor Statistics Bulletin*, p. 386, 1925.

Tannenbaum, D. *People with Problems: Seeking Help in an Urban Community.* Toronto: University of Toronto, Center for Urban and Community Studies, 1975.

Temporary State Commission on Living Costs and the Economy. *Report on Nursing Homes and Health Related Facilities in New York State.* Albany, N. Y., April 1975.

Thomas, W. C. *Nursing Homes and Public Policy: Drift and Decision in New York State.* Ithaca, N. Y.: Cornell University Press, 1969.

Tolkoff-Rubin, N. E., et al. "Coordinated Home Care: The Massachusetts General Experience." *Medical Care.* 16, 453, 1978.

Townsend, P. "The Effects of Family Structure on the Likelihood of Admission to an Institution in Old Age: The Application of General Theory." In Shanas, E., and Streib, G., Eds., *Social Structure and the Family Generational Relations*, pp. 170–178. Englewood Cliffs, N. J.: Prentice-Hall, 1965.

U.S. Department of Commerce, Bureau of the Census. *1976 Survey of Institutionalized Persons: A Study of Persons Receiving Long-Term Care.* Current Population Reports, Special Studies, Series P–23, No. 69. Washington, D.C.: USGPO, June 1978.

U.S. Department of Health, Education, and Welfare. Public Health Service. *Areawide Planning of Facilities for Long-Term Treatment and Care.* Report of the Joint Committee of the American Hospital Association and Public Health Service. PHS Pub. NO 930–B–1. Washington, D. C. : USGPO, 1963.

————. Health Resources Administration. *Health: United States, 1976–1977.* Washington, D.C.: USGPO, 1977.

————. National Center for Health Statistics. *The Nation Nursing Home Survey: 1977 Summary for the United States.* Vital and Health Statistics, Series 13, No. 43. Washington, D.C.: USGPO, 1979a.

————. Federal Council on Aging. *Mental Health and the Elderly.* DHEW

Pub. No. (OHOS) 80–20960. Washington, D.C.: USGPO, 1979b.

————. National Center for Health Statistics. *Inpatient Health Facilities as Reported from the 1976 MFI Survey.* Vital and Health Statistics, Series 14, No. 23. Washington, D.C.: USGPO, 1980.

U.S. Senate. *Developments in Aging 1977.* Part 2. USGPO, p. 56–57, 1977.

Vladeck, B. *Unloving Care: The Nursing Home Tragedy.* New York: Basic Books, 1980.

Wagner, D. L. "Social Interaction of the Urban Elderly." In O'Brien, J. D., and Alexander, R., Eds., *A Longitudinal Study of High Risk Urban Elderly Population: An Analysis of the Environmental, Social, Economic and Personal Aspects of Everyday Life.* A Report to the Social Security Administration. Available from Institute on Aging, Portland State University, Portland, Oregon, pp. 257–303, December 1978.

Weissert, W. G. "Two Models of Geriatric Day Care: Findings from a Comparative Study." *The Gerontologist 16,* 420, 1976.

————. "Adult Day Care Programs in the United States: Current Research Projects and Survey of 10 Centers." *Public Health Reports,* 92, 49, 1977.

————. "Long Term Care: An Overview" In *Health: United States, 1978.* Department of Health, Education and Welfare Pub. No. 78–1232, Washington, D.C.: USGPO, 1978.

Weissert, W. G., et al. *Effects and Costs of Day Care and Homemaker Services for the Chronically Ill: A Randomized Experiment.* Washington, D.C.: Department of Health, Education and Welfare, Office of the Assistant Secretary for Health, National Center for Health Services Research, 1979.

Wetle, T. *Coordination in Social Service Systems: The Area Agency on Aging as a Case Study.* Portland: Institute on Aging, Portland State University, 1976.

Wetle, T., and Whitelaw, N. "Person Centered Service Delivery." In Rifai, M. A., Ed., *Justice and Older Americans.* Lexington, Massachusetts: Lexington Books, D.C. Heath, pp. 103–107, 1977.

Williams, T. F., and Hill, J. G. *Evaluation-Placement of the Chronically Ill and Aged.* Report No. NCHSR 78–155. Rochester, N. Y.: Genessee Region Health Planning Council, 1977.

Wylie, C. M. "Health Projections of an Aging Kind." *PAS Reporter, 16,* 1, 1979.

9

Mental Health Services

Lorrin M. Koran

Expenditures for mental health services were estimated at $17 billion in 1977, 11% of the nation's expenditures for health care. Over half this expenditure paid for care in public mental hospitals and nursing homes (President's Commission on Mental Health, Vol. II, p. 530; Koran, 1976). Mental disorders indirectly cost the nation an additional $20 billion due to total disability, premature death, and lost productive time while receiving care. These dollar estimates can only begin to suggest the magnitude of human suffering that mental disorders represent.

Despite great progress in the past quarter-century, the delivery of mental health care, like the delivery of general health care, is beset by many difficulties. The pluralistic nature of the service delivery system leads to: inequitable access based on geography, class, and diagnosis; inadequate coordination of different phases of care; fragmented planning, evaluation, and regulation; and insufficient coordination with such other human services as general medicine, education, and welfare. Other difficulties stem from our inability to cure many mental disorders, from limited manpower, and from inadequate community-based treatment facilities. The social stigma attached to mental patients and public apathy toward them also hamper care. Finally, mental health professionals often deal with extraordinarily complex problems, especially when working with groups affected by poverty and racism.

The challenge of the 1980s and 1990s is to find ways to resolve these difficulties. To help the reader participate in the search, this chapter will discuss the forms of mental disorder; the kinds of mental health care; the history of that care in the United States; the prevalence of mental disorders; mental health manpower; the delivery of services; insurance coverage; and legal issues.

The Forms of Mental Disorder

After five years of intensive work, the American Psychiatric Association (1980) published the third edition of its *Diagnostic and Statistical Manual of Mental Disorders*, or DSM-III. The manual includes more than 200

235

mental disorders grouped in 17 categories. This new edition improves upon earlier editions in several ways: the term "mental disorder" is carefully defined; diagnostic criteria are given for each disorder in order to increase the reliability of diagnoses, and new diagnostic entities have been created to take into account discoveries in the last 20 years regarding the causes, natural history, and treatment responsiveness of many forms of mental disorder. The 17 major diagnostic classes in DSM-III are:

1. *Disorders usually first evident in infancy, childhood, or adolescence*—including intellectual, behavioral, emotional, physical, and developmental disorders
2. *Organic mental disorders*: disorders caused by or associated with impairment of brain tissue function
3. *Substance use disorders*, including alcohol, drugs, and tobacco
4. *Schizophrenic disorders* (more narrowly defined than in DSM–II)
5. *Paranoid disorders*
6. *Affective disorders*—mood disorders with manic, depressive, or mixed symptomatology
7. *Psychotic disorders not elsewhere classified*: psychotic disorders that do not meet the criteria for organic, schizophrenic, paranoid, or affective disorders
8. *Anxiety disorders*, including phobias and obsessive compulsive disorders
9. *Somatoform disorders*: physical symptoms suggesting physical disorders but without organic findings
10. *Dissociative disorders*, including multiple personality and psychogenic amnesia
11. *Psychosexual disorders*, including homosexuality where the individuals are "either disturbed by, in conflict with, or wish to change their sexual orientation"
12. *Factitious disorders*—disorders deliberately simulated by the individual for psychological gain. Malingering is excluded because it aims at environmental gains.
13. *Disorders of impulse control not elsewhere classified*, including pathological gambling and kleptomania
14. *Adjustment disorders*—maladaptive reactions to psychosocial stress
15. *Personality disorders*: enduring, maladaptive patterns of relating to, perceiving, and thinking about the environment and oneself that cause significant impairment of social or occupational functioning or subjective distress
16. *Psychological factors affecting physical condition*

17. *Conditions not attributable to a mental disorder*, including malingering, adult antisocial behavior, and marital problems.

The placement of adult antisocial behavior in the category "Conditions not attributable to a mental disorder" is representative of the attempt in DSM-III to avoid labeling all socially deviant behavior as "mental disorder." Although a few mental health professionals believe all mental disorders are social myths (Szasz), the reasoning and evidence to the contrary are powerfully convincing (Murphy; Kendall).

Kinds of Mental Health Care

The term "mental health care" encompasses diverse preventive, therapeutic, and rehabilitative activities. Preventive mental health care aims to promote mental health and prevent specific mental disorders. Promoting mental health is an objective that is difficult to attain because it is vague— few people agree on exactly what "mental health" is. Efforts to prevent specific mental disorders have met with some success; syphilitic dementia and pellagrinous psychoses, for example, now rarely occur. The effectiveness of efforts to prevent functional mental disorders such as neuroses and alcoholism through school programs and other means remains unproven (Zusman).

Therapeutic mental health services include individual, family, and group psychotherapies; hypnosis; psychodrama; milieu therapy; medications; electroconvulusive therapy; and psychosurgery. Psychotherapies rely primarily on structured conversation to change patients' attitudes, feelings, beliefs, defenses, personality, and/or behavior. The therapist's procedures vary with his school of psychotherapy and with the nature of the patient's problem. Psychoanalysis, for example, employs techniques such as free association and interpretations based on psychoanalytic theory to bring about personality restructuring. Most forms of psychotherapy, however, have much in common (Frank). Psychotherapy, hypnosis, and psychodrama are generally used to treat mental disorders other than psychoses and organic brain syndromes. Milieu therapy involves arranging the physical setting and social organization of an inpatient ward to encourage socially acceptable and responsible behavior. Most drugs effective in treating mental disorders have been available less than 25 years. These include phenothiazines and other drugs for schizophrenia; tricyclic antidepressants and monoamine oxidase inhibitors (MAOI) for treating depression; lithium for manic-depressive psychosis; and benzodiazepines for anxiety states. Amphetamine has been used to treat hyperactive children since the 1930s. Electroconvulsive therapy, which is effective in treating certain forms of depression, schizophrenia, and mania, was introduced in

1938 (Fink). Psychosurgery, neurosurgical operations for mental disorders, was widely used to treat schizophrenia in the late 1940s and early 1950s, but is rarely used today for any mental disorder, and then usually as a treatment of last resort (Sweet; Bernstein et al.)

Rehabilitative mental health care includes occupational therapy and reeducation to help the patient return to normal living patterns. It may begin in an inpatient setting with patient-government and social activities, and can progress through transitional settings such as halfway houses, group homes, or supervised apartments. Rehabilitative care is usually required only for patients with psychoses, drug addiction, or alcoholism.

Brief History of Mental Health Care in the United States

The mentally disordered in colonial America were slightly better treated than their European counterparts: fewer were tortured, burned, hanged, or drowned as witches. The Salem witch trials of 1691–1692, during which 250 persons were tried and 19 executed, were an exception, not the rule. Throughout the colonial period, most mentally ill people were kept at home or wandered from town to town where they were lodged in jails or almshouses (workhouses). This remained the pattern until the 1840s (Shryock).

As early as 1756, however, mentally ill patients were admitted to the newly established Pennsylvania Hospital, and in 1773 the first American mental asylum was established under government auspices in Williamsburg, Virginia. These two institutions marked the beginnings of humanitarian treatment of mentally disordered patients in America, although some treatments administered within their walls until the 1800s seem barbaric; for example, bloodletting, purges, and emetics.

In the early 1800s, the Quakers and American physicians exposed to European psychiatry encouraged the view that mental illness was treatable and espoused kind and sympathetic methods. Partly as a result, a few mental hospitals were opened where "moral treatment" (combining work, recreation, education, and kind but firm management) was predominant (Bockoven). Violent patients, however, were segregated in separate wards, and in most of the country mentally disordered paupers and blacks were sent to workhouses and jails (Mora). In 1841, Dorothea Dix began her successful 30-year crusade to encourage states to build hospitals specifically for the care of the mentally ill. Many mental hospitals were built, usually in rural areas, since the countryside was believed to provide refuge from noxious urban and familial influences. Despite Dix's successes, the quality of care in state mental hospitals rapidly declined. Outright neglect and poor custodial care were fostered by the overcrowding of the hospitals with criminals, alcoholics, vagrants, and state paupers; by a tendency to build larger institutions to keep expenditures down; and by an increasing pessimism regarding the curability of mental disorders. Since mental hospitals were located away from population centers, the dismal conditions within them were easily ignored for a time. In the 1870s and 1880s a wave of reform began, with criticisms of commitment procedures, the use of restraints, and the low level of staff training (Deutsch). Between 1890 and 1900, New York State reformed its institutions for mental patients, but its example was not widely followed.

In 1908, Clifford Beers, a former mental patient, exposed the cruel conditions in public and private asylums in his autobiography, *A Mind That Found Itself*. Together with William James, Adolf Meyer, and others, Beers helped launch the National Committee for Mental Hygiene, which lobbied on behalf of the mentally disordered and carried out a national census of institutionalized mental patients until the Bureau of the Census took over in 1923. During World War I, the Surgeon General's Office asked the National Committee to organize the psychiatric branch of the Army Medical Corps. For many years the committee surveyed conditions in mental hospitals. (Inspection and accreditation of mental hospitals was not undertaken by the Joint Committee on Accreditation of Hospitals, the accrediting body for general hospitals, until 1958.)

At the beginning of this century, mental health care was primarily hospital-based, and biological approaches dominated theories of cause and treatment of mental disorders. During World War I, however, the contributions of psychological and social influences to cause and treatment were forcibly brought home to professionals and public alike. Thousands of men were rejected for service because of psychoneuroses. War neuroses ("shell shock") accounted for a large proportion of psychiatric casualties. Psychiatrists saw that situational stress could precipitate a mental disorder in "normal" individuals as well as in those with "psychopathic constitutions." Psychological and social influencing techniques were soon widely employed by military psychiatrists to treat war neuroses and return soldiers to the front (Strecker). Early intervention prevented chronic disability. These lessons were lost on the military until World War II, but psychiatrists carried them back into civilian life.

In the 1920s, the mental hygiene movement, nurtured by the National Committee for Mental Hygiene and strengthened by the psychological theories of Freud and experience gained in World War I, captured the popular imagination. As Deutsch writes:

Enthusiasm for mental hygiene swept the social work field . . . [There was an] accelerated trend toward organizing mental hygiene clinics in the community. Most of them were connected with mental hospitals; some were attached to outpatient departments of general hospitals or to social agencies, courts, and correctional institutions; some were independently created . . . the movement was oversold by overenthusiastic converts who advanced mental hygiene as a sure cure for practically every ill that beset the world. . . . (pp. 362–363)

In the 1930s, the mental hygiene movement slowed under the weight of the Depression, the limited scientific knowledge regarding prevention of mental disorders, and conflicts among various schools of psychiatric theory.

Between 1910 and World War II, psychoanalysis gradually came to dominate psychiatric training, outpatient care, and popular views of the nature of man. It did little, however, for severely disturbed individuals who, for the most part, remained in poorly funded, sparsely staffed, biologically oriented, custodial state institutions. In the 1930s, new hope for these severely disturbed patients was raised by the discovery of new biological treatments: insulin coma, cardiazol convulsive treatments, electroconvulsive therapy, and psychosurgery. The Public Works Adminstration added more than 60,000 beds to state and local mental institutions.

World War II again focused public attention on mental disorders: 1.75 million men were rejected for service because of mental or emotional disturbances and a large number of veterans returned with emotional problems. In 1946, Congress passed the National Mental Health Act, which established the National Institute of Mental Health (NIMH) and gave new federal support for mental health services, training, and research. The Veterans Administration established psychiatric hospitals and outpatient clinics. Most inpatient treatment, however, still took place in state institutions, whose deplorable conditions were graphically described by two journalists, Mike Gorman and Albert Deutsch. Partly to compensate for limited professional manpower, institutions and outpatient clinics began to use group psychotherapy, which allowed one professional to treat many patients at once.

By the mid-1950s, the number of persons hospitalized in state and county mental hospitals reached its peak, 558,900. At the same time, however, effective drugs for treating schizophrenia and mania were discovered (reserpine and chlorpromazine). These drugs replaced insulin coma and psychosurgery and allowed many patients to behave more acceptably in institutions, to leave them, or to avoid hospitalization entirely. Effective drug treatment stimulated the introduction of milieu therapy, halfway houses, and aftercare.

In 1955, Congress established the Joint Commission on Mental Illness and Health, representing 36 organizations, to examine American mental health care. The Commission's 1961 report, *Action for Mental Health*, concluded that half the patients in the state mental hospitals were not receiving active treatment. The Commission's recommendations set the stage for the emphasis on community mental health that marked the 1960s. The Commission recommended establishing one fully staffed community mental health clinic per 50,000 citizens, limiting the bed complement of psychiatric hospitals to a maximum 1,000, and employing only brief and local inpatient care.

Many of the Commission's recommendations were incorporated in a 1963 Message to Congress by President John F. Kennedy, the first presidential message Congress had ever received on behalf of the mentally ill and the mentally retarded. Congress responded with the Mental Retardation Facilities and Community Mental Health Centers Construction Act, which, in part, created federal support for community-based mental health services delivered by community mental health centers. The 1960s also saw the introduction of additional effective drug treatments for mental disorders—benzodiazepines for anxiety, tricyclic antidepressants and MAOI drugs for certain depressions, and lithium for manic-depressive psychosis. Behavior therapy became popular for treating certain neuroses and behavior disorders, and research to identify the effective elements in various psychotherapies blossomed. Congress continued to expand the NIMH financial support for psychiatric and behavioral science research, psychiatric education in medical schools, residency training of psychiatrists, and community mental health centers.

The 1970s saw a decline in federal support for mental health research and training and slow growth in funding community mental health centers. The Carter Administration renewed presidential interest in mental health, and in 1977 President Carter appointed a President's Commission on Mental Health, with Mrs. Carter as Honorary Chairperson. The Commission's 1978 Report included an extensive review of the magnitude of the nation's mental health problems and of the resources available to meet them. Detailed recommendations were made for increasing community services for chronic mental patients; improving access to care for underserved groups (children, minorities, rural citizens, and the aged); improving insurance coverage for mental health services; targeting federal manpower training support to underserved areas and population groups; increasing public understanding of mental disorders; protecting patients' rights; and expanding the knowledge base through increased federal support of research (President's Commission on Mental Health, Volume I).

The Commission's recommendations came at a time when the mental health care system had effective treatments, experience with community-based service, and a cadre of research scientists to offer. There is good evidence that some forms of psychotherapy are effective for specific mental disorders (Bergin; Malan; Smith and Glass). Effective drugs are available for treating many mental disorders (Barchas et al.). Techniques for assessing community needs for services, integrating a spectrum of services in single or multiple agencies, and evaluating the quality and outcome of care have been pioneered in community mental health centers and other settings. Despite these assets, however, the mental health care system is dwarfed by the amount of mental disorder revealed by epidemiological studies.

The Prevalence of Mental Disorders

Epidemiological studies of the prevalence of mental disorders have encountered the same problems as epidemiological studies of somatic diseases meet—deciding what constitutes a "case," establishing operational diagnostic criteria, choosing a method of case-finding. For these reasons, prevalence estimates for mental disorders have varied widely. A review of community surveys of mental disorders carried out before 1960 found one-day prevalence rates ranging from 3,640 to 33,300 per 100,000 population (Plunkett and Gordon, p. 90). A later review found estimates of psychiatric morbidity in North American and European studies ranging from about 1% to 64% of the population (Dohrenwend and Dohrenwend, p. 10). Estimates of the prevalence of psychoses like schizophrenia vary less widely, perhaps because the diagnostic criteria, though variable, are considerably less variable than those for "mental disorder" in general. Estimates of the prevalence of schizophrenia in a variety of populations range from 0.7 to 7.0 per 1,000 population, with most estimates much nearer the 0.7 figure (Gruenberg and Turns).

Based on a review of epidemiological studies and the experience of the nation's only psychiatric case register, the 1978 President's Commission concluded that at least 15% of the American population suffer from a mental disorder encompassed in the *International Classification of Diseases, Adapted for Use in the United States*. This figure excludes persons experiencing mere "problems in living" and transient emotional symptoms. Of the estimated 32 million persons in the U.S. with mental disorders in 1975, the Commission estimated that approximately 20% received treatment in the mental health sector, 3% in the general hospital inpatient/nursing home sector, 57% in the primary care/outpatient medical sector, and 20% either received no treatment or were seen by other human-service providers such as clergymen or social welfare agencies. Thus, only 1 in 5 persons with a mental disorder receives treatment from a mental health professional (Regier et al.)

Mental Health Manpower

Mental health professionals serving the mentally disordered include psychiatrists, nonpsychiatric physicians, psychologists, social workers, and registered nurses. In addition, services are provided by vocational rehabilitation counselors, occupational therapists, teachers, and other health

Table 9.1

Distribution of Staff Positions by Discipline and Status, U.S. Mental Health Facilities, January 1976

Discipline	All Staff	Full-Time	Part-Time	Trainee
Psychiatrists	13.2%	6.3%	25.9%	30.1%
Nonpsychiatric physicians	3.0	2.0	6.1	3.9
Psychologists	11.6	10.1	13.1	17.7
Social workers	17.7	18.9	13.3	18.2
Registered nurses	25.6	29.4	16.9	18.1
Other mental health professionals	22.4	26.2	17.6	9.9
Physical health professionals	6.5	7.1	7.1	2.1
Total professional patient-care staff	100.0%	100.0%	100.0%	100.0%

Source: NIMH, "Staffing of Mental Health Facilities, United States—1976." *Mental Health Statistics,* Series B, No. 14. USDHEW Publication No. (ADM) 78–522. Washington, D.C. USGPO, 1978, Table G.

workers such as licensed practical nurses. In January 1976, an NIMH survey identified 479,000 filled staff positions in 3,800 mental health facilities in the United States (National Institute of Mental Health, 1978a).* The distribution of mental health professionals working in these facilities is shown by profession in Table 9.1. Slightly more than one-third were professional patient-care staff, about 30% other patient-care staff, and about 30% nonpatient-care staff. Combining part-time and full-time staff into full-time equivalent (FTE) staff, about half of FTE professional patient-care staff were employed in state and county mental hospitals (33%) or community mental health centers (17%).

Psychiatrists

Psychiatrists are physicians with postgraduate training, usually a year's medical or other internship followed by three years of psychiatric residency training. Before being certified by a psychoanalytic institute, psychoanalytic psychiatrists (analysts) undergo additional years of part-time didactic education, a personal psychoanalysis, and supervision of their analytic treatment cases. About 10% of psychiatrists are psychoanalysts. About 50% have passed examinations entitling them to be certified in psychiatry by the American Board of Psychiatry and Neurology.

*All data cited in this chapter are those available at the time of writing early in 1980.

Table 9.2

**Distribution of All Positions by Discipline and Type of Facility,
U.S. Mental Health Facilities, January 1976**

Facility	Psychiatrist	Psychologist	Social Worker	Registered Nurse
State & county mental hospitals	28.4%	19.9%	23.0%	38.4%
Private mental hospitals	8.9	3.7	3.0	8.6
VA psychiatric services	9.6	8.2	6.3	13.5
General hospital psychiatric services	25.6	8.9	9.7	24.0
Free-standing outpatient clinics	9.4	24.3	22.2	2.1
CMHCs	14.9	29.9	26.1	11.6
Residential treatment centers	1.0	2.8	6.9	0.8
Others	4.4	4.8	5.6	2.0
All facilities	100.0%	100.0%	100.0%	100.0%

Source: NIMH, "Staffing of Mental Health Facilities, United States—1976." *Mental Health Statistics,* Series B, No. 14. USDHEW Publication No. (ADM) 78–522. Washington, D.C.: USGPO, 1978, Table 3.

By 1977, about 21,500 psychiatrists had completed training in adult psychiatry and an additional 3,358 were trained in child psychiatry (Center for Health Services Research and Development, p. 61). The growth in the number of psychiatrists will slow markedly in the next two decades unless recruitment trends change. In 1970, 12% of medical students chose psychiatric careers; by 1979, this figure had fallen to 3% (Pardes). The primary professional activity of about half of psychiatrists was office-based practice, with the other half devoting most of their time to full-time hospital work, or to a mixture of teaching, research, and administration. The distribution of psychiatrist and other professional positions in mental health facilities is shown in Table 9.2. While almost half of full-time psychiatrist positions in 1971 were in state and county mental hospitals, this percentage had decreased to 28% by 1976, primarily because of an increase in psychiatric positions in community mental health centers and private psychiatric hospitals.

Like other physicians, psychiatrists are unevenly distributed geographically, ranging in 1977 from one psychiatrist per 4,500 people in New York to one per 31,800 in North Dakota (Kole). Within states, psychiatrists are more concentrated in urban areas than is the general population. They are somewhat more maldistributed across the 50 states than pediatricians, internists, and surgeons (Marmor, p. xiv).

Psychologists

Psychologists are nonmedical professionals who may have either a master's or doctorate degree in one of many kinds of psychology, including experimental, social, general, or clinical (Shakow). Only psychologists trained in clinical psychology programs must have supervised clinical experience. Because most states license individuals generically as psychologists, any psychologist, regardless of training, can open a private practice (Meltzer). Private practice has not been the primary professional activity of most clinical psychologists (National Center for Health Statistics, 1974, p. 268). Nonetheless, psychologists are lobbying the federal and state governments for legislation to allow third-party payments to psychologists without requiring physician referral or supervision (Meltzer). In 1976, approximately 22,000 psychologists (including 15,000 clinical psychologists) were providing mental health services in mental health facilities, schools, community agencies, and private practice (National Center for Health Statistics, 1979a, p. 233).

Psychologists working in mental health facilities carry out psychotherapy, diagnostic testing, research, teaching, and administrative duties, and offer consultation to other human service agencies. Some strain exists between psychiatrists and psychologists regarding the qualifications necessary for practicing psychotherapy. On the one hand, a medical education is not needed to be a skilled psychotherapist or to counsel or treat physically well individuals whose mental disorders do not require medications. But only physicians can prescribe indicated psychotherapeutic drugs, knowledgeably treat the large proportion of psychiatric patients who suffer from both organic illnesses and mental disorder (Hall et al.; Koranyi; Babigian and Odoroff), and be relied upon to recognize organic diseases masquerading behind mental symptoms (Lishman).

Social Workers

Social workers may have a bachelor's, master's, or doctorate degree in social work. In 1976, 73% of social workers in psychiatric facilities had a master's or doctorate degree (National Center for Health Statistics, 1979a, p. 247). Social work programs are accredited by the Council on Social Work Education; by 1977, however, only 12 states licensed social workers (National Center for Health Statistics, 1979a, p. 247).

Psychiatric social work received great impetus from the mental hygiene movement and child guidance clinics of the 1920s and 1930s. The social worker obtained diagnostic information concerning the child, his parents, and environment from the child's parents, pooled this information with the psychologist and psychiatrist, and then carried out therapy with the child's parents (Modlin). Today, psychiatric social workers bring resources of community health and welfare agencies to bear on their patients' problems; continue in their diagnostic and therapeutic roles; offer consultation to human service agencies; and, to a limited degree, engage in research, teaching, and administration.

Registered Nurses

Some training in psychiatric nursing is part of all general nursing programs. A small percentage of registered nurses pursue specialized training in psychiatric nursing or other fields at the master's or doctorate level. Psychiatric nursing education was stimulated by the availability of federal funds under the 1946 Mental Health Act and by the introduction of psychotherapeutic drugs in the 1950s (O'Toole). By 1972, registered nurses were the largest group providing professional patient care in mental health facilities (National Institute of Mental Health, 1973d). Approximately 11,000 mental health nurses with master's or doctorate degrees worked in mental health facilities in 1976 (Kole).

The roles of psychiatric nurses include surpervising patients' interactions on the ward; administering medications; assisting in somatic treatments; assisting patients with activities of daily living; and, in some instances, engaging in individual, group, or family therapy. Psychiatric nurses with advanced training participate in research, teaching, and administration and offer consultation to nurses and others working in medical wards and public health agencies (O'Toole).

Training Mental Health Manpower

In 1947, when the federal government began NIMH funding of mental health manpower training, there were only 3,000 psychiatrists in the United States. By 1977, there were 25,000. In 1970, the Nixon Administration concluded that there were enough mental health professionals of all kinds and announced its intention to phase our federal training support. The mental health professions, supported by lay mental health organizations, argued before Congress against this policy decision. Barton (1972) pointed out that if federal support for psychiatry training were withdrawn, almost half the psychiatric residency positions in medical schools would be lost. Psychiatry cannot generate substantial training funds, as do most other medical specialties, from insurance benefits for care because insurance coverage for psychiatric services is much more limited. The Ford Administration continued attempts to phase out federal support for mental health manpower training, but the Carter Administration largely reversed these actions and tied support more closely to increasing the number of mental health professionals serving underserved groups.

Are more mental health professionals needed? Certain observations suggest that they are—the high prevalence of mental disorders, together with estimates of the number of patients a psychiatrist can treat in a year (Sharfstein et al.); the disparity in patient-care staffing ratios between public and private mental health facilities (National Institute of Mental Health, 1978a); and the observation that four out of five mentally disordered Americans receive treatment outside the mental health care system. But assessing manpower needs remains a thorny task: simply increasing the numbers of mental health professionals will not correct geographic maldistribution and inadequate staffing of public facilities. The current pattern of financial incentives, prestige, career opportunity paths, and conditions of work must also be changed. Moreover, the number and kinds of mental health professionals needed will be influenced by any governmentally mandated changes in the health care delivery system. Other methods of decreasing mental illness morbidity, such as mandating insurance coverage and increasing funds for preventive services and research, may be more cost-effective than attempting to redistribute manpower (Koran, 1979).

Delivery of Services

Both the public and private sectors of mental health care underserve certain groups more than others: children, the mentally retarded, the brain-damaged, alcoholics, ethnic minorities, the elderly, rural citizens, and individuals in correctional facilities (Talkington). As a result, services for these groups are receiving increased federal attention, especially through the CMHC Program discussed below.

Private Practice

In mid-1973, the American Psychiatric Association performed the first nationwide study of a random sample of private-practice psychiatrists, defined as psychiatrists spending 15 hours or more per week in private practice (Marmor). The sample, 440 psychiatrists, was skewed toward psychoanalysts. Almost all psychoanalysts are in private practice, whereas nonanalytic psychiatrists may not be. The private-practice psychiatrists saw an average of 32 patients per week, most in individual psychotherapy (including use of medications), but some in group therapy, family therapy, or couple therapy. The average fee was $35 for a 45- to 60-minute visit. Psychoanalysts estimated that 60% of their patients would require 100 or more visits to achieve the goals of therapy, whereas nonanalysts estimated that only 16% of their patients would require this many visits.

Who seeks private psychiatric treatment? The APA survey (Marmor) found that:

> . . . Professional and managerial workers are quite disproportionately represented in the private offices of psychiatrists as compared to blue- and

white-collar workers. . . . The percentage of lawyers, physicians, and social
workers receiving private psychiatric treatment ranges from 12 to 19 times
higher than their actual percentage in the work force. (pp. 38–39)

Although most of this differential can be attributed to the expense of
private care, psychiatric treatment is also socially more acceptable among
better-educated groups. (The fact that uninsured and insured patients had
the same average number of visits per year shows that expense is not the
only determining factor.) Despite common stereotypes to the contrary,
more than three-quarters of the psychiatrists' patients were rated moderately or severely functionally impaired; and the proportion of women in
private treatment (57%) did not differ significantly from the proportion
seen in public treatment settings. The 1975 National Ambulatory Medical
Care Survey produced similar results (National Center for Health Statistics, 1978a).

Outpatient Psychiatric Clinics

Over the last two decades, use of outpatient psychiatric clinics has greatly
increased: clinic outpatient care episodes in 1975 accounted for 70% of all
patient care episodes (inpatient, outpatient, and day care) recorded by
NIMH, compared to 23% in 1955. The number of outpatient care episodes
in 1975 was 12 times the number in 1955, a rise traceable to an increase in
the number of mental health professionals; the provision of services to less
severely disabled patients; the emphasis on aftercare; and the insurance
coverage for outpatient care (National Institute of Mental Health, 1977b).
In clinics that are not affiliated with inpatient facilities, the increased
volume of care has meant more care rendered by social workers and
psychologists, who constitute most of the staff; in 1976 psychiatrists
accounted for only 16% of staff in these clinics (National Institute of Mental
Health, 1978a). The nearly 2,300 outpatient psychiatric clinics operating in
1975 varied considerably in diagnostic groups served, hours of operation,
and treatment modalities offered—for example, some offered only individual psychotherapy (National Institute of Mental Health, 1973b).
  Although patients seen in outpatient clinics in 1975 resembled in sex
distribution those seen in private-practice psychiatry, there were striking
differences in terms of socioeconomic status and race. Only 9% of patients
seen in private psychiatric practice in 1977 were nonwhite, compared to
16% in outpatient psychiatric clinics in 1975 (President's Commission on
Mental Health, Vol. II, pp. 103, 110). On the other hand, the cost of a visit
to an outpatient clinic was about the same as the cost of a visit to a private
psychiatrist (National Institute of Mental Health, 1973b; American Medical Association). The difference was in the mixture of government, insur-

ance, philanthropic, and out-of-pocket dollars that paid for the services. Despite the emphasis on organized mental health care settings in many national health insurance bills considered by Congress in the 1970s, no evidence exists that services in these settings are more cost-effective than those delivered in private psychiatric practice. To legislate in favor of organized care settings in the absence of such evidence would be less than rational public policymaking.

State and County Mental Hospitals

Since the mid-1950s, state and county mental hospitals have played a progressively smaller role in the total delivery of mental health care. These hospitals accounted for half the patient care episodes recorded by NIMH in 1955, but for only 14% in 1975 (National Institute of Mental Health, 1977c). The number of resident patients declined by 60% between 1955 and 1975 (National Institute of Mental Health, 1978b; President's Commission, Vol. II, p. 94), despite an increase in admission rate every year from 1950 to 1972. As noted above, there are several reasons for the decline: the introduction of antipsychotic drugs in the mid-1950s; the proliferation of nursing and personal care homes to provide custodial care for the mentally disordered elderly; the increased availability of outpatient care and after-care; the growing efforts to prevent inappropriate admissions; the establishment of community mental health centers; and the reorganization of large mental hospitals into smaller units responsible for particular geographic areas (National Institute of Mental Health, 1974a, Statistical Note 77).

State departments of mental health have welcomed the decrease in the resident population, since fewer patients mean a higher staff-patient ratio for the same staffing costs, which should facilitate more humane and effective care. Moreover, since antipsychotic drugs were introduced, mental health professionals have come to believe that shorter hospital stays are preferable to longer stays for most patients: longer stays are associated with increased loss of social skills and family and community roles and cost the state more than shorter stays. In general, care in state mental hospitals is more expensive for the state than care in local public outpatient facilities, where federal and local funds contribute.

The decline in use of state hospitals has had negative effects, however. Many patients have been discharged into communities that are ill-prepared to provide the therapeutic and rehabilitative services they need, such as halfway houses, aftercare clinics, sheltered workshops, and rehabilitation centers (Talbott). The board and care homes to which many patients are discharged may be unlicensed and uninspected. As Greenblatt and Glazier note: "Without appropriate standards and monitoring procedure, the chronically mentally ill may be prey to incompetent or mercenary caregivers" (p. 1137). This deficiency of local services raises the readmission rate. (Low community tolerance and, in some instances, family tolerance for socially disruptive or ineffective behavior, and the tendency of psychoses to recur despite treatment, also contribute to readmissions.) Aged mentally disordered patients may receive less humane care in nursing and personal care homes, which often use untrained staff, than in state mental hospitals.

Patients with a diagnosis of schizophrenia continue to be the largest group of state hospital admissions—almost 34% in 1975. Patients with alcohol disorders are the next-largest group, about 28% in 1975, and, together with drug abuse patients, were a rapidly growing segment of the state and county mental hospital population in the 1960s and early 1970s (National Institute of Mental Health, 1978c). Many other mental health facilities refused to treat these patients.

Despite the drop in resident population, state and county mental hospitals face a number of problems. First, they have trouble convincing most state legislatures to place a high priority on funds for mental health care (National Institute of Mental Helath, 1972a). Second, they cannot easily attract well-trained staff since they cannot compete with many other facilities or with private practice in terms of location, prestige, working conditions, or income. As a result, state hospitals rely heavily on foreign medical graduates, who are handicapped by limited psychiatric training in their medical schools, by limited educational opportunities in most state hospital psychiatric residency programs, and by language and cultural barriers (Miller et al.). State hospitals have the smallest percentage of professionals (doctors, nurses, psychologists, and social workers) on their staff of any kind of mental health facility (National Institute of Mental Health, 1978a).

A third problem is how to use buildings and staff now that the resident population has declined and the emphasis is on community care. One answer is to help urban state and county hospitals provide a range of mental health services designed around community needs. In addition, state and county hospitals can serve patients with special treatment and rehabilitative needs, e.g., chronic patients with no families, alcoholic patients, and patients dangerous to themselves or others (Demone and Schulberg.)

A fourth problem—the difficulty in finding low-cost or publicly supported aftercare services to decrease the need for readmission—is being addressed in part by the federal government's support for community mental health centers, many of which are administratively coordinated with state hospitals.

Community Mental Health Centers

The federal Community Mental Health Centers (CMHC) program was established to improve the delivery of mental health services to the entire U. S. population by eventually creating 1,500 to 2,000 centers. Each center was responsible for providing services to all residents of a geographic area, or "catchment area," that included a population of from 70,000 to 200,000 people. Centers had to provide the requisite services (inpatient care; outpatient care; 24-hour emergency service; partial hospitalization; and consultation and education services to community agencies and professional personnel). In addition, centers were encouraged to develop diagnostic, rehabilitative, precare and aftercare services (e.g., home visits and halfway houses); training activities; research and evaluation programs; and an administrative organization fostering continuity of care, accessibility of services, and community participation in planning and operating the center (Koran and Brown).

By 1975, 590 federally funded CMHCs provided 29% of the total patient care episodes in mental health facilities. The patient population treated in CMHCs contained more low-income and minority group individuals than the general population, and inner city CMHCs had much higher utilization rates than suburban or rural ones (National Institute of Mental Health, 1974a, Statistical Note 87; 1976). Patients with diagnoses of neuroses and personality disorders were the largest group admitted to care (21%), with substance abusers (13%) and depressed patients (13%) next (President's Commission, Vol. II, p. 319).

CMHCs were designed to remedy in mental health care some of the deficiencies long recognized in the U.S. health care delivery system; however, the achievement of this laudable aim has been blocked by various obstacles. Growth of nonfederal sources of funding has been slower than expected, leading Congress in 1970 to extend staffing grants from 51 months to eight years. Part of the difficuty stems from limited coverage for partial hospitalization, outpatient care, and sheltered living arrangements in most insurance policies. Some CMHCs have had difficulty in obtaining provider status under state Medicaid plans and some states have limited their participation in Medicaid. In addition, local governments often can allocate very little support to CMHCs, particularly in poverty areas. Moreover, some CMHCs aroused local opposition when, in attempts at preventing mental disorders, they plunged into local political conflicts about resource allocation. Unfortunately, CMHCs were not able to cure social inequities and injustices rooted in economics, politics, and racism (Musto). Finally, nongovernmental funds are rarely available to support preventive services like consultation and education. Nonetheless, older CMHCs depend less on federal funds than younger ones (National Institute of Mental Health, 1974a, Statistical Note 91).

The Nixon and Ford administrations attempted to limit the CMHC program to a demonstration program (Koran et al.). In the Community Mental Health Centers Amendments of 1975 (Title III of Public Law 94–63), passed over President Nixon's veto, Congress renewed its commitment to a nationwide network of centers and addressed problems identified in the first decade of the CMHC program's existence (Ochberg). The 1975 Amendments required centers to establish services for children, the elderly, drug addicts, alcoholics, and chronically and severely handicapped patients. Bilingual staff were required if non-English-speaking patients were served. The Amendments also provided grants to support consultation and education services and required centers to create utilization review and other evaluation procedures. Governing bodies of new centers were required to be consumer-dominated and to have power to select a center director and approve the budget. Unfortunately, Congressional appropriations for carrying out these mandates have been quite limited.

The Carter Administration introduced legislation designed to increase the flexibility of federal requirements for funding local mental health services (The Mental Health Systems Act), but its passage and ultimate form are uncertain. The declining participation of psychiatrists in providing services and in administering CMHCs, together with the falling percentage of CMHC caseloads that represent servere, disabling mental disorders, have led some to question whether CMHCs may evolve into social agencies rather than providers of mental health care (Fink and Weinstein; National Institute of Mental Health, 1979a). Nonetheless, the experiences of CMHCs with catchment area responsibility, multiagency agreements, continuity of care, consumer participation, and local, state, and federal politics provide a rich record to be consulted by those interested in planning improvements in general health care service delivery.

General Hospital Psychiatric Inpatient Units

The number of general hospitals with separate psychiatric inpatient services has increased dramatically since World War II, and patient-care episodes in these units more than doubled between 1955 and 1971. But because of the vast increase in outpatient patient-care episodes, inpatient units accounted for a slightly smaller percentage of all patient-care episodes in 1975 (16%) than they did in 1955 (21%) (National Institute of Mental Health, 1971, Statistical Note 23; 1977c).

General hospital psychiatric inpatient units have increased in number for several reasons (National Institute of Mental Health, 1972b). Insurance coverage for treatment of mental disorders in general hospitals gradually increased; in the 1960s, limited Medicare and Medicaid coverage for mental illness provided incentives to treat indigent psychiatric patients and to correct the classification of psychiatric patients previously given nonpsychiatric diagnoses so they could qualify for private health insurance reimbursements. In addition, the 1961 report of the Joint Commission on Mental Illness recommended that every general hospital of 100 beds or more have a psychiatric unit; federal Hill-Burton hospital construction funds were released for construction of psychiatric beds; and NIMH training grants greatly increased the number of mental health professionals.

General hospital psychiatric inpatient units offer several advantages over state mental hospitals. The ratio of full-time equivalent patient-care staff per patient is much higher (National Institute of Mental Health, 1973d; 1978a). Patients are treated close to their homes. Outpatient psychiatric services are frequently available in the same hospital or from private psychiatrists who utilize the inpatient unit. Psychiatric inpatients who have associated or coincidental physical illnesses can readily obtain medical consultation. And psychiatric units provide a base from which psychiatrists can provide consultations for medical and surgical patients with psychiatric disturbances (Lipowski). On the other hand, general hospital inpatient psychiatric units are usually not equipped to meet the vocational rehabilitation and other needs of chronically disabled mental patients.

In psychiatric units of nonpublic general hospitals, patients with depressive disorders are the largest diagnostic group, a reflection both of the treatability of depressive disorders and of these patients' ability to pay. In Veterans' Administration (VA) and public nonfederal general hospitals, patients with schizophrenia are the largest diagnostic group; because schizophrenia is more chronically disabling, these patients are less able to pay for care. In VA hospitals, patients with alcohol disorders are the second-largest diagnostic group (National Institute of Mental Health, 1973a, Statistical Note 68). The higher prevalence of alcohol disorders in the armed forces compared to the general population has not stimulated adequate preventive measures (Gunderson and Schuckit).

Private Mental Hospitals

With the rise of general hospital psychiatric inpatient units and other facilities, the contribution of private mental hospitals to mental health care has gradually declined. In 1975, these hospitals accounted for only 3% of all patient-care episodes and 18 states had no private mental hospitals (National Institute of Mental Health, 1977a; 1977c). This small percentage belies the influence of private mental hospitals on mental health care. Books written by staff psychiatrists in these hospitals—Fromm-Reichman (1950), Sullivan (1953), Stanton and Schwartz (1954), and Menninger (1963)— have strongly influenced psychiatric practice since the early 1950s.

Like psychiatric units in nongovernmental general hospitals, private mental hospitals most frequently admit patients with depressive disorders (about 42% of admissions); schizophrenic patients are the second-largest group (President's Commission, Vol. II, p. 102).

The ratio of full-time equivalent patient-care staff in private nonprofit mental hospitals is somewhat higher than in psychiatric units in general hospitals, but in private for-profit hospitals it is lower (National Institute of Mental Health, 1973d). No studies are available to indicate whether the profit motive is creating care that is more efficient or less complete.

Public Institutions for the Mentally Retarded

Persons with intelligence quotients (IQs) more than two standard deviations below the mean score of 100 on the Revised Stanford-Binet Tests of Intelligence are defined as mentally retarded. Since intelligence scores follow a normal statistical distribution, about 2.5% of the United States population is mentally retarded by this definition.

In 1975, there were 168,000 residents in public institutions for the mentally retarded, less than 3% of all mentally retarded persons (Nelson and Crocker). Of all mentally retarded persons, 5% are profoundly re-tarded and unable to take care of themselves; among institutionalized mentally retarded persons, however, almost 70% are this severely dis-abled. The number of institutionalized retarded began to decline in the 1970s and standards of medical care were promulgated by the Joint Com-mission on Accreditation of Hospitals and the U.S. Department of Health, Education and Welfare. Class-action suits, brought primarily by parents groups, have led to some improvements in funding and care, but institu-tions for the mentally retarded face the same or greater difficulties in attracting political support and professional staff as do state mental hospi-tals. Large size and the mixing of patients of all ages and degrees of mental and physical handicap also hamper treatment efforts (Cytryn and Lourie). Many institutions remain understaffed human warehouses.

Mentally retarded persons receive care in a variety of settings. Of some 123,000 patient-care episodes recorded by NIMH in 1971 involving men-tally retarded persons, about one-third took place in the mental institutions and hospitals mentioned above, about 5% in other inpatient settings, about 20% in the outpatient service of a CMHC, and about 40% in other outpa-tient settings (National Institute of Mental Health, 1973c). Both the federal and state governments support many programs, in addition to mental health care, designed to aid the mentally retarded. Among them are special education, vocational training, day care, foster care, and funds for research and training. Nonetheless, the needs of mentally retarded persons are not being adequately met (President's Commission, Vol. IV, p. 2001).

Residential Psychiatric Facilities for Children and Adolescents

Residential psychiatric facilities for children and adolescents in 1975 included 331 residential treatment centers (RTCs) for emotionally disturbed children and 24 psychiatric hospitals for children (CPHs), but no facilities such as training schools for juvenile delinquents (National Institute of Mental Health, 1972c; 1977b). RTCs provide inpatient services primarily to moderately or seriously disturbed children under 18 years of age. The programs and physical facilities are usually designed to meet patients' daily living, schooling, recreational, socialization, and routine medical care needs. Because of the large number and variety of staff needed, costs are high. Treatments include milieu therapy, psychotherapy, behavior modification, psychotropic drugs, and special education (Lewis and Solnit). CPHs differ from RTCs in serving more severely disturbed children and in relying more heavily on psychiatric and medical treatments. As a result, fewer of their staff are educators and more are mental health professionals.

There were 16,000 children under age 18 in RTCs at the beginning of 1975 and an additional 12,000 children admitted during the year. By way of comparison, 25,000 children under age 18 were admitted to state and county mental hospitals, and 43,000 to general hospital psychiatric inpatient units, most of which are not specifically designed to meet children's needs (President's Commission, Vol. II, p. 101). Moreover, RTCs and CPHs do not attempt to treat all serious mental problems of children. For example, three-quarters of RTCs and one-quarter of CPHs will not admit children who are "heavy drug users."

Day Treatment

Day-treatment patients spend most of the day at the treatment facility in structured activities, but return home in the evenings. Day-treatment services—including psychotherapy, pharmacotherapy, and occupational therapy—are used as an alternative to inpatient care, as a transition from inpatient to outpatient care or to discharge, or as a locus for rehabilitating or maintaining long-term patients. Most day-treatment facilities are affiliated with psychiatric hospitals, psychiatric units in general hospitals, or CMHCs, but some are affiliated with outpatient clinics or other mental health facilities (National Institute of Mental Health, 1974a, Statistical Note 96). Day-treatment services have grown in number in response to the increased number of patients discharged from mental hospitals in improved condition, even if not fully recovered, on antipsychotic drugs. Between 1962 and 1971, for example, the number of day-treatment settings increased sevenfold and the number of persons treated increased fourteenfold (National Institute of Mental Health, 1974a, Statistical Note 96).

Despite this impressive growth, expansion of day-treatment services has been slowed by the widespread failure of insurance policies to cover day treatment. In rural areas, long travel times also impede the use of day-treatment facilities. Day treatment accounted for only 3% of patient-care episodes in mental health facilities in 1975 (National Institute of Mental Health, 1977c).

Psychiatric Halfway Houses

Psychiatric halfway houses are nonmedical residential facilities that provide room and board in a homelike atmosphere for mentally disturbed individuals who cannot live independently, but who can work or occupy themselves productively during the day if given some support and supervision. Where they exist, halfway houses allow patients a graded transition from the extreme dependency of hospital life to the full responsibility of independent living. Like day-treatment services, halfway houses grew in number in the 1950s and 1960s to meet the needs of discharged patients partly recovered on antipsychotic drugs. In 1973, NIMH identified 209 halfway houses for psychiatric patients (with 6,000 residents). State and local governments are the largest source of funds for these halfway houses (National Institute of Mental Health, 1975).

Because patients in halfway houses are not fully recovered, residential neighborhoods usually resist the establishment of a halfway house. Fears about felonious sexual or aggressive behavior of mental patients, for which the empirical evidence is contradictory (Gulevich and Bourne; Rubin), and reasonable fears about the effects of a halfway house on property values make establishing these desirable facilities difficult (Ozarin).

Nursing Homes and Personal-Care Homes

The number of senile or otherwise mentally disordered persons in nursing homes and personal-care homes increased dramatically after the passage of Medicare legislation in 1965. Since federal Medicaid covers care in these homes for psychiatric disorders on the same basis as for general medical disorders, but limits coverage of psychiatric care in state mental hospitals, states had a clear financial incentive to transfer patients to nursing homes and personal-care homes. For example, 75% of persons aged 65 or over who were resident in long-term institutions in 1969 with diagnoses of senility or other mental disorders were in nursing homes and personal-care homes; only 23% were in state and county mental hospitals. Nonetheless, many homes did not accept mentally disordered patients (National Institute of Mental Health, 1974b).

In 1976, 20% of the 1.3 million persons in nursing homes carried a primary diagnosis of mental disorder or senility without psychosis. But when all diagnoses (primary and other) are considered, more than 415,000 were suffering from senility, about 325,000 from chronic brain syndromes, 150,000 from mental disorders, and 80,000 from mental retardation (National Center for Health Statistics, 1979b, p. 32–33). Almost 77,000 nursing-home residents had resided in mental hospitals prior to admission to the nursing home and many of the 420,000 persons transferred from general hospitals came from the psychiatric wards of these hospitals.

Because staff of nursing and personal care homes usually lack extensive training in the care of mentally disordered persons, many patients do not receive active or appropriate treatment, especially individuals in personal-care homes without nursing services. It remains to be demonstrated that these patients would not benefit from treatment, and that these homes offer a socially more economical and humane custodial care than state mental hospitals (Epstein and Simon). A growing body of evidence indicates that many elderly institutionalized mentally disordered patients can be returned to their communities if active treatment and supportive community services are available. Recommendations for preventing prolonged institutionalization include more community-based services in CMHCs, halfway houses, and psychiatric clinics; greater availability of home health care services; greater use of active treatments in institutions; and greater cooperation between disparate community agencies that serve the elderly (National Institute of Mental Health, 1974b; President's Commission, Vol. III, pp. 1117–1154).

Insurance Coverage for Mental Disorders

In 1975, approximately 73% of the noninstitutionalized population were covered by fee-for-service private health insurance and 3% were members of prepaid group health plans (National Center for Health Statistics, 1978b). As of 1978, only ten states required insurers to include a minimum level of mental health benefits in policies, and only ten others required insurers to offer such benefits (National Institute of Mental Health, 1979b). Mental health services were included, however, in more than 90% of plans, but frequently less completely than health services for physical disorders. A 1974 survey of 148 employee health benefit packages (Reed et al.) found that 32% of plans provided lesser inpatient coverage and 53% provided lesser outpatient coverage for mental health services than for physical health services. In 1974, insurance accounted for twice the percentage of expenditures for physical illness (25%) as for mental disorders (12.5%), further evidence of the discrimination against mental health services in private insurance (National Institute of Mental Health, 1979b).

These differences in coverage arose in the 1920s and 1930s, when hospital insurance began to be written. Hospital treatment for mental disorders then occurred largely in state-funded mental hospitals or in private mental hospitals used primarily by the wealthy. When nonhospital services began to be covered in the 1950s, psychoanalysis was the most common outpatient treatment for mental disorders; it was very costly and was given to individuals functioning well in the community (for example, members of the intelligentsia) as well as to the seriously disturbed. Although treatments and treatment settings have changed, these restrictions have remained because of rising health care costs, the absence of strong consumer demand for mental health coverage, and insurers' continuing fear of the potential cost of this coverage. A recent comprehensive study of utilization experience concluded, however, that mental health payments account for about 7% of total health payments when they are included in benefit packages (National Institute of Mental Health, 1979b). Further study is needed regarding the effects of benefit limitations and effects of the composition of covered populations on utilization. Unemployed persons and blue-collar workers were underrepresented in the NIMH study. The effects of omitted, uncovered costs, e.g., costs of care in state mental hospitals, also require further study (Allison and Volz). Thus, definitive conclusions about the cost of broad coverage for mental health care cannot be drawn. Yet cost should not be the determining consideration: "One does not cover a service because the cost is high or low, but rather, because the service is an essential and desirable one . . ." (Reed, 1974, p. 974). Are people with mental disorders less in need of care than people with somatic illnesses?

Detailed utilization and cost data are available for the interested reader (Goldensohn and Fink; Hustead and Sharfstein; Reed, 1975; Reed et al.; Spiro et al.; Sharfstein and Magnas). For illustrative purposes, information concerning Medicare, Medicaid, and Blue Cross/Blue Shield for federal employees is summarized here.

Medicare

The general benefits and costs to the beneficiary of Medicare, a federal program in which some health care costs of persons aged 65 and over are covered through the Social Security system, are described in Chapter 10. Under Part A (hospital insurance), benefits for inpatient treatment in a psychiatric hospital are limited to 190 days in a lifetime. Only 150 of these days (90 benefit-period days plus 60 lifetime-reserve days) can be used in any one benefit period. Benefits for psychiatric care in a certified general hospital or extended care facility are the same as for any other form of medical care. This provision has increased the use of general hospitals to provide psychiatric care for the elderly.

Under Part B (supplementary medical insurance), benefits for physicians' outpatient care for mental illness are limited to 50% of the charges or $250, whichever is less. Benefits for physicians' inpatient care for mental illness are the same as for other illnesses, i.e., not limited. One hundred home visits are also covered and may be provided by mental health agencies.

In 1975, Medicare reimbursements for mental health services under Part A were 2% of all reimbursements, and under Part B were 1% (President's Commission, Vol. II, p. 517). In comparison with the prevalence of mental disorders among the elderly, these percentages are strikingly low. After reviewing these and other data, the President's Commission on Mental Health recommended increased mental health benefits under Medicare as well as national standards for minimum mental health benefits and other service expansions and improvements under Medicaid (President's Commission, Vol. II, p. 517–526).

Medicaid

Medicaid, also described in detail in the next chapter, is a combined federal-state program to cover certain health care costs for eligible persons with incomes falling below stated levels. Eligibility standards vary from state to state. However, in no state is care of patients under age 65 in mental institutions included; the federal government views this as a responsibility long borne by the states through their own mental hospitals. Although no other restrictions by diagnosis are permitted, states can and have limited the amounts of care they will cover; for example, the number of hospital days.

Few utilization data are available, since states are not required to keep record by diagnosis. It has been noted, however, that " . . . a comprehensive program of services for the mentally ill, with emphasis on ambulatory care, is not at present a Medicaid requirement and is not included in the Medicaid plans of a number of states" (Reed et al., p. 144). This deficiency reflects the priority given by both the federal and state governments to the mental health care needs of the poor.

Blue Cross and Blue Shield Plans for Federal Employees

Hustead and Sharfstein have provided utilization data for these plans for 1973, when more than 4 million persons were covered under high-option benefits. The high-option benefits provide relatively comprehensive benefits for mental conditions. Under the high-option basic hospital and medical-surgical benefits, mental health benefits included 365 days of inpatients care per year in general hospitals or Blue Cross member hospitals, together with in-hospital psychotherapy, electroconvulsive therapy, drugs, X-rays, and laboratory services. Supplemental benefits covered other medically necessary services and supplies in or out of the hospital; the plan covered 80% of the cost of these after a deductible of $100.

Over the decade 1961–1962 to 1972, mental health services took an increasing percentage of benefit payments, rising from 3.9% to 7.1%. This increase supported the belief of some insurance planners that unlimited mental health care benefits would lead to an ever-increasing percentage of benefits being paid out for mental health services. Recent statistics tend to prove this assumption wrong; mental health benefits reached a plateau in 1973 and 1974, when they accounted for 7.3% and 7.2%, respectively, of benefit payments (Sharfstein and Magnas). The 1962–1971 increase resulted from elimination of benefit restrictions for mental disorders, and probably also reflected a greater willingness to seek psychiatric care and the more widespread availability of services.

Mental Health Care Coverage Under National Health Insurance

The broad issues in National Health Insurance (NHI) are treated in Chapter 15. Insurance coverage of mental health care under NHI can be considered in the following categories: costs, indications for and effectiveness of treatments; services and service providers that should be covered; needs for research; and consumer demand.

Insurance carriers and government officials continue to fear the costs and degree of utilization of mental health care benefits. Previously cited studies (National Institute of Mental Health, 1979b; Reed et al.; Spiro et al.; Reed, 1975; Sharfstein and Magnas), although not definitive because of benefit and population limitations, suggest that mental health services can be covered at a reasonable cost per subscriber and as a small proportion of benefits paid. Moreoever, studies suggest that when mental health care is available, utilization of other health care services decreases (Jameson, et al.). Access to costly treatments such as long-term psychoanalysis may or may not need to be limited (Sharfstein and Magnas), but similar restrictions should also apply to such costly medical or surgical procedures as long-term renal dialysis. The potential effects of different methods of cost-control should be carefully studied before they are incorporated in large-scale insurance plans (Muller and Schoenberg). Cost-control, if unwisely implemented, can seriously damage the quality of health or mental health care.

Some health insurance experts have questioned mental health coverage on the grounds that the indications for and effectiveness of psychiatric treatments are not well documented and agreement regarding diagnoses and diagnostic criteria is more limited than in other health care fields (Hall). These experts seem unaware that the indications for and effectiveness of medical and surgical treatments are constantly being tested and debated in the medical literature (Ingelfinger et al.; Koran, 1975a; Varco and Delaney). These tests and debates create medical progress. Yet treatments whose benefits are uncertain (Banta and Behney), such as tonsillectomy, coronary artery bypass surgery (Kloster et al.), certain drug treatments of cancers (Chalmers et al.), and care in coronary care units (Hiatt), have not been denied insurance coverage. If coverage were limited to those medical and surgical treatments for which incontrovertible evidence of effectiveness exists, far fewer treatments would be covered. In any case, the effectiveness of many pharmacological treatments in psychiatry is not in question (Barchas, et al.) and evidence for the effectiveness of psychotherapy is overwhelming (Bergin; Malan; Smith and Glass).

Insurers and public policymakers must be helped to understand that "effectiveness" does not mean "cure." Even today, physicians can only hope "to cure sometimes, to relieve often, to comfort always" (Strauss, p. 410). Diabetes, hypertension, multiple sclerosis, and a host of other diseases are treated, not cured. Furthermore, physicians other than psychiatrists often disagree regarding signs and symptoms, diagnostic criteria, and diagnoses (Koran, 1975b). Diagnostic disagreements, which DSM III should do much to diminish, do not justify limiting insurance coverage of mental disorders or of physical illnesses; they merely reflect the imperfect but progressing state of medical science.

A variety of mental health service providers should be covered to assure high-quality mental health services (President's Commission, Vol. II, p. 497–544). Coverage for ambulatory care services, partial hospitalization, and consultation with another health practitioner or community agency should be included. Covering services of nonphysicians is most important. Questions concerning indications for and duration of treatment by nonphysicians can perhaps be met by requiring physician referral and periodic consultation. The social services often required for adequate mental health care must be financed even if insurance is not the mechanism chosen (Muller and Schoenberg). Mental health care in halfway houses has not been well covered by insurance, although it should be. Although few people would dispute that alcohol and drug abuse frequently create disorders that necessitate physical and mental health care, full insurance coverage of these disorders remains controversial, perhaps because they are often chronic and because they bear a moral stigma.

To plan mental health service coverage most intelligently, we need to study the effects of various cost-control and quality-assurance mechanisms on utilization rates and on the level of mental health in covered populations. Research is also needed on the cost-effectiveness of treatments rendered in different settings—private practice versus public outpatient clinics, for example.

Finally, public demand would be a powerful force for bringing about adequate coverage for mental health services. Continued educational efforts to combat the stigma and myths surrounding the mentally disordered and the treatments available to them are sorely needed (Rabkin; Glasser et al.).

Legal Issues

Laws and their interpretations change with the times, and laws regulating the delivery of mental health services are no exception. In the 1960s and 1970s, legal issues receiving attention in the courts included commitment procedures, the right to treatment, the right to refuse treatment, and confidentiality (Brooks; Stone).

Civil commitment to a mental institution deprives a mentally disordered person of his liberty in exchange for treatment. The grounds for civil commitment vary in different states, but include judgments that the person is dangerous to himself or others, unable to care for physical needs, or needs care or treatment. The trend in recent years had been toward restricting the grounds for civil commitment; reducing the length of time a person can be committed by physicians without judicial review; abolishing indeterminate stays during which the patient could not initiate discharge or release; and requiring commitment through the courts with due process guarantees for longer-term commitments. In addition, the civil and personal rights of committed and voluntary patients have been given increasing statutory recognition. These rights include the right to communicate with persons outside the institution; to keep clothing and personal effects; to practice religion freely; to receive independent psychiatric examination; to manage or dispose of property; to retain licenses, permits, or privileges established by law; to enter into contracts; to marry; and to sue and be sued (McGarry and Kaplan). The Mental Health Law Project, sponsored by the American Civil Liberties Union Foundation, the American Orthopsychiatric Association, and the Center for Law and Social Policy, has been engaging in litigation and consulting with legislatures and mental health organizations to help secure these and other patient rights. Because of this attention to procedures and rights, seriously disturbed individuals are being given more humane care. But the conflicts between a patient's right to liberty, his need for care or treatment, and the state's interests in protecting his welfare and in preventing harm to others remain unresolved (Roth).

A constitutional right to treatment for involuntarily committed patients was first recognized by a court in *Wyatt* v. *Stickney* (1972). Guardians of involuntarily committed patients sued the Alabama mental health commissioner, charging that inadequate care was rendered in a state mental hospital. The federal district court judge agreed that patient had a right to treatment that included certain standards of care. With the aid of medical and psychiatric consultations, he defined these standards to include individual evaluation, active treatment, minimum staffing ratios, detailed nutritional and physical standards, and compensation for work performed. But the judgment had certain limitations: it did not apply to voluntary patients, and it set no penalty for noncompliance. The psychiatrist mental health commissioner, who did not contest the inadequacy of care at the state institutions, was fired and replaced by a finance officer. Although Alabama increased its daily per-patient expenditure, qualified mental health professionals, particularly psychiatrists, have not come forward to work in the state system because of continuing low salaries and poor working conditions.

Still, in time, *Wyatt* v. *Stickney* and similar cases may force the state legislatures to allocate more resources to institutional care of the mentally disordered and to community-based care in order to prevent costly admissions and readmissions (Kaufman). Right-to-treatment cases on behalf of the mentally retarded have had some success in this regard (McGarry and Kaplan). Right-to-treatment litigation does raise the dangerous possibility that lawyers and judges rather than mental health professionals may begin determining the details of hospital administrative practices and the adequacy of individual treatment plans. If courts intrude too far on the decision-making prerogative of mental health professionals working in state institutions and departments of health, even fewer will work there than do now (Robitscher).

The right of committed patients to refuse treatments is not well recognized. Since the committed patient is deprived of his liberty in exhange for treatment presumably in his best interest, to allow him to refuse it would seem contradictory. On the other hand, the state's coercive power must be restrained to prevent capricious application. The committed patient is usually regarded as legally incompetent to decide whether to accept particular treatments, although exceptions are made for electroconvulsive therapy and psychosurgery in a few states, on the grounds that these treatments may harm the patient or change him irrevocably. Electroconvulsive therapy, however, is much safer than many common surgical procedures, is not known to cause permanent brain damage, and brings about well-documented benefits (Fink). Committed patients' only grounds for refusing medications is religious principle (*Winters* v. *Miller*), which is now recognized by the Supreme Court. With additional litigation and statutory change, reasonable rights to refuse treatments will be ensured in all states, without erecting unnecessary legal barriers to treatment of seriously disturbed individuals.

The confidentiality of patient-psychotherapist communications has important bearings on treatment. If therapists' records or memories can be subpoenaed when a patient introduces a medical or psychiatric condition into a civil litigation (such as a divorce), the public may hesitate to consult psychiatrists or to confide in them. Moreover, the patient may be tempted to exaggerate or prolong his symptoms in therapy to aid his legal case (Dubey). Relying on the evaluation of an independent court-appointed psychiatrist has been suggested to prevent abuse of therapeutic communications, but it has not been widely written into law. Reporting to insurance companies to allow patients to obtain benefits is another area wherein a method for balancing the need for confidentiality against an outside agency's need for information has yet to be satisfactorily devised (Grossman). Protection of confidentiality will be vital in the context of national health insurance.

Conclusion

Mental health care has come a long way in the past 75 years. Asylums and private care have been supplemented by new outpatient clinics, psychiatric wards in general hospitals, day-care programs, halfway houses, and a federally mandated network of community mental health centers. Moreover, many new, effective treatments have been discovered. Still, opportunities abound for improving the delivery of mental health care and for increasing our understanding of mental disorders. Only 300 of the nation's 25,000 psychiatrists are intensively engaged in research. Adequate insurance coverage of mental disorders, legal rights of patients, and legal duties of care-giving institutions remain unresolved issues. Mental health professionals and members of the general public must still participate in the political process to generate government support for mental health services, training, and research. We hope that some readers will wish to take up these challenges in the closing decades of the 20th century.

References

Allison, T., and Volz, F. A. "Health Insurance and Psychiatric Care: Utilization and Cost." *Inquiry, 10,* 77, 1973.
American Medical Association. *Profile of Medical Practice—1973*. Chicago: American Medical Association, 1973.
American Psychiatric Association. *The Diagnostic and Statistical Manual of Mental*

Disorders (DSM-III). Washington, D.C.: American Psychiatric Association, 1980.

Babigian, H. M., and Odoroff, C. L. "The Mortality Experience of a Population with Psychiatric Illness." *American Journal of Psychiatry, 126*, 470, 1969.

Banta, H. D., and Behney, C. J. *Assessing the Efficacy and Safety of Medical Technologies*. Washington, D.C.: Office of Technology Assessment, 1978.

Barchas, J. D., et al. Eds. *Psychopharmacology: From Theory to Practice*. New York: Oxford University Press, 1977.

Barton, W. "Federal Support of Training of Psychiatrists." *Psychiatric Annals, 2*, 42, 1972.

Beers, C. W. *A Mind That Found Itself*. New York: Doubleday, 1939.

Bergin, A. E. "The Evaluation of Therapeutic Outcomes." In Bergin, A. E., et al., Eds., *Handbook of Psychotherapy and Behavior Change*. Chapter 7. New York: Wiley, 1971.

Bernstein, I. C., et al. "Lobotomy in Private Practice: Long-Term Follow-Up." *Archives of General Psychiatry, 32*, 1041, 1975.

Bockoven, J. S. *Moral Treatment in Community Mental Health*. New York: Springer Publishing Co., 1972.

Brooks, A. D. *Law, Psychiatry and the Mental Health System*. Boston: Little, Brown and Co., 1974.

Center for Health Services Research and Development. *Physician Distribution and Medical Licensure in the U. S., 1977*. Monroe, Wisconsin: American Medical Association, 1979.

Chalmers, T. C., et al. "Controlled Studies in Clinical Cancer Research." *New England Journal of Medicine, 287*, 75, 1972.

Cytryn, L., and Lourie, R. S. "Mental Retardation." In Freedman, A. M., et al., Eds., *Comprehensive Textbook of Psychiatry II*. Chapter 20.1. Baltimore: Williams and Wilkins, 1975.

Demone, H. W., and Schulberg, H. C. "Has the State Mental Hospital a Future as a Human Service Resource?" In Zusman, J., and Bertsch, E. F., Eds., *The Future Role of the State Hospitals*. Chapter 1. Lexington, Massachusetts: Heath, 1975.

Deutsch, A. "The History of Mental Hygiene." In Hall, J. K., et al., Eds., *100 Years of American Psychiatry*, p. 325. New York: Columbia University Press, 1947.

Dohrenwend, B. P., and Dohrenwend, B. S. *Social Status and Psychological Disorder: A Causal Inquiry*. New York: Wiley, 1969.

Dubey, J. "Confidentiality as a Requirement of the Therapist: Technical Necessities for Absolute Privilege in Psychotherapy." *American Journal of Psychiatry, 131*, 1093, 1974.

Epstein, L. J., and Simon, A. "Alternatives to State Hospitalization for the Geriatric Mentally Ill." *American Journal of Psychiatry, 124*, 955, 1968.

Fink, M. *Convulsive Therapy: Theory and Practice*. New York: Raven Press, 1979.

Fink, P. J.; and Weinstein, S. P. "Whatever Happened to Psychiatry? The Deprofessionalization of Community Mental Health Centers." *American Journal of Psychiatry, 136*, 406, 1979.

Frank, J. D. "Common Features of Psychotherapy." *Australian and New Zealand Journal of Psychiatry*, 6, 34, 1972.

Fromm-Reichmann, F. *Principles of Intensive Psychotherapy*. Chicago: University of Chicago Press, 1950.

Glasser, M. A., et al. "Obstacles to Utilization of Prepaid Mental Health Care." *American Journal of Psychiatry*, 132, 7, 1975.

Goldensohn, S. S., and Fink, R. "Mental Health Services for Medicaid Enrollees in a Prepaid Group Practice Plan." *American Journal of Psychiatry*, 136, 160, 1979.

Greenblatt, M., and Glazier, E. "The Phasing Out of Mental Hospitals in the United States." *American Journal of Psychiatry*, 132, 1135, 1975.

Grossman, M. "Insurance Reports as a Threat to Confidentiality." *American Journal of Psychiatry*, 128, 64, 1971.

Gruenberg, E. M., and Turns, D. M. "Epidemiology." In Freedman, A. M., et al., Eds., *Comprehensive Textbook of Psychiatry II*. Chapter 6.1. Baltimore: Williams and Wilkins, 1975.

Gulevich, G. D., and Bourne, P. G. "Mental Illness and Violence." In Daniels, D. N., et al., Eds., *Violence and the Struggle of Existence*. Chapter 11. Boston: Little, Brown and Co., 1970.

Gunderson, E. K. E., and Schuckit, M. A. "Hospitalization Rates for Alcoholism in the Navy and Marine Corps." *Diseases of the Nervous System*, 36, 681, 1975.

Hall, C. P. "Financing Mental Health Services Through Insurance." *American Journal of Psychiatry*, 131, 1079, 1974.

Hall, R. C. W., et al. "Physical Illness Presenting as Psychiatric Disease." *Archives of General Psychiatry*, 35, 1315, 1978.

Hiatt, H. H. "Protecting the Medical Commons: Who Is Responsible." *New England Journal of Medicine*, 293, 235, 1975.

Hustead, E. C., and Sharfstein, S. S. "Utilization and Cost of Mental Illness Coverage in the Federal Employees Health Benefits Program, 1973." *American Journal of Psychiatry*, 135, 315, 1978.

Ingelfinger, F. J., et al., Eds. *Controversy in Internal Medicine II*. Philadelphia: W. B. Saunders, 1972.

Jameson, J., et al. "The Effects of Outpatient Psychiatric Utilization on the Costs of Providing Third-Party Coverage." *Medical Care*, 16, 383, 1978.

Joint Commission on Mental Illnes and Health. *Action for Mental Health*. New York: Basic Books, 1961.

Kaufman, E. "The Right of Treatment Suit as an Agent of Change." *American Journal of Psychiatry*, 136, 1428, 1979.

Kendall, R. E. "The Concept of Disease and Its Implications for Psychiatry." *British Journal of Psychiatry*, 127, 305, 1975.

Kloster, F. E., et al. "Coronary Bypass for Stable Angina." *New England Journal of Medicine*, 300, 149, 1979.

Kole, D. M. "Report of the ADAMHA Manpower Policy Analysis Task Force." Alcohol, Drug and Mental Health Administration, May 1978. Rockville, Maryland. Unpublished document. (Mimeographed.)

Koran, L. M. "Controversy in Psychiatry and Medicine." *American Journal of Psychiatry, 132,* 1064, 1975a

————. "The Reliability of Clinical Methods, Data and Judgments." *New England Journal of Medicine, 239,* 642, 695, 1975b

————. "Mental Health Services in the Public and Private Sectors." *American Journal of Psychiatry, 135,* 1052, 1976.

————. "Psychiatric Manpower Ratios: A Beguiling Numbers Game?" *Archives of General Psychiatry, 36,* 1409, 1979.

Koran, L. M., and Brown, B. S. "The Community Mental Health Center." In Corey, L., et al., Eds., *Medicine in a Changing Society.* Chapter 12. St. Louis, Missouri: C. V. Mosby, 1974.

Koran, L. M., et al. "The Federal Government and Mental Health." In Hamburg, D. A., and Brodie, H. K. H., Eds., *American Handbook of Psychiatry.* Chapter 43. New York: Basic Books, 1975.

Koranyi, E. K. "Morbidity and Rate of Undiagnosed Physical Illnesses in a Psychiatric Clinic Population." *Archives of General Psychiatry, 36,* 414, 1979.

Lewis, M., and Solnit, A. J. "Residential Treatment." In Freedman, A. M., et al., *Comprehensive Textbook of Psychiatry II.* Chapter 40.4. Baltimore: Williams and Wilkins, 1975.

Lipowski, Z. J. "Review of Consultation Psychiatry and Psychosomatic Medicine. II. Clinical Aspects." *Psychosomatic Medicine, 29,* 201, 1967.

Lishman, W. A. *Organic Psychiatry.* London: Blackwell Scientific Publications, 1978.

McGarry, A. L., and Kaplan, H. A. "Overview: Current Trends in Mental Health Law." *American Journal of Psychiatry, 130,* 621, 1973.

Malan, D. H . "The Outcome Problem in Psychotherapy Research." *Archives of General Psychiatry, 29,* 719, 1973.

Marmor, J. *Psychiatrists and Their Patients.* Washington, D.C.: American Psychiatric Association, 1975.

Meltzer, M. L. "Insurance Reimbursement a Mixed Blessing." *American Psychologist, 30,* 1150, 1975.

Menninger, K. A. *The Vital Balance.* New York: Viking, 1963.

Miller, M. H., et al. "Foreign Medical Graduates: A Symposium" *American Journal of Psychiatry, 130,* 435, 1973.

Modlin, H. C. "Psychiatric Social Service Information." In Freedman, A. M., et al., Eds., *Comprehensive Textbook of Psychiatry II.* Chapter 12.6. Baltimore: Williams and Wilkins, 1975.

Mora, G. "Historical and Theoretical Trends in Psychiatry." In Freedman, A. M., et al., Eds., *Comprehensive Textbook of Psychiatry II.* Chapter 1.1. Baltimore: Williams and Wilkins, 1975.

Muller, C., and Schoenberg, M. "Insurance for Mental Health: A Viewpoint on Its Scope." *Archives of General Psychiatry, 31,* 871, 1974.

Murphy, J. "Psychiatric Labelling in Cross Cultural Perspective." *Science, 191,* 1019, 1976.

Musto, D. A. "Whatever Happened to 'Community Mental Health'?" *Public Interest*, No. 39, 53, 1975.

National Center for Health Statistics. *Health Resources Statistics—1974*. DHEW Publication No. 74–1509. Washington, D. C.: Government Printing Office, 1974.

National Center for Health Statistics. *Office Visits to Psychiatrists: National Ambulatory Medical Care Survey, United States, 1975–76, Advance Data*. No. 38, DHEW Publication No. (PHS) 78–1250. Washington, D.C.: USGPO, 1978a.

National Center for Health Statistics. "Sociodemographic and Health Characteristics of Persons by Private Health Insurance Coverage and Type of Plan: United States, 1975." *Vital and Health Statistics Advance Data*. No. 32. USDHEW Publication No. (PHS) 78–1250. Washington, D.C.: USGPO, 1978b.

National Center for Health Statistics. *Health Resources Statistics—1976–1977*. DHEW Publication No. (PHS) 79–1509. Washington, D.C.: USGPO, 1979a.

National Center for Health Statistics. *The National Nursing Home Survey: 1977 Summary for the United States*. Vital and Health Statistics, Series 13 No. 43. DHEW Publication No. (PHS) 79–1794. Washington, D.C.: USGPO, 1979b.

National Institute of Mental Health. Statistical Notes 1–25. Rockville, Maryland: National Institute of Mental Health, 1971.

————. "Private Mental Hospitals 1969–1970." *Mental Health Statistics Series A*, No. 10. HEW Publication HSM 72–9089. Washington, D.C.: Government Printing Office, 1972a.

————. "Psychiatric Services in General Hospitals, 1969–70." *Mental Health Statistics Series A*, No. 11. HEW Publication HSM 72–9139. Washington, D.C.: Government Printing Office, 1972b.

————. "Residential Psychiatric Facilities for Children and Adolescents: United States, 1971–72." *Mental Health Statistics Series A*, No. 14. HEW Publication ADM 74–78. Washington, D.C.: Government Printing Office, 1972c.

————. Statistical Notes 51–75. Rockville, Maryland: National Clearinghouse for Mental Health Information, 1973a.

————. "Outpatient Psychiatric Services 1971–1972." *Mental Health Statistics Series A*, No. 13. HEW Publications ADM 74–69. Washington, D.C.: Government Printing Office, 1973b.

————. "Utilization of Mental Health Facilities 1971." *Mental Health Statistics Series B*, No. 5. HEW Publication NIH 74–657. Washington, D.C.: Government Printing Office, 1973c.

————. "Staffing of Mental Health Facilities United States 1972." *Mental Health Statistics Series B*, No. 6. HEW Publication ADM 74–28. Washington D.C.: Government Printing Office, 1973d.

————. Statistical Notes 76–100. HEW Publication OM 2799. Washington, D.C.: Government Printing Office, 1974a.

————. "Patterns in Use of Nursing Homes by the Aged Mentally Ill."

Statistical Note 107. HEW Publication ADM 74–69. Washington, D.C.: Government Printing Office, 1974b.

—————. "Halfway Houses Serving the Mentally Ill and Alcoholics, United States, 1973." *Mental Health Statistics Series A*, No. 16. USDHEW Publication No. (ADM) 76–264. Washington, D.C.: USGPO, 1975.

—————. *Addition Rate to Federally Funded Community Mental Health Centers, United States, 1973.* Statistical Note 126. USDHEW Publication No. (ADM) 76–158. Washington, D.C.: USGPO, 1976.

—————. "Private Psychiatric Hospitals, 1974–75." *Mental Health Statistics Series A*, No 18. USDHEW Publication No. (ADM) 77–380. Washington, D.C.: USGPO, 1977a.

—————. *Residential Treatment Centers for Emotionally Disturbed Children 1975–76.* Statistical Note 135. USDHEW Publication No. (ADM) 78–158. Washington, D.C.: USGPO, 1977b.

—————. *Provisional Data on Patient Care Episodes in Mental Health Facilities—1975.* Statistical Note 139. USDHEW Publication No. (ADM) 77–158. Washington, D.C.: USGPO, 1977c.

—————. "Staffing of Mental Health Facilities, United States—1976." *Mental Health Statistics Series B*, No. 14. USDHEW Publication No. (ADM) 78–522. Washington, D.C.: USGPO, 1978a.

—————. *Changes in the Age, Sex and Diagnostic Composition of the Resident Population of State and County Mental Hospitals, United States, 1965–1975.* Statistical Note 146. USDHEW Publication No. (ADM) 78–158. Washington, D.C.: USGPO, 1978b.

—————. *Changes in the Age, Sex and Diagnostic Composition of Additions to State and County Mental Hospitals, United States, 1969–1975.* Statistical Note 148. USDHEW Publication No. (ADM) 78–158. Washington, D.C.: USGPO, 1978c.

—————. "CMHC Staffing: Who Minds the Store." *Mental Health Statistics Series B*, No. 16. DHEW Publication No. (ADM) 78–686. Washington, D.C.: USGPO, 1979a.

—————. *Analysis of State Programs Which Mandate Mental Health Benefits Under Private Health Insurance.* Final Report of Contract #278–78–0040 MH. Rockville, Maryland: June 1979b.

Nelson, R. P., and Crocker, A. C. "The Medical Care of Mentally Retarded Persons in Public Residential Facilities." *New England Journal of Medicine, 299,* 1039, 1978.

Ochberg, F. M. "Community Mental Health Center Legislation: Flight of the Phoenix." *American Journal of Psychiatry, 133,* 56, 1976.

O'Toole, A. W. "Psychiatric Nursing." In Freedman, A. M., et al., Eds., *Comprehensive Textbook of Psychiatry II.* Chapter 47. Baltimore: Williams and Wilkins, 1975.

Ozarin, L. D. "Community Alternatives to Institutional Care." *American Journal of Psychiatry, 133,* 69, 1976.

Pardes, H. "Future Needs for Psychiatrists and Other Mental Health Personnel." *Archives of General Psychiatry, 36,* 1401, 1979.

Plunkett, R. J., and Gordon, J. E. *Epidemiology and Mental Illness*. New York: Basic Books, 1960.

President's Commission on Mental Health. *Report to the President—1978*, Volumes I–IV. Washington, D.C.: USGPO, 1978.

Rabkin, J. "Public Attitudes Toward Mental Illness: A Review of the Literature." *Schizophrenia Bulletin*, 10, 9, 1974.

Reed, L. S. "Utilization of Care for Mental Disorders Under the Blue Cross and Blue Shield Plan for Federal Employees, 1972." *American Journal of Psychiatry*, 131, 964, 1974.

————. *Coverage and Utilization of Care for Mental Conditions under Health Insurance—Various Studies, 1973–74*. Washington, D.C.: American Psychiatric Association, 1975.

Reed, L. S., et al. *Health Insurance and Psychiatric Care: Utilization and Cost*. Washington, D.C.: American Psychiatric Association, 1972.

Regier, D. A., et al. "The DeFacto U. S. Mental Health Services System." *Archives of General Psychiatry*, 35, 685, 1978.

Robitscher, J. "Implementing the Rights of the Mentally Disabled: Judicial Legislative and Psychiatric Action." In Ayd, F. J., Jr., et al., Eds., *Medical, Moral and Legal Issues in Mental Health Care*. Chapter 9. Baltimore: Williams and Wilkins, 1974.

Roth, L. H. "A Commitment Law for Patients, Doctors and Lawyers." *American Journal of Psychiatry*, 136, 1121, 1979.

Rubin, B. "Prediction of Dangerousness in Mentally Ill Criminals." *Archives of General Psychiatry*, 27, 397, 1972.

Shakow, D. "Clinical Psychology." In Freedman, A. M., et al., Eds., *Comprehensive Textbook of Psychiatry II*. Chapter 46. Baltimore: Williams and Wilkins, 1975.

Sharfstein, S. S., and Magnas, H. L. "Insuring Intensive Psychotherapy." *American Journal of Psychiatry*, 132, 1252, 1975.

Sharfstein, S. S., et al. "Private Psychiatry and Accountability: A Response to the APA Task Force Report on Private Practice." *American Journal of Psychiatry*, 132, 43, 1975.

Shryock, R. H. "The Beginnings: From Colonial Days to the Foundation of the American Psychiatric Associaton." In Hall, J. K., et al., Eds., *100 Years of American Psychiatry*. New York: Columbia University Press, 1947.

Smith, M. L., and Glass, G. V. "Meta-Analysis of Psychotherapy Outcome Studies." *American Psychologist*, 32, 752, 1977.

Spiro, H. R., et al. "Fee-for-Service Insurance versus Cost Financing, Impact on Mental Health Care Systems." *American Journal of Public Health*, 65, 139, 1975.

Stanton, A. H., and Schwartz, M. S. *The Mental Hospital*. New York: Basic Books, 1954.

Stone, A. A. *Mental Health and Law: A System in Transition*. National Institute of Mental Health, HEW Publication 75–176, 1975.

Strauss, M. B., Ed. *Familiar Medical Quotations*, Boston: Little, Brown, and Co., 1968.

Strecker, E. A. "Military Psychiatry: World War I 1917–1918." In Hall, J. K., et al.,

Eds., *100 Years of American Psychiatry*. New York: Columbia University Press, 1947.

Sullivan, H. S. *The Interpersonal Theory of Psychiatry*. New York: W. W. Norton, 1953.

Sweet, W. H. "Treatment of Medically Intractable Mental Disease by Limited Frontal Leucotomy—Justifiable?" *The New England Journal of Medicine*, *289*, 1117, 1973.

Szasz, T. S. *The Myth of Mental Illness*. New York: Hoecker–Harper, 1961.

Talbott, J. A., Ed. *The Chronic Mental Patient*. Washington, D.C.: American Psychiatric Association, 1978.

Talkington, P. C. *Delivering Mental Health Services: Needs, Priorities and Strategies*. Washington, D.C.: American Psychiatric Association, 1975.

Varco, R. L., and Delaney, J. P. *Controversy in Surgery*. Philadelphia: Saunders, 1976.

Winters v. *Miller* 446 F 2nd 65 (2nd Cir 1971).

Wyatt v. *Stickney* 344 F Supp. 373 (MD Ala 1972).

Zusman, J. "Secondary Prevention." In Freedman, A., et al., Eds., *Comprehensive Textbook of Psychiatry II*. Chapter 43.3 Baltimore: Williams and Wilkins, 1975.

10

Financing for Health Care

Carol McCarthy

Introduction

Up until now we have been discussing the people and institutions involved in the health care delivery system; we have seen that they interact in complex ways. These relationships are brought about by the medium of money and its exchange for goods and services. In this chapter we turn our attention to the financing of health care delivery: what the money buys, where it comes from, how it is paid out, and how the medical marketplace works. Since constantly rising expenditures have been a feature of the U. S. health care delivery system since such data were first collected in 1929 (except for a few years during the Depression), this topic will also receive attention.

As Table 10.1 shows, it has been estimated that in the calendar year 1978, $192.4 billion was spent for health purposes in the United States (Gibson, 1979), representing 9.1% of that year's Gross National Product (GNP). In 1950, health expenditures had totaled only $12.7 billion, 4.5% of the GNP; in 1965, $43 billion, 6.2% of the GNP. Since 1965, outlays for health have risen, on the average, more than 12% each year. Per capita, in 1978, the United States spent about $863 on health services in comparison with a 1929 expenditure of about $30. Since 1929, the population has almost doubled, while expenditures for health care increased fiftyfold. In terms of contribution to the national income, by 1977 the health services industry was the fifth largest in the country, following retail trade, real estate, wholesale trade, and construction (Bureau of the Census, 1978, Table 721).

What Does the Money Buy?

Until 1979, statistics on health care financing were gathered by the Office of Research and Statistics of the Social Security Administration (SSA) and published in the Social Security Bulletin. That year, the Office of Research, Demonstrations and Statistics of the Health Care Financing Administration (HCFA) took over the task, and recent statistical compilations are published in the HCFA series, *Health Care Financing Review*.

Table 10.1

Aggregate and Per Capita National Health Expenditures, by Source of Funds and Percent of Gross National Product, Selected Calendar Years, 1929–1978

Calendar year	GNP¹	Total Health Expenditures			Private Health Expenditures			Public Health Expenditures		
		Am't.¹	Per capita	% of GNP	Am't.¹	Per capita	% of total	Am't.¹	Per capita	% of total
1929	$ 103.1	$ 3.6	$ 29.49	3.5	$3.2	$ 25.49	86.4	$ 0.5	$ 4.00	13.6
1935	72.2	2.9	22.65	4.0	2.4	18.30	80.8	0.6	4.34	19.2
1940	99.7	4.0	29.62	4.0	3.2	23.61	79.7	0.8	6.03	20.3
1950	284.8	12.7	81.86	4.5	9.2	59.62	72.8	3.4	22.24	27.2
1955	398.0	17.7	105.38	4.4	13.2	78.33	74.3	4.6	27.05	25.7
1960	503.7	26.9	146.30	5.3	20.3	110.20	75.3	6.6	36.10	24.7
1965	688.1	43.0	217.42	6.2	32.3	163.29	75.1	10.7	54.13	24.9
1966	753.0	47.3	236.51	6.3	34.0	169.81	71.8	13.3	66.71	28.2
1967	796.3	52.7	260.35	6.6	33.9	167.61	64.4	18.8	92.74	35.6
1968	868.5	58.9	288.17	6.8	37.1	181.40	63.0	21.8	106.76	37.0
1969	935.5	66.2	320.70	7.1	41.6	201.83	62.9	24.5	118.87	37.1
1970	982.4	74.7	358.63	7.6	47.5	227.71	63.5	27.3	130.93	36.5
1971	1,063.4	82.8	393.09	7.8	51.4	244.12	62.1	31.4	148.97	37.9
1972	1,171.1	92.7	436.47	7.9	57.7	271.78	62.3	35.0	164.69	37.7
1973	1,306.6	102.3	478.38	7.8	63.6	297.17	62.1	38.8	181.22	37.9
1974	1,412.9	115.6	535.99	8.2	69.0	319.99	59.7	46.6	216.00	40.3
1975	1,528.8	131.5	604.57	8.6	75.8	348.61	57.7	55.7	255.96	42.3
1976	1,700.1	148.9	678.79	8.8	86.6	394.73	58.2	62.3	284.06	41.8
1977	1,887.2	170.0	768.77	9.0	100.7	455.27	59.2	69.3	313.50	40.8
1978²	2,107.6	192.4	863.01	9.1	114.3	512.62	59.4	78.1	350.40	40.6

Source: R. M. Gibson, "National Health Expenditures, 1978," *Health Care Financing Review, 1,* Summer 1979, Table 1.
¹ In billions of dollars.
² Preliminary estimates (See Appendix I, A13.)

National health care expenditures are considered under two categories: (1) research and medical facilities construction and (2) payments for health services and supplies. Personal health care expenses constitute the bulk of the latter, $167.9 billion in 1978 (Gibson, 1979, Table 3). Five types of personal health care expenditure accounted for about 80% of the total 1978 dollar outlay (see Table 10.2): 39.5% went to hospitals, approximately 18% to physicians, 8% for nursing home care, another 8% for drugs and drug sundries, and 7% for dentists' services. The other categories of expenditures are: "other professional services," such as podiatry and private speech therapy, 2.2%; eyeglasses and appliances, 2%; "other health services," 2.3%; administrative expenses, 5.2%; government public health activities, 2.6%; and construction, 2.7%. The costs of medical education are not included in these Health Care Financing Administration figures, except insofar as they are inseparable from hospital expenditures and biomedical research.

Thus, hospital services are the greatest drain on the health care dollar. Most appropriately, since the 1976 amendments to the Social Security Act (P. L. 90–248), interest has focused on the development of programs for reimbursing hospitals through federal payment and private insurance mechanisms that incorporate incentives for economy while maintaining quality of care (Bauer; McCarthy; Sigmond; Wolkstein). It is also worth noting the relatively low rate of increase over the years in expenditures for drugs, given that some of the major advances against morbidity and mortality in this century are attributable to the discovery and application of such therapeutic agents (Fuchs, 1974, pp. 105–121).

Where the Money Comes From

Ultimately, of course, the people pay all health care costs. Thus, when we say that health care monies come from different sources, we really mean that dollars take different routes on their way from consumers to providers of care. The three major routes are direct payment from consumer to provider; through government; and through private insurance companies, profit and nonprofit. In 1978, approximately 33% of expenditures were directly out of pocket ($55.3 billion); the public share was about 39% (about $65 billion), with the federal government bearing almost three-fourths of that; and 27% was paid through insurance companies (over $45 billion). The balance, 1.3% ($2.2 billion), was provided by philanthropy and by industry for in-plant health services (Gibson, 1979, Table 7.)

Public Outlays

The amount transferred by the public sector in 1978 ($65 billion, 39% of the total) compares with 24.8% in 1966, 22.4% in 1950, 14.7% in 1935, and 9% in 1929 (Gibson, 1979, Table 7.) The increase is largely due to greater federal expenditures. Proportionately, state and local government outlays have remained rather constant over time, in the 11%–13% range. They accounted for 11% of the total in 1978. In contrast, the federal share of outlays rose from 12.9% in 1966 to 20.8% in 1967, to almost 28% in 1978 (Gibson, 1979, Table 7.) This significant rise in federal spending is accounted for by the Medicare and Medicaid programs, Titles XVIII and XIX, respectively, of the Social Security Act.

Medicare. Medicare was inaugurated on July 1, 1966. It provided a limited range of medical care benefits for persons aged 65 and over who were covered by the Social Security system. In July 1973, benefits were extended to the disabled and their dependents, and those suffering from chronic kidney disease (Russel et al., p. 49). Part A of the program, financed by payroll taxes collected under the Social Security system, provides coverage for care rendered in a hospital, an extended care facility, or the patient's home. Part B, a voluntary supplemental program that pays certain costs of doctors' services and other medical expenses, is supported in part by general tax revenues and in part by contributions paid by the elderly (Somers and Somers, p. 15). Neither Part A nor Part B of Medicare, however, offers comprehensive coverage. Built into the program are deductibles (set amounts the patient must pay for each type of service each year before Medicare begins to pay) and co-payments (a percentage of charges paid by the patient). Limitations on the amount of coverage exist as well. Hospital benefits cease after 90 days if the patient has exhausted his lifetime reserve pool of 60 additional days; extended-care facility benefits end after 100 days. Home health care visits are limited to 100 (Russel et al., p. 51).

The 1972 amendments to the Social Security Act also extend benefits to persons 65 and over who do not meet the criteria for the regular Social Security program but who are willing to pay a premium for both Part A and Part B coverage. The amendments provide as well for the establishment of Professional Standards Review Organizations (PSROs) to monitor the quality and quantity of institutional services delivered to Medicare and Medicaid recipients.

Medicare was intended to stimulate the use of less costly mechanisms for acute care services. Reimbursement was therefore made available on a limited basis to home health care programs and extended care facilities (ECFs). Payments to nursing homes occur in instances where those homes qualify as ECFs (Coe et al.). For a further discussion of the principles of Medicare and Medicaid, see Chapter 15.

In brief, Medicare provides the elderly with some protection in time of illness but does not pay the whole bill. Spending under Medicare rose from $3.2 billion in 1967 to $18.3 billion in 1977, but as Table 10.3 shows, only 44.3% of the $41.3 billion dollars that went for personal health care for the

Table 10.2

Aggregate and Per Capita Amount and Percentage Distribution of National Health Expenditures, Selected Calendar Years 1970–1978

Type of expenditure	1970	1971	1972	1973	1974	1975	1976	1977	1978¹
				Aggregate amount in (millions of dollars)					
Total	$74,740	$82,764	$92,679	$102,345	$115,610	$131,465	$148,870	$169,994	$192,448
Health services and supplies	69,449	76,773	86,210	95,627	108,306	123,211	140,064	161,247	183,007
Personal health care expense	65,723	72,115	79,870	88,471	100,885	116,297	132,127	149,139	167,911
Hospital care	27,799	30,769	34,974	38,585	44,857	52,138	59,806	67,914	76,025
Physicians' services	14,340	15,918	17,162	19,075	21,245	24,932	27,658	31,242	35,250
Dentists' services	4,750	5,068	5,625	6,531	7,366	8,237	10,131	11,650	13,300
Other professional services	1,595	1,628	1,802	1,973	2,230	2,619	3,202	3,700	4,275
Drugs and drug sundries	8,406	8,745	9,344	10,050	11,038	11,812	12,809	13,810	15,098
Eyeglasses and appliances	2,100	2,035	2,215	2,480	2,706	2,981	3,201	3,455	3,879
Nursing-home care	4,677	5,629	6,151	7,088	8,355	9,886	11,452	13,364	15,751
Other health services	2,058	2,323	2,597	2,690	3,088	3,691	3,868	4,005	4,333
Expenses for prepayment and administration	2,286	2,854	4,300	4,897	4,664	3,717	4,204	7,844	10,022
Government public health activities	1,440	1,804	2,040	2,259	2,757	3,198	3,733	4,264	5,073
Research and medical facilities construction	5,291	5,991	6,469	6,718	7,304	8,254	8,806	8,746	9,441
Research	1,862	1,983	2,227	2,402	2,632	3,186	3,552	3,714	4,287
Construction	3,429	4,008	4,242	4,316	4,672	5,068	4,254	5,032	5,154

Per capita amount [2]

Total	$358.63	$393.09	$436.76	$478.38	$535.99	$604.57	$678.79	$768.77	$863.01
Health services and supplies	333.25	364.64	406.00	446.98	502.12	566.61	638.64	729.22	820.68
Personal health care expense	315.25	342.52	376.14	413.53	467.72	534.82	602.45	674.46	752.98
Hospital care	133.39	146.14	164.71	180.35	207.97	239.77	272.69	307.13	340.93
Physicians' services	68.81	75.60	80.82	89.16	98.49	114.66	126.11	141.29	158.08
Dentists' services	22.79	24.07	26.49	30.52	34.15	37.88	46.19	52.69	59.64
Other professional services	7.65	7.73	8.49	9.22	10.34	12.04	14.60	16.73	19.17
Drugs and drug sundries	40.33	41.54	44.00	46.98	51.17	54.32	58.40	62.45	67.70
Eyeglasses and appliances	10.07	9.67	10.43	11.59	12.55	13.71	14.60	15.62	17.40
Nursing-home care	22.44	26.74	28.97	33.13	38.73	45.46	52.22	60.44	70.64
Other health services	9.87	11.03	12.23	12.57	14.32	16.97	17.64	18.11	19.43
Expense for prepayment and administration	10.93	13.56	20.25	22.89	21.62	17.09	19.17	35.47	44.94
Government public health activities	6.91	8.57	9.61	10.56	12.78	14.71	17.02	19.28	22.75
Research and medical facilities construction	25.39	28.45	30.47	31.40	33.86	37.96	40.15	39.55	42.34
Research	8.93	9.42	10.49	11.23	12.20	14.65	16.19	16.80	19.23
Construction	16.45	19.04	19.98	20.17	21.66	23.31	23.96	22.76	23.11

Source: R. M. Gibson "National Health Expenditures, 1978," Health Care Financing Review, 1, Summer 1979, Table 3.

[1] Preliminary estimates (see Appendix I, A13).

[2] Based on July 1 population estimates including outlying territories, armed forces and federal employees overseas, and their dependents.

aged in fiscal 1977 was paid for by Medicare. Nor was coverage uniform: 74% of hospital care costs was covered; 56% of physicians' charges; 52% of "other professional services," and only 3% of nursing home expenses. Even after other government programs and supplementary private health insurance were taken into account, 1977 per capita out-of-pocket expense for the elderly was $613, approximately 35% of costs (Gibson and Fisher, 1979). The dimensions of the problem emerge when data from the 1970 census are presented: 58% of elderly individuals were in families with less than $5,000 income; only 18% had family incomes over $10,000.

Medicaid. Unlike Medicare, Medicaid is a program run jointly by federal and state governments: the name is more or less a blanket label for 49 different state progams. (Arizona has no Medicaid program.) Designed specifically to serve the poor, Medicaid provided, as of January 1967, federal funds to states on a cost-sharing basis (according to each state's per capita income), so that welfare recipients could be guaranteed medical services. Payment in full was to be afforded to the aged poor, the blind, the disabled, and families with dependent children if one parent was absent, unemployed, or unable to work. Four types of care were covered: (1) inpatient and outpatient hospital care; (2) other laboratory and X-ray services; (3) physician services; and (4) skilled nursing care for persons over 21. By July 1970, home health services and early and periodic detection and treatment of disease for persons under 21 were also covered.

The 1972 Social Security Act amendments added family planning to the list of "musts." Prescriptions, dental services, eyeglasses, and care in an "intermediate facility" (institutions that do not qualify as skilled nursing homes or those serving the mentally retarded) are allowable "optionals," as is coverage of the medically indigent (those who are self-supporting except for medical care costs). Under the 1972 amendments, coverage of the medically indigent is, by law, tied to their payment of monthly premiums, the amount being graduated by income. Deductibles and co-payments are also allowed on all services for the medically indigent and on optional services for welfare recipients (Russel et al., p. 53).

Those who pass a means test proving that their income is below state-established poverty levels must be supplied with the basic services without charge in any state participating in the Medicaid program. Limits on covered benefits are, however, left to the individual state, which, along with the variety of options allowed, has resulted in a wide diversity of operative programs. New York and California, for instance, established such broad programs that in 1976 they received 34% of total Medicaid expenditures (USDHEW, 1978).

There has been a continuing increase in spending for Medicaid. In 1968, federal outlays for the program totaled $1.8 billion. By 1978, total federal,

Table 10.3

Estimated Amount and Percentage Distribution of Personal Health Care Expenditures for Persons Aged 65 and Over, by Type of Expenditure and Source of Funds, Year Ending September 1977 [1]

Type of expenditure	Amount (in millions) of dollars						Percentage distribution				
			Public					Public			
	Total	Private	Total	Medicare	Medicaid	Other	Private	Total	Medicare	Medicaid	Other
Total	$41,256	$13,624	$27,631	$18,282	$6,890	$2,459	33.0%	67.0%	44.3%	16.7%	6.0%
Hospital care	$18,185	$2,140	$16,045	$13,533	$638	$1,874	11.8%	88.2%	74.4%	3.5%	10.3%
Physicians' services	7,145	2,889	4,255	3,975	221	60	40.4	59.6	55.6	3.1	.8
Dentists' services	1,022	976	46	......	31	15	95.5	4.5	......	3.1	1.4
Other professional services	816	325	490	425	61	4	39.9	60.1	52.1	7.5	0.5
Drugs and drug sundries	2,859	2,423	436	......	418	18	84.7	15.3	......	14.6	0.6
Eyeglasses and appliances	312	303	9	......	9	9	97.2	2.8	......	......	2.8
Nursing-home care	10,536	4,535	6,001	349	5,325	328	43.0	57.0	3.3	50.5	3.1
Other health services	381	33	348	......	196	152	8.8	91.2	......	51.3	39.9

Source: R. M. Gibson and C. R. Fisher "Age Differences in Health Care Spending, Fiscal Year 1977," *Social Security Bulletin, 42*, January 1979, Table 6. (See Appendix I, A12, 13.)
[1] Preliminary estimates.

state, and local expenditures under Medicaid had reached $18.4 billion, about 56% of it federal (Gibson, 1979, Table 6). These monies provided services for approximately 23 million American eligible poor. Excluded from benefits were most working poor, childless couples, the medically indigent in 27 states, and in 26 states, low-income families with an unemployed father present (Russel et al., pp. 54–56, 64). Estimates made in 1974 by the Office of Research and Statistics of the Social Security Administration indicate that 9 million persons officially designated as "poor" were still excluded from Medicaid coverage (Mueller).

In 1978, Medicaid and Medicare accounted for two-thirds of public outlays for personal health care services. The next-largest expenditure category, state and local government dollar support for their own hospitals, totaled $5.5 billion in 1978—up 6% from the previous year (Gibson, 1979, derived from Table 6). Included here are funds used to operate psychiatric hospitals and other long-term care facilities, as well as acute-care general hospitals at the county and municipal levels.

Other public expenditures. There are four remaining significant personal health care categories for which government monies are spent: (1) federal outlays for hospital and medical services for veterans ($4.9 billion in 1978, 7.6% of public personal health care expenditures); (2) provision of care by the Department of Defense for the armed forces and military dependents (in 1978, $3.6 billion, 5.6%); (3) workmen's compensation medical benefits ($3.1 billion, 4.7%); and (4) other federal, state, and local outlays for personal health care ($3.5 billion, 5.4% in 1978), including support for maternal and child health programs, vocational rehabilitation, Public Health Service and other federal hospitals, the Indian Health Service, temporary disability insurance, and the Alcohol, Drug Abuse, and Mental Health Administration. In contrast, all government public health activities are recorded as costing only $5.1 billion in 1978. It must be noted, however, that while federal prevention and control operations are included in toto in this figure, excluded are funds expended by other than health departments at the state and local levels for air and water pollution control, sanitation, and sewage treatment (Gibson, Table 6, p. 18).

The relatively low level of government funding for public health activities deserves special attention in view of the growing recognition of the relationship between the environment and health and the importance of preventive care and health promotion. Unfortunately, as experience in all fields shows, voiced interest without dollar support seldom moves beyond the interest stage.

The programs of the Veterans' Administration and the Department of Defense are described in Chapter 11. The programs for general hospital and medical care of the United States Public Health Service and Indian

Health Service, state mental and tuberculosis hospitals, and local government hospitals, primarily for the poor, are described in Chapters, 7, 9, and 11.

Workmen's compensation is an insurance system operated by the states, each with its own law and program, which provides covered workers with some protection against the costs of medical care and loss of income resulting from work-related injury and, in some cases, sickness (U.S. National Commission on State Workmen's Compensation Laws; Congressional Research Service; Price, 1979a, 1979b). The first workmen's compensation law was enacted in New York in 1910; by 1948, all states had enacted such laws. The theory underlying workmen's compensation is that all accidents, irrespective of fault, must be regarded as risks of industry, and that the employer and employee shall share the burden of the loss: the employer by paying in money and the employee by losing a portion of his/her wages. As of 1977, $7.2 billion, including $2.5 billion in hospital and medical benefits, were paid out under state programs. In addition, $1.5 billion was paid out by the federal government to persons including its own employees and beneficiaries of the Black Lung program (Bureau of the Census, 1979, Table 522).

On July 31, 1972, the National Commission on State Workmen's Compensation Laws reported on the status of such laws. The commission recognized the important role the states had played, but found the protection given by such laws to be inadequate and inequitable. The commission made 84 recommendations, of which 19 have been considered "essential" by the Department of Labor. These include compulsory, universal coverage, full coverage for occupational diseases, no limitations on medical care and rehabilitative services, standards for the amount of benefits for death and for permanent and temporary total disability, and principles relating to extraterritorial coverage (coverage for injuries suffered while working for U.S. companies outside of the U.S.). The commission also recommended including all its recommendations as mandates in federal legislation applicable to all employers. There have been several attempts in Congress to pass legislation putting the commission's regulations into effect. Primarily due to opposition from industry, no bills on the subject had made it out of committee by 1980. The Department of Labor does keep tabs on the states' own efforts to implement the commission's recommendations. As of 1980, on the average nationally among the states, about 65% of the "essential" recommendations had been implemented at least to some extent (U.S. Department of Labor).

For research and facilities construction, public spending in the late 1970s was also on the rise. Dollars devoted to construction totaled approximately $1.9 billion in 1978. Public outlays for research totaled almost $4 billion in 1978, with the federal government the source for all but $312

million (Gibson, 1979, Table 4). Another $296 million for research came
from private sources. Although expenditures for biomedical research represent a small percentage of total health outlays (2.2%), their effects are
far-reaching. Federal research dollars not only increase the probability of
advancements in disease prevention and control but also provide about
one-quarter of medical school revenues (American Medical Association,
Table 29).

Private Health Care Expenditures

The bulk of private health care expenditures comes from two sources: the
individual receiving treatment and the private insurer making payment on
his behalf. In 1978, their combined contributions totaled $100.6 billion,
59.9% of all personal health care expenditures. In 1965, prior to the advent
of Medicare and Medicaid, their share was 76.9%; in 1935, 82.4%; in 1929,
88.4% (Gibson, 1979, Table 7). This decline in the private share of total
expenditures is due primarily to the sharp drop in out-of-pocket payments
that is associated with increased federal spending. In 1965, for example,
53% of personal health care expenditures was paid directly by the patient;
in 1978, only 33%. Unfortunately, however, because of inflation and other
factors, the per capita dollar amount paid directly in 1978 was 2½ times
what it was in 1965 (Gibson, 1979, p. 14).

Private insurers have paid between 20% and 28% of personal health care
costs since 1965. Their share was $45.3 billion in 1978, 27% of the total
(Gibson, 1979, Table 7). But it is not the dollar figure alone that focuses
attention on the private insurance industry. Medicare, and Medicaid to a
limited extent, utilize the industry in a middle-man capacity, as a "fiscal
intermediary." Several of the major national health insurance plans proposed are based on the private insurance mechanism, as discussed in
Chapter 15.

Americans questioned on health care problems more often than not cite
the expense, confusion, or inadequacies of their insurance policies (Strick-
land). Commentators like Sylvia Law (1974) charge the not-for-profit Blue
Cross operation with lack of public responsiveness and accountability.
Private insurance is both an important and a controversial part of the
American system of payment for health care.

Before considering private health insurance in any depth, the manner in
which the term "insurance" is used in the health care industry should be
clarified. "Insurance" originally meant, and still usually refers to, the
contribution by individuals to a fund for the purpose of providing each
contributor with protection against financial losses following the occurrence of a relatively unlikely but damaging event. Thus, there is insurance
against fire, theft, death at an early age. All of these events occur within a

group of people at a predictable rate but are rare occurrences for any one individual in the group.

Medical insurance, when it began, was in this tradition. From 1847, when the first commercial insurance plan designed to defray the costs of medical care was organized, to the 1930s, health insurance consisted essentially of cash payments by commercial carriers to offset income losses resulting from disability attributable to accidents. Sickness benefits (cash payments during sickness) began as an extra, a "frill" on accident insurance policies. As with accident insurance, emphasis was on the replacement of income lost, in this instance as a result of contracting certain specified and catastrophic communicable diseases—typhoid, scarlet fever, smallpox, and the like (Health Insurance Institute, 1975). With the origin of Blue Cross and Blue Shield, a new policy developed: reimbursing health care costs in general.

Health care utilization is not a rare occurrence. On the average, each person in the United States visits a physician five times a year. One out of every seven Americans is admitted to a hospital at least once a year. Other than coverage for catastrophic illness, a fairly rare event, health insurance has become a mechanism for offsetting expected rather than unexpected costs. The experience of the many is pooled in an effort to reduce expected outlays to manageable prepayment size. Perhaps the term "assurance" more appropriately describes the health care payment system that has evolved. In Britain, "assurance" is used to denote coverage for contingencies that must eventually happen (life assurance); "insurance" is reserved for coverage of those contingencies like fire and theft, which may not occur (*Encyclopaedia Britannica,* 1970, Vol. 12, p. 337).

Blue Cross and Blue Shield. The establishment of payment mechanisms to defray in general the costs of illness can be traced to the Great Depression. Previously, hospitals had sought to assure reimbursement for their services through public education campaigns directed at encouraging their users, middle-income Americans, to put money aside for unpredictable medical expenses (Law, p. 6). When hard times proved the inadequacy of the savings approach, attention turned to the development of a stable income mechanism. A model was at hand in the independent prepayment plan pioneered in 1929 at Baylor University Hospital in Texas to assure certain area schoolteachers of some hospital coverage. Under the plan, 1,250 teachers prepaid half a dollar a month to provide themselves with up to 21 days of semiprivate hospitalization annually.

Like Baylor's, most early plans were for single hospitals. Then, in the early 1930s, nonprofit prepayment programs offering care at a number of hospitals were organized in several cities. The American Hospital Association vigorously supported the growth and development of these plans, soon to be named Blue Cross, and the special insurance legislation that was required for their establishment in each state (Law, pp. 7–8). The AHA set standards for plans and then offered its seal of approval to plans meeting the standards. A provider-insurer partnership was firmly established. Indeed, not until 1972 did national Blue Cross formally separate from the American Hospital Association.

Like Blue Cross, Blue Shield was a child of provider interests born of the Depression. In this instance, the provider was the physician: the professional organization, the state medical society. In 1917, county medical societies in Washington and Oregon had established "medical bureaus" to compete with private doctors and clinics for medical service contracts covering employees of railroads and lumber companies. In 1939, generally recognized as the year Blue Shield began, state medical societies sponsored plans in California and Michigan. Eight additional states followed suit in the period from 1940 to 1942, and in 1943, the American Medical Association established a Council on Medical Service and Public Relations in order to formulate standards and approve state and local Blue Shield plans (Somers and Somers, p. 319). The growth of Blue Shield was less dramatic than that of Blue Cross following the Depression because physicians in general were in less dire financial circumstances than hospitals were (Anderson, p. 119). Instead, the period of greatest growth for Blue Shield was between 1945 and 1949, when the medical profession sought to stave off movements for federal and state health insurance (Somers and Somers, p. 321).

In other respects, however, Blue Shield mirrors Blue Cross. For example, both are local or statewide undertakings organized for the most part under special state enabling acts. They are incorporated as not-for-profit charitable organizations and therefore relieved of the obligations facing stock and mutual insurance companies—namely, the maintenance of substantial cash reserves and the payment of state and federal taxes (Anderson, p. 123). In most states, the Department or Commissioner of Insurance supervises the Blues, issuing or approving their certificates of incorporation, reviewing their annual income and expenditure reports, monitoring the rates subscribers pay into the program and the rates the programs pay to the providers (Law, pp. 13–18).

In line with their not-for-profit status, both programs, at least initially, were committed to "community rating." Under such a policy, a set of benefits is offered at a single rate to all individuals and groups within a community, regardless of age, sex, or occupation of community members. In essence, the rate represents an averaging out of high- and low-cost individuals and groups so that the community as a whole can be serviced with adequate benefits at reasonable cost (Somers and Somers, p. 309). When commercial for-profit insurance companies entered the field,

however, they did so with a policy of "experience rating," charging different individuals and population subgroups different premiums based on
their use of services. Low-risk goups could secure benefits at a lower
premium. As a result, the Blues also decided to offer a multiplicity of
policies with differing rate and benefit structures, and often had to go to
experience rating. Had they not, adverse risks alone would have comprised
their health insurance portfolios (Krizay and Wilson, p. 40).

Finally, it is the Blues that, by and large, serve as the fiscal intermediaries between the federal and state governments in the Medicare and
Medicaid programs (Somers and Somers, pp. 34–35). The role of intermediary is a key one. Under Medicare, for example, the intermediary:
(1) determines how much the provider is to be paid; (2) makes the payment;
(3) audits the provider's books; and (4) assists in the development and
maintenance of utilization review systems designed to check unnecessary
costs. In 1977, 68 Blue Cross/Blue Shield plans served as fiscal intermediaries under Medicare. In contrast, only five private health insurance
companies were intermediaries for Part A of Medicare and only 12 for part
B (Health Insurance Institute, 1979).

Commercial insurance. The profit-making commercial insurance
companies (Aetna, Metropolitan Life, etc.) entered the general health
insurance market cautiously. They had realized losses on income-
replacement policies during the Depression; they were leery of the Blues'
initial emphasis on comprehensive benefits. However, a Supreme Court
decision recognizing fringe benefits as a legitimate part of the collective
bargaining process, following as it did upon the freezing of industrial wages
during World War II, proved too much of a temptation. Business was
shopping for insurance carriers, and the commercials responded (Somers
and Somers, pp. 262–263). By the end of 1977, over 700 for-profit companies were offering insurance of one sort or another against the cost of
illness (Health Insurance Institute, 1979).

In the main, Blue Cross offers hospitalization insurance; Blue Shield,
coverage of in-hospital physician services and a limited amount of office-
based care. The commercials offer both. As in the case of the Blues,
commercial hospital and hospital physician coverage is primarily provided
to groups through employee fringe-benefit packages negotiated through
collective bargaining. Individual coverage can be purchased, but it is
usually quite expensive or has limited coverage. The commercials also sell
major-medical and cash-payment policies. The former, directed primarily
at catastrophic illness, pay all or part of the treatment costs beyond those
covered by basic plans. They are sold on both a group and an individual
basis. (Blue Cross and Blue Shield also sell group major-medical policies.
In 1977, they had more than a third of such coverage [Carroll and Arnett].
Cash-payment policies pay the insured a flat sum of money per day of hos-

pitalization, and are usually sold directly to individuals, often through mass advertising campaigns. Although the daily cash-payment sum is usually small, it can help defray costs left uncovered by other insurance.

Like the Blues, the commercials are subject to supervision by state insurance commissioners, although such supervision does not include rate regulation. The one requirement is that commercials establish premium rates high enough to cover claims made under the insurance they provide. Solvency of the insurer is the principal aim of insurance commission surveillance (Krizay and Wilson, p. 44).

The independent plans. In addition to Blue Cross/Blue Shield and the commercials, a number of so-called independent insurance plans have been established. Kaiser-Permanente, located primarily on the West Coast; the Health Insurance Plan of Greater New York; and the Group Health Cooperative in Washington State are among them. These have been discussed to a certain extent in Chapter 6. Most combine a prepayment mechanism with a captive medical group practice, although Independent Practice Associations (see Chapter 6) and Group Health Insurance in New York use individual practices. Some plans cover inpatient and ambulatory services; some, ambulatory services alone. Sponsors may be industry, employees/unions, community groups, or providers.

In sum, most independent plans combine to some extent the functions of insurance carrier and provider (Somers and Somers, p. 340–343): in exchange for premium payments, plan enrollees are entitled to medical services provided by physicians contracting with or employed by the plan. At times, care is provided at sites owned or leased by the plan or in institutions with whom the plan has contracted for services for its enrollees.

Some Health Maintenance Organizations (HMOs), if they provide their own prepayment mechanisms rather than using Blue Cross or a commercial carrier, are also classified by the Social Security Administration (SSA) in the independent plan group.* However, while sponsors include medical schools, hospitals, unions, consumer groups, government, and other organizations, health insurers are in the vanguard of activity (Salmon). In mid-1976, Blue Cross and private insurers were involved in 103 HMO

---

*In arriving at insurance statistics, the Social Security Administration has included in the category of "independent plans" HMOs sponsored by consumer groups, physician groups, hospitals, medical schools, labor unions, and private corporations, when such sponsors are at major financial risk for prepaid care. When the HMO is sponsored by the Blues or a commerical carrier that has accepted financial responsibility for failure, that HMO is included in statistics on the Blues or commercial carriers.

operations (Goldberg and Greenberg). Primarily, insurers are engaged in financial backing, consultation, administrative management, marketing, coverage for hospitalization and/or out-of-area emergency care, reinsurance, and acceptance of risk in the event of failure (Health Insurance Institute, 1975.)

Their involvement is an effort to advance the establishment of alternative, less costly delivery systems, utilizing in diverse ways the present insurance framework. Some observers believe that the commercial insurance companies see the development of Health Maintenance Organizations as a positive strategy ultimately leading to the corporate takeover of the health care delivery system (Salmon). (See also Chapter 15.)

Extent of Insurance Coverage in the United States.

Private health insurance coverage for Americans is extensive but uneven. In 1977, approximately three out of every four Americans had at least some coverage for hospital services, surgical physician care, outpaitent X-ray and laboratory examinations, prescribed drugs, and nursing services, according to the Health Care Financing Administration (whose figures are slightly lower than those of the Health Insurance Association of America). Moreover, 56% of Americans were covered for some home and office physician visits; 23% for some dental services; and 31% for some nursing-home care (Carroll and Arnett, p. 3).

The proportions of persons with some private health insurance have been increasing over time. By 1962, the proportions of the population having some coverage for hospitalization and physicians' services already stood at a fairly high level: 70% and 65%, respectively (Mueller and Piro, Table 7). However, the same was not true of the proportions of the population covered for other services. In 1962, for example, some nursing-home coverage was held by only 3% of the population, while for dental care the figure was 0.5%. From 1960 to 1977, the number of Americans with some major-medical coverage increased from 31 to 162 million (Carroll and Arnett, p. 5). In private insurance, however, deductibles and co-payment abound, as do benefit limits and exclusions. An examination of the proportions of total consumer expenditures met by private insurance for various types of care tells the story. As we noted above, in 1978, expenditures made through private health insurance amounted to about 27% of the total. The same was true in 1977 (Gibson, 1979, Table 5). Table 10.4 translates that percentage for 1977 and prior years into the proportions of expenditures met for the several categories of health care covered by such insurance. It is obvious that although many people have some coverage for drugs, doctors' office visits, and "other" services, the coverage does not go very far.

Table 10.4

Percentage of Consumer Health Expenditures Met by Private Health Insurance, 1950–1977

Year	Total	Hospital care	Physicians' services	Prescribed drugs (out-of-hospital)	Dental care	Other types of care
1950	12.2%	37.1%	12.0%	*	*	*
1960	27.8	64.7	30.0	*	*	5.0%
1965	30.5	70.1	34.0	2.4%	1.6%	2.0
1966	30.4	71.0	34.0	2.7	2.0	2.2
1967	31.8	76.7	36.7	3.5	2.5	3.4
1968	34.5	78.8	40.5	3.6	3.1	3.8
1969	35.5	77.7	41.1	4.0	3.9	4.7
1970	37.2	77.7	43.7	3.9	5.3	4.9
1971	39.1	80.9	43.7	4.9	6.3	5.3
1972	39.0	76.5	45.8	5.0	7.2	5.4
1973	39.0	75.4	46.0	5.6	8.1	6.1
1974	41.4	77.3	49.8	6.2	11.0	7.2
1975	45.0	82.6	51.3	6.7	15.8	7.2
1976	47.0	84.6	53.1	7.9	19.6	8.2
1977	45.5	79.3	52.9	7.9	20.2	8.8

Source: M. S. Carroll and R. H. Arnett, III, "Private Health Insurance Plans in 1977: Coverage, Enrollment and Financial Experience," *Health Care Financing Review, 1,* Fall 1979, p. 14. (See Appendix I, A13.)
*Data not available for this year.

Retention of Premiums in Private Insurance

The cost to the consumer for insurance coverage—premiums or subscription charges—reached $47.1 billion in 1977. That same year, benefit expenditures by all private insurers totaled $41.6 billion, 88.3% of premium income. The total operating expenses for the industry were almost $6 billion. Therefore the industry suffered what is called an underwriting loss—the sum of benefit claims and operating expenses exceeded premium income by almost $500 million (Carroll and Arnett, 1979). However, different methods of allocation of administrative costs to health insurance are used by different kinds of insurance companies. For example, it is thought that some commercial insurance companies allocate to health insurance their sales costs for other kinds of insurance sold to the same beneficiaries. This could considerably alter the "underwriting loss" picture, as could return on investment of premiums, discussed below.

The share of the premium dollar returned in benefits varies widely among the different types of carriers and different types of insurance. In

1977, for example, Blue Cross and Blue Shield returned 91.7% and 86.6%, respectively, of monies taken in; commercial carriers, 85% (90.8% on group and 53.7% on individual policies); and the independents, 96.6% (Carroll and Arnett, 1979, Table 8).

All insurance companies have the opportunity to make money by investing premium income while they have it. Assuming a going concern, with fairly steady rates of premium income and benefit payments, $1 billion in premium income annually means about $1 billion in the pot at any one time. That money can be invested. An analysis of the financial experience of 20 of the 30 leading insurance companies is displayed in Table 10.5. As the table indicates, the companies realized a net gain in every year examined except for 1975.

It is also interesting to compare the difference in operating costs among the different insurers. Blue Cross spent 5.1% of premium income in 1978; Blue Shield spent 10.7%; the commerical insurers for group policies spent 13.6%; for individual policies, 45.8%; and the independent plans, 7%

Table 10.5

Financial Statistics of Selected Commercial Health Insurers,[1] 1974–1977

| Item | Amounts (in millions of dollars) | | | |
	1974	1975	1976	1977
Income, total	$10,658.9	$11,948.8	$13,309.4	$14,841.3
Premiums	10,326.4	11,590.0	12,874.6	14,269.2
Investment income	309.6	301.8	343.5	414.6
Other income	22.9	57.0	91.3	157.5
Benefit expense, total	8,744.4	10,227.3	11,032.0	11,929.2
Benefits incurred	8,648.8	10,231.0	10,723.7	11,556.1
Increases in reserves	184.8	192.7	153.7	463.3
Other loss items	16.1	17.3	232.1	(27.1)
Transfers	(75.3)	(213.7)	(77.5)	(63.1)
Operating expense	1,567.7	1,744.6	1,947.8	2,165.3
Gain before dividends	346.7	(23.1)	329.6	746.8
Dividends	97.2	71.7	169.1	324.8
Gain after dividends before income taxes	249.5	(94.8)	160.5	422.0
Income tax	76.5	69.5	109.2	146.9
Net gain	173.0	(164.3)	51.3	275.1
Aggregate reserves	2,451.6	2,645.6	2,769.5	2,701.5

Source: M. S. Carroll and R. H. Arnett, III, "Private Health Insurance Plans in 1977: Coverage, Enrollment and Financial Experience," *Health Care Financing Review, 1,* Fall 1979, p. 9. (See Appendix I, A13.)
[1]20 of top 30 commercial health insurers, representing 56% of the industry, based on earned premiums for 1977. (*National Underwriter,* June 17, 1978.)

(Carroll and Arnett, 1979, Table 8). Most notable is the difference in the cost of handling individual as opposed to group policies. The reasons become evident when the functions included under operating costs are outlined: (1) claims handling; (2) statistical services: (3) marketing, including costs of selling and advertising; (4) billing and collection; (5) investment management; and (6) special taxes, licenses, and fees (Krizay and Wilson, p. 45). When the insurance carrier is issuing a single policy to a large group as opposed to diverse individual policies, the costs associated with the first four functions are obviously quite a bit less. However, the question must be raised: are individual policies, which return such a low proportion of premiums to the policyholders as a group, really justified?

For the independent plans, administrative costs are often reduced by employing physicians on a salaried or contract basis to provide a full range of services in return for a set annual payment by enrollees. In such instances, there is no need for billing and collection after each episode of care. Statistical data are more easily collected. Blue Cross and Blue Shield operate at lower cost than the commercials do because they are exempt from state premium taxes in certain instances and because they pay lower salaries on the average (Krizay and Wilson, p. 46). Finally, Blue Cross, it can be hypothesized, has the administrative-cost edge over all other carriers because it deals *directly* with the *institutional* provider, thereby eliminating the high claims volume characteristic of indirect plans (via cash payments to the insured) and individual provider plans (Blue Shield). Once reimbursable services and charges have been determined and incorporated, after negotiation, in the hospital's reimbursement formula, Blue Cross simply pays the hospital the costs of allowable services used by Blue Cross subscribers.

The several insurers hold different shares of the private health care insurance market. In 1977, in all categories of insurance except nursing home care (a small category indeed), commercial carriers served as insurers for over half the Americans covered (Carroll and Arnett, Table 4). Although Blue Cross/Blue Shield is most often the target of criticism for failure to utilize the insurance mechanism to promote health care cost-control (Law), that operation captured 39% or less of persons insured for hospital, physician, dental, drug, and nursing services. The commercials are first in premium income too, taking 49%, compared to 42% for the Blues and 9% for the independents (Carroll and Arnett, pp. 7, 10). The order of market dominance—commercials, Blues, then independents—has held since 1950. For those over age 65, however, it is Blue Cross/Blue Shield, rather than the commerical carriers, that play the largest role, issuing policies, for the most part, that cover the gaps in Medicare. For the rest, "cash policies" are made available, providing the elderly with specified weekly or monthly payments during periods of hospitalization.

The private health insurance industry is extremely influential in the U.S. health care delivery system. In addition to its independent role as a financial agent, which we have analyzed in some detail, its role as the Medicare—and in certain states, Medicaid—fiscal intermediary cannot be forgotten. Its potential as a deliverer of service under national health insurance in the United States is discussed in Chapter 15. Nevertheless, it must be remembered that although more than 75% of Americans have *some* private hospitalization insurance, private insurance covers only 35% of expenditures for hospitalization and slighlty more than 25% of *all* expenditures. Is it possible that the industry is being accorded authority to determine future directions for U.S. health care out of proportion to its true importance in the system?

How the Money Is Paid Out
Paying Providers

Health care is a labor-intensive industry, as has been discussed in Chapter 4. About 70% of all expenditures are for personnel (Kramer and Roemer, p. 57). The vast majority of health workers are paid by wages or salary. However, about 500,000 dentists, physicians, osteopaths, optometrists and opticians, chiropractors, psychologists, social workers, speech pathologists, and physicial and occupational therapists, among others, are paid on a fee-for-service basis by their patients or third parties—private insurers or government.

Fee for service. The fee-for-service system has provoked a great deal of controversy. It has been vigorously attacked (Jonas, 1979, 1980; Lium; Roemer, 1962, 1971) and just as vigorously defended (Sade). Proponents of the fee-for-service system usually argue, especially in relation to fee-for-service reimbursement for physicians, that direct payment cements the necessary bond between provider and patient, a bond on which effective treatment often hinges; that it gives the provider an incentive to work that is not present under any other system; that it is justified by the special life-and-death responsibility that physicians, in particular, must accept.

Opponents claim there is no "natural" justification for the fee-for-service system: it is simply a product of the guild status of physicians, since the majority of health care providers are paid by salary. They point out that the fee-for-service approach creates the two-class system of medical care in the United States about which there is so much complaint. If fees, which some people cannot afford, were not charged at the time of service, then there would be no need to have one set of health care facilities for those who can afford to pay the doctor and a second for those who cannot.

Further, opponents for fee-for-service see the cash exchange as a barrier to utilization and as an interference rather than a help in the provider-patient relationship. As for the argument based on the life-and-death relationship, opponents say that the provider is not usually in a life-and-death relationship with his patient. But even if he were, the airplane pilot does not collect a fee for service, and he certainly has a life-and-death relationship to his passengers. The fireman does not request personal payment before he turns on the water or even after he has put out the fire. Indeed, when a fireman undertakes a life-and-death responsibility for a person in a burning building, he does not ask for a fee, even though he risks his own life, which doctors rarely, if ever, do.

Finally opponents argue that with fee-for-service reimbursement, costs go up more rapidly than with other payment mechanisms. They point to the national health insurance experience of other countries such as Canada (Korcok); Australia ("Amendments to Australia's Act"); and Japan (Jonas, 1975). Thinking along the same lines, William Glaser (Chapter 7) cites the unnecessary work so frequently attendant on the fee-for-service system— encouraging the paying patient to return when he wishes, ordering inpatient rather than ambulatory services, and the like. In addition, he indicates that, given the choice of two or more, the practicitioner more often chooses the higher-paid procedure when payment is on a fee basis.

Capitation and salary. The alternative forms of provider reimbursement are capitation and salary. The latter approach is self-explanatory. As indicated earlier, its use as a payment mechanism for health professionals is widespread. Certainly, from the employer's point of view, a salary system has the merit of administrative simplicity. When the employer is the government, there is the added benefit of flexibility: the movement of providers into areas of medical scarcity and unpopular jobs is more easily accomplished under a salary system than under other payment mechanisms. From the provider's point of view, he or she has an income protected from sudden fluctuations in supply and demand, is free of bill collection problems, and, usually, benefits from extensive fringe benefits (Roemer, 1962). In a survey conducted by Goldberg, 40% of the physicians interviewed mentioned shorter work weeks, time off to study, rests or vacations without income loss, liberal pension plans, and paid life, health, and malpractice insurance as significant compensations in a salaried system. Finally, salaried providers tend to utilize less costly diagnostic and treatment procedures and to avoid unnecessary utilization of services (Densen et al.; Williams; Roemer, 1962).

However, payment by salary is not without drawbacks. The provider, for example, is faced with a limit on his lifetime income. The comparatively high salaries marking his early years of practice are balanced by the fact that his earnings peak more quickly than the fee-for-service practitioner's (*Harvard Law Review*; Goldberg). In addition, he is subject to administrative constraints on such matters as schedules and vacations and to peer review regarding his performance. Often, he must abandon individual goals in order to conform with his employer's objectives (Shinefield and Smillie; Hayt). To the extent that fee-for-service stimulates quality work, the employer, in turn, must increasingly rely upon the individual physician's dedication, his desire to give fully of his attention and skill to all his patients (Ricketts). From the patient's vantage point, the salary system provides few incentives against undertreatment. The physician receives the negotiated salary regardless of the amount of services provided.

Under the capitation arrangement—which is used primarily for physicians providing ongoing care—the physician receives a flat annual fee for each person who agrees to be under his care, again regardless of the frequency with which his services are utilized. Like salary, capitation promotes administrative simplicity—unless, of course, financial incentives are added to base payments to encourage care of the chronic or time-consuming patient. Capitation too removes barriers to care raised by fee requirements for each treatment episode and offers the physician no incentive to undertake more costly rather than less costly medical procedures. In addition, the capitation system advances continuity of care and, thus, an improved provider-patient relationship (Glaser, Chapter 10).

But there are drawbacks in this system too. With barriers to care reduced, the provider may have to cope with unnecessary calls for treatment. There is also an incentive to increase the number of patients served even if such an increase should result in too little time to offer comprehensive care and needed emotional support (Roemer, 1962).

Paying Hospitals

As stated earlier, payments to hospitals constitute the largest single category of national health expenditures. There are four major modes of hospital reimbursement. The first, oldest, and most rapidly disappearing, is that based on *charges*. This method is used by private, profit, and not-for-profit hospitals. A price (which may or may not bear some relationship to the cost of that service) is put on each item of service—a day in bed, use of the operating room, a lab test—and the patient, and/or his insurer under cash-indemnity plans, is billed for that price, usually called a charge.

A more sophisticated reimbursement mode is based on cost. The determination of cost never involves individual patients. It is a matter for negotiation between hospitals and the major insurance companies in their areas. In certain states, the Insurance Department and/or Department of Health may be a party to the negotiations in either an advisory or approval capacity. Cost reimbursement is used when insured patients receive their benefits as *services* rather than as dollar indemnities. (Almost all group health insurance policies in the United States now provide service benefits rather than dollar indemnities.) In the usual approach, one of several accounting techniques determines the cost of various services per unit of service; the hospital is reimbursed for those costs as it provides the services. Thus, if the agreed bed-day cost figure is $150 for each day of care provided to a patient with Blue Cross insurance, the hospital will receive $150 from Blue Cross. This method is sometimes called "retrospective cost reimbursement."

A still more sophisticated approach, "prospective reimbursement" (Dowling, 1974, 1979; Drake; McCarthy), is used in certain parts of the country. An insurer and/or public agency attempts to predict, on the basis of previous experience and current rates of cost-increase, what costs will be for the coming year. (Hospital influence on the process depends upon the extent to which the process is voluntary or mandated by state law.) The hospital then receives that rate per service (or, in some instances, per hospital stay or even per time-period without relation to the number of units of service actually provided), regardless of its actual cost. There is an obvious stimulus for hospitals to attempt to control costs, because under prospective reimbursement they receive a given amount of money for providing a given service without regard to the service at the time it is rendered. This method, particularly when applied to the total hospital budget, obviously approaches annual budgeting for hospitals as related to total program, rather than to individual units of service. However, in most cases reimbursement to the hospitals is still based on the number of items of service delivered.

Finally, government hospitals at all levels operate on total annual budgets, and have always done so. The costs of various inputs, salaries, and expenses are determined and a budget is prepared that is not related to units of service in any way. Although some third-party payments, primarily Medicaid/Medicare, are available to them with reimbursement rates calculated on a cost basis, for most government hospitals the proportion is small. The bulk of government hospital monies comes from tax revenues (Falk et al.). Thus, government hospital budgets are subject to other considerations besides costs and programs. As health care expenditures, particularly for hospitals, continue to rise at a high rate, and as we move toward national health insurance, it is likely that prospective reimbursement or annual budgeting will be applied to increasing numbers of hospitals outside of the public sector in an attempt to control costs, if nothing else.

The Medical Marketplace

Ours is predominantly a market-directed economy: the basic economic questions of what to produce, how, and for whom, are most often answered through the exchange decisions on factors (land, labor, and capital) and products made by individual producers and consumers acting in response to price. According to Samuelson (pp. 44–45) and a host of other noted economists, the distribution of goods and services that results in such instances is difficult to improve upon. Given the way income is apportioned, someone cannot be made better off without making someone else worse off. A condition of optimality is said to exist.

Understood, of course, is a market that, in economic terms, is "perfect" and "competitive"—a situation that rarely, if ever, exists in the health care industry. The industry is, on the contrary, replete with instances of market failure.

Today's medical care cost picture makes it all the more imperative to take a closer look at those failures. When the health care expenditures data presented in the preceding pages are placed against the cost implications for the economy as a whole of employee health care fringe-benefit packages and the knowledge that direct income is foregone to gain protection against the possible cost of illness, the dimensions of the prevailing cost problem emerge. The bulk of private insurance, for example, is obtained through one's place of employment, but employer contributions to employee health plans are not simply written off. The costs involved, allocated from what would otherwise be wages, are passed along to the general public in the form of higher prices for goods and services.

What, then, is a "perfect" market? What are the prerequisites for a "competitive" market? In what specific ways does the medical care market fall short of these ideals that lead to economic efficiency? The requirement for a "perfect" market is simply stated: buyers and sellers must have complete knowledge of market conditions. Price, quantity, quality, and any changes in the same are immediately known to the participants and can be acted upon by them. For a market to be "competitive," three conditions must prevail: (1) there must be a multitude of participants with none so large or powerful that he can exert significant influence on the market itself or on other competitors; (2) there must be no restriction on entry into the market; and (3) the commodity exchanged must be homogeneous—that is, there must be no difference between one seller's product and another's. If conditions one and two are met but not three, one can still speak of "imperfect competition," for price will remain the major determinant of supply and demand (Haveman and Knopf, pp. 140–143).

In the health care industry, however, price is a poor regulator of production and consumption (Fuchs, 1972, pp. 5–8; Mushkin; Klarman, 1965, p. 10–19). First, unlike the consumer in the general marketplace, the patient is dependent upon the seller, the health care provider, for information about the product he is purchasing, and, in many circumstances, for information about his need for it. At any one time, the patient does not have at his disposal data on the quantity and quality of services offered at a particular price, much less information on changes in quantity, quality, and price. Moreover, he is in no position to make an independent judgment about the most important variable, quality.

The technical nature of medicine, the tremendous uncertainty regarding medical practice outcomes, professional sanctions against advertising, the relative infrequency with which any of the diverse services available are purchased—all work to keep the patient uninformed. In any case, it must be remembered that for the most part, it is the physician, not the patient, who determines what services will be purchased and in what amounts (Fuchs and Kramer, p. 2). Even if one discounts the proven correlation between the number of practicing physicians and the number of per capita physician visits per year (Wasyluka), it is impossible to disregard the central role played by the physician in prescribing drugs, other professional services, and hospital and nursing home care. This point has been stressed by the President's Council on Wage and Price Stability (Dyckman).

Just as there is no "perfect" market, there is no "competitive" market. Because of the skills involved, one appendectomy or tonsillectomy is not necessarily the same as another. Because of physical facilities, equipment, and manpower resources, a stay at Hospital A may vary considerably from a stay at Hospital B for an identical ailment. Moreover, although on a national basis there is a multiplicity of "sellers" with none large enough to control the market, in smaller geographic regions both institutions and providers of care may be so few that they dominate the health care delivery system. In some commercial health care operations, for example, the drug industry, even nationwide market control exists. By product category, the four largest drug firms often account for 50% to 60% of output, with the result that prescription drug prices are seldom responsive to changes in supply and demand (Fuchs, 1974, pp. 105–121).

Finally, as discussed further in Chapter 14, monopolies in the area of education, certification, and licensure of health professions restrict the mobility of manpower both into and within the industry. Licensing prerequisites for physicians, for example, are essentially determined by organized medicine. One of the primary prerequisites is graduation from an approved school. Such schools are those accredited by the Liaison Committee on Medical Education, composed of representatives of the American Medical Association and the Association of American Medical Colleges. The requirements of institutional accreditation and/or licensure, in turn, place limitations on a hospital's entry into the market.

Even if a "perfect" and "competitive" medical care market existed, however, other industry characteristics would prevent conditions of economic optimality. In the first place, it is largely need rather than demand that occasions the purchase of health services. Those in pain seldom choose health care by rationally weighing the relative merits of all available goods and services. Consider the relation between a family's medical care expenditures and income when illness strikes and stays. When the need factor is added to physician control over the ordering of services, it is easy to understand why a weak relationship exists between consumer demand and price in the medical care industry. Moreover, that relationship is weakened even further by the role of the third-party payor, a role that might be traced, at least in part, to the belief that need should indeed occasion service because health care is a right, as was discussed in Chapter 2. The more frequently and extensively a third party pays, the less often the cost of care enters into decisions of whether or not to seek service (Andersen and Anderson, pp. 136–140). Second, a large segment of the industry—particularly the voluntary hospitals—is operated on a not-for-profit basis. Under such circumstances, capital does not flow in and out of the industry in response to market signals. Often, investments are made and resources allocated for other than economic reasons—to improve the quality, availability, and accessibility of care, for example, or because a generous donor wants a particular kind of hospital built or service offered. Third, at certain times, an individual expenditure in the health care market involves a social utility. Immunization against contagious diseases or treatment for syphilis, for example, benefits the community as a whole. As Mushkin indicates, in instances such as these involving "extra buyer benefits," market price underestimates the total value derived.

The Rising Costs of Health Care

The continually rising cost of health care is one of the most serious problems facing the United States health care delivery system. This problem plagues most capitalist countries (Abel-Smith). The system has long been viewed as expensive. In 1932, the Committee on the Costs of Medical Care was very concerned with a $3 billion annual rate of expenditure (p. 2), around 4% of the GNP. In 1948, the Director of the Montefiore Hospital in the Bronx, N.Y., was worried because a patient-day of care cost $12 and hospital capital construction costs were prorated at $20,000 per bed (Bluestone). In 1978, the patient-day cost at Montefiore was over $200; the prorated cost of constructing a teaching hospital bed was recorded at almost $200,000 at the University Hospital, State University of New York at Stony Brook.

Between 1965 and 1978, health care costs increased at an annual rate of between 10% and 14% (see Table 10.6). The usual increase was in the 11%–13% range. The low occurred in 1973, when a government price

Table 10.6

National Health Care Expenditures, Annual Percentage Increase, and Annual Percentage of GNP, 1965–1978

Year	Amount (in billions)	% increase over previous year	% GNP
1965	$43.0	————	6.2%
1966	47.3	10.0%	6.3
1967	52.7	11.4	6.6
1968	58.9	11.8	6.8
1969	66.2	12.4	7.1
1970	74.7	12.8	7.6
1971	82.8	10.8	7.8
1972	92.7	12.0	7.9
1973	102.3	10.3	7.8
1974	115.6	13.0	8.2
1975	131.5	13.7	8.6
1976	148.9	13.2	8.8
1977	170.0	14.2	9.0
1978[1]	192.4	13.2	9.1

Source: R. M. Gibson, "National Health Expenditures, 1978," *Health Care Financing Review, 1,* Summer 1979. Derived from Table 1. (See Appendix I, A13.)
[1]Preliminary estimates.

control system, the Economic Stabilization Program (ESP), was in full effect. With the end of the ESP health care cost controls, the rate of increase began an inexorable climb.

Another way to evaluate health care spending is as a percentage of the GNP. This rose continually from 1965, dropping off a bit only under the ESP. Health care costs can also be considered in relation to the Consumer Price Index (CPI), a Department of Labor indicator (see Table 10.7). During the decade 1968–1978, the price index for all medical services rose about 19% faster than did the CPI as a whole. The index for physicians' fees rose about 24% faster. The drug index rose above one-third the rate of the CPI between 1968 and 1977, the last year for which consistent drug data are reported. However, the index of hospital semiprivate room rates rose at almost twice the rate of overall health care costs and 104% faster than did the CPI during the 1968–1978 period. It is obvious that the cost of hospitalization contributes the most to rising health care costs.

There are five major theories used to explain rises in health care costs in general and hospital costs in particular (Davis and Foster, Chapter 1; Davis, 1972a, 1972b, 1973a, 1973b). The "demand-pull" theory attributes increases to rising income and the growth of insurance, which have en-

Table 10.7

Consumer Price Index* for Medical Care Items in the United States, 1968–1978

Calendar year	All medical care items	Physician fees	Dentist fees	Optometric exam and eyeglasses	Hospital room	Prescrip-tions and drugs
1968	106.1	105.6	105.5	103.2	113.6	100.2
1969	113.4	112.9	112.9	107.6	128.8	101.3
1970	120.6	121.4	119.4	113.5	145.4	103.6
1971	128.4	129.8	127.0	120.3	163.1	105.4
1972	132.5	133.8	132.3	124.9	173.9	105.6
1973	137.7	138.2	136.4	129.5	182.1	105.9
1974	150.5	150.9	146.8	138.6	201.5	109.6
1975	168.6	169.4	161.9	149.6	236.1	118.8
1976	184.7	188.5	172.2	158.9	268.6	126.0
1977	202.4	206.0	185.1	168.2	299.5	134.1
1978	219.4	223.3	199.3	**	331.6	**

Source: U.S. Department of Labor, Bureau of Labor Statistics, *CPI Detailed Report.*
*For urban and clerical workers.
**Revisions to CPI prevent presentation of indices for these categories that are comparable to prior years.

larged the fund of purchasing power and created new or increased demand on a relatively inelastic suppply (Feldstein, 1971). The "labor cost-push" theory states that expenditures rise in response to increased hospital wages and/or lagging productivity gains in the hospital industry. According to the "scientific progress" theory, new, costlier methods of care force prices up. The "waste" theory says that prices rise because of capital investment in costly, expensive-to-maintain facilities that already exist in sufficient supply. Finally, the "cost-reimbursement" theory states that increases in supply, equipment, and salary expenditures have occurred with the growth in the number of insurance plans reimbursing at cost. Hospital administrators, it is alleged, have little reason to operate efficiently when costs can be passed on to third-party payors. In fact, the evidence suggests that all five factors contribute to increasing hospital costs. Let us try to determine which are the most important.

The average cost per day in community hospitals increased from $15.62 in 1950 to $194.34 in 1978, or 1,144%. During that same period payroll costs rose slightly more, from $8.86 per patient day to $111.06, or 1,153%. As M. Feldstein found in his study period (1955–1968), the bulk of this latter increase is attributable to a rise in wages and salaries (Feldstein,

1971). More specifically, from 1950 to 1978, the number of full-time equivalent employees (FTE) per average daily census increased from 2.03 to 3.24, or 60%, while the average annual earnings per FTE were up 325%, from $2,563 to $10,896 (American Hospital Association, 1966, pp. 427–428; American Hospital Association, 1979, pp. ix–xi).

Although acceleration in payroll costs is unmistakable, the reason for the acceleration is less clear. Available studies on changes in the skill-mix of hospital personnel predate Medicare; moreover, their conclusions are contradictory (Feldstein, 1971; Davis and Foster). Some researchers cite unionization as a key factor in hospital wage increases (Lee; Elkin); others dismiss the unions as a causative agent (Bunker). Some credence can be given to the "catch-up" theory—namely, that over time, hospital wages have risen sharply in an effort to bring them more in line with industry as a whole. From 1969 to 1978, for example, the hourly earnings of non-supervisory hospital workers—91% of total private hospital employees—increased at an annual rate exceeding that of nonsupervisory employees in nonfarm, service, and manufacturing occupations (Freeland, et al.). There is also some support for the belief that if hospitals had done more to substitute less costly capital for more costly labor, personnel costs could and would have risen less dramatically (Lytton; Klarman, 1969a; Feldstein, 1971).

However, sharp increases in hospital productivity could not alone have reversed the upward trend in hospital costs. Jeffers and Siebert (1974) show, for example, that with labor productivity rising at an annual rate of almost 10%, hospital costs per day would still increase 8% a year. Indeed, even total control over personnel expenditures would not provide the complete answers, for labor costs as a proportion of total hospital expenses have been declining steadily since 1962. In 1978 payroll represented only 49.7% of dollar outlays in community hospitals (American Hospital Association, 1979, p. xi). Moreover, nonlabor inputs and their prices have been on the rise.

Assuming that prices paid by community hospitals for nonlabor inputs rose at the same rate as wholesale prices in general, Waldman calculated an average annual rate of increase of 6.4% in nonlabor inputs and 2.4% in their prices from 1951 to 1970. Waldman estimated increases in labor inputs over the same period at 2.9% annually, wage rates at 5.8%. HEW's hospital input price index (Table 10.8) reveals the continuing significance of nonlabor factors in overall cost increases in the 1970–1978 period. Malpractice insurance, food, fuel, surgical and medical supplies, and capital costs, among others, have been growth categories.

The rise in importance of nonlabor inputs is attributed to changes in the resources applied to a day of care—increased use of ancillary services (lab tests, X-rays, etc.) per day of care, and the advent of new and more expensive types of services (Gibson and Fisher). Klarman (1964), for example, links one-fourth of the dollar increase in patient-day cost in the 1950s to medical advances as reflected in ancillary service use. Davis cites the following "supply" factors as major forces behind hospital cost increases from 1962 to 1968: the creation of new expensive services like open-heart surgical theaters and intensive-care units; the addition of new employees to staff them; and the increase in the cost of money for capital expansion itself (Davis, 1972a, 1972b, 1973a, 1973b). In her analysis of hospital expenditures from 1950–1953, Nancy Worthington found that "real nonlabor inputs"—that is, new services, often reflecting technological changes—are the major determinant of cost increases. Increases in the number of employees, in the prices of goods and services hospitals must buy, and in hospital utilization were found to be less important (Worthington, 1975b).

It is certainly true that facilities and services unavailable in 1960 or found only in medical centers are now offered in a substantial number of community hospitals. In 1960, for instance, 10% of community hospitals had intensive-care units, in which bed costs per day are often double that in a semiprivate room (Worthington, 1975b); in 1978, almost 68% of community hospitals had them (American Hospital Association, 1979, Table 12A).

Supporters of the "scientific progress" theory consider cost increases resulting from advances in or greater use of medical technology as the necessary price of improvements in health care, if not health. Opponents suggest that a substantial portion of such increases is totally unnecessary. They link a proportion of the increase in ancillary service usage to physician fear of exposure to malpractice claims. Similarly, they charge a percentage of the increase in capital investments per se to wasteful duplication of services. And just as data on longer life span and improved functioning support the "scientific progress theory," the literature contains a number of assessments that lend strength to the "waste" theory. In the early 1960s, for example, the DeBakey Commission reported that 30% of the 770 hospitals equipped for open-heart surgery had not had cases in the year under study and 87% of those with cases performed less than one operation per week (Newhouse). The situation had changed little by 1967. At that time, 31% of hospitals with open-heart surgery facilities had not used them in a year (USDHEW). Commenting on the situation in Philadelphia in 1975, Tresnowski averred that only five of the 16 hospitals with open-heart surgery capabilities had a utilization rate high enough to assure either cost/effectiveness or quality care (U.S. Council on Wage and Price Stability). Goldstein reported similar underutilization of other sophisticated medical facilities in 1973. To separate the relative contributions of duplication and

Table 10.8

Percentage Change in the National Hospital Input Price Index, by Expense Category, 1970–1981

Expense category	Relative weight, 1977	Historical percentage changes									Forecasted percentage changes [1,2]		
		1970	1971	1972	1973	1974	1975	1976	1977	1978	1979	1980	1981
Total	100.00	7.5	6.4	5.8	6.0	10.1	10.6	8.8	8.1	8.4	9.0	8.5	8.5
Payroll expenses and employee benefits	58.91	9.0	8.1	7.8	5.8	7.8	10.1	10.0	8.7	8.8	8.5	9.1	9.0
Payroll expenses (wages and salaries)	51.69	7.5	6.4	6.7	5.3	7.5	9.3	9.0	8.0	8.4	7.9	8.5	8.3
Employee benefits	7.22	32.8	31.5	19.1	11.0	11.2	17.3	18.4	14.0	12.0	12.6	12.9	13.6
Professional fees	4.98	7.4	6.9	3.5	3.6	9.0	11.9	10.8	9.1	8.8	9.6	9.6	8.3
Medical	4.46	7.5	6.9	3.1	3.3	9.2	12.3	11.3	9.3	8.9	9.8	9.7	8.2
Other	0.52	6.7	7.1	6.5	6.2	8.0	8.3	7.3	7.6	8.1	8.5	8.9	8.9
Capital	6.02	8.6	3.1	3.5	6.2	9.0	5.1	4.2	5.6	7.9	9.2	4.6	5.5
Depreciation	4.01	4.5	5.2	5.5	5.5	6.7	9.0	8.8	8.5	9.0	8.8	7.6	8.0
Building & fixed equipment	2.58	5.7	6.5	6.8	7.1	8.9	11.0	10.1	9.4	9.6	9.1	7.9	8.7
Movable equipment	1.43	2.8	3.4	3.5	3.2	3.4	5.7	6.6	6.9	7.8	8.2	7.1	6.8
Interest	2.01	15.1	0.0	0.5	7.4	12.5	-0.8	-3.4	0.2	5.9	10.1	-1.6	0.0
Working capital	0.41	14.0	-21.7	-17.3	25.4	49.7	-6.9	-23.3	-6.5	21.2	36.6	-1.2	2.7
Capital debt	1.60	15.6	9.0	5.8	3.2	2.0	1.8	4.1	2.1	1.9	2.0	-1.7	-1.0
Hospital malpractice insurance premiums	2.00	29.9	27.8	15.2	21.3	87.5	100.0	33.3	20.0	15.0	15.0	10.0	10.0
Food	3.13	5.0	2.6	4.8	17.9	14.6	7.6	0.2	5.2	9.4	12.0	8.2	7.5
Purchases at early stages of distribution	1.57	4.4	2.2	5.5	22.6	15.4	6.8	-2.5	4.5	8.9	12.3	7.9	7.4
Purchases at later stages of distribution	1.56	5.5	3.1	4.2	13.2	13.8	8.4	3.1	6.0	9.9	11.7	8.4	7.6

	Weight												
Fuel and other utilities	2.42	4.6	7.2	3.4	8.1	28.4	11.8	9.2	12.2	7.8	10.5	11.0	9.7
Fuel oil and coal	0.94	3.9	6.2	0.5	15.3	58.4	8.1	7.2	13.3	6.0	15.6	13.0	10.7
Electricity	0.67	3.3	6.7	4.9	4.9	18.3	13.1	6.4	6.6	7.5	3.9	8.3	7.3
Natural gas	0.50	5.4	7.2	5.2	4.4	12.7	19.8	16.6	19.1	9.9	12.0	11.9	10.3
Water and sanitary services	0.31	7.7	10.8	3.8	5.4	6.0	9.8	11.1	10.8	10.7	7.1	8.9	10.2
Other	22.54	4.5	3.4	2.4	4.8	12.5	10.2	6.5	6.0	6.7	9.0	7.6	7.7
Drugs	2.48	−0.1	−0.4	0.1	0.8	4.3	8.6	6.3	4.2	5.1	7.8	6.0	8.0
Chemicals and cleaning preparations	1.88	2.4	1.9	0.0	5.6	33.5	23.5	3.2	3.0	3.2	8.1	7.5	6.3
Surgical and medical instruments and appliances	1.78	5.2	4.5	2.3	5.2	16.1	15.9	7.7	7.6	10.0	9.9	7.0	7.1
Rubber and miscellaneous plastics	1.62	2.9	0.7	0.2	2.9	12.1	10.3	6.0	5.3	4.3	9.3	7.8	7.0
Business travel and motor freight	1.51	5.2	5.2	1.2	3.2	11.2	9.4	9.9	7.1	4.7	10.3	9.4	9.0
Apparel and textiles	1.45	1.0	1.8	4.2	9.0	12.3	−0.8	7.4	3.9	3.8	4.3	3.3	6.9
Business services	4.12	8.1	5.6	3.8	4.2	9.4	9.6	8.2	7.7	8.6	9.0	8.6	8.4
All other miscellaneous expenses	7.70	5.9	4.3	3.3	6.2	11.0	9.2	5.7	6.5	7.7	9.8	8.1	7.7
Consumer Price Index, all items, all urban		5.9	4.3	3.3	6.2	11.0	9.2	5.7	6.5	7.7	9.8	8.1	7.7

Source: M. S. Freeland et al., "National Hospital Input Price Index," *Health Care Financing Review, 1,* Summer 1979, Table 3. (See Appendix I, A13.)

[1] Data Resources, Inc., provided all forecasts presented here, except for "malpractice insurance premiums," which was forecast by HEW.

[2] Historical employee compensation variables for 1970–1978 are internal to the hospital industry:

Wages—average payroll expense per full-time equivalent community hospital worker (American Hospital Association)

Employee benefits—employee benefits per full-time equivalent community hospital worker (American Hospital Association).

Forecasted employee compensation variables for 1979–1981 are external to the hospital industry:

Wages—average hourly earnings of service industry workers (Bureau of Labor Statistics)

Employee benefits—supplements to wages and salaries per employee on nonagricultural payrolls (Bureau of Economic Analysis and Bureau of Labor Statistics).

medical progress to increases in nonlabor inputs, however, requires a more extensive research base than presently exists. Proponents of the cost-reimbursement theory would consider such a distinction unnecessary, as they would any attempt to assign weights to the labor and nonlabor components of rising hospital costs. Both, they concede, have been inflationary factors. At fault is the method of health care financing that assures the hospital administrator that his costs, as long as they fall under the definition of "allowable," will be reimbursed.

With the advent of Medicare, it is estimated that the volume of service paid for at cost increased 75% or more (Klarman, 1969b). Thus, statistical support for the cost-reimbursement theory is found in a comparison of pre- and post-Medicare costs. Before 1965, patient-day costs in community hospitals increased at an annual rate of 6.5%; after Medicare went into effect, the rate doubled to 13%. Coupled with the rise in physicians' fees, this upward shift resulted in an annual increase of 10% or more in total health care expenditures, despite the Economic Stabilization Program (Klarman, 1974).

A study by Davis (1973a), however, failed to establish any relation between hospital costs and the extensiveness of cost-reimbursement. Using data from 1965, 1967, and 1968, Davis examined the joint effect of Blue Cross cost-reimbursement plans and Medicare and Medicaid. In her analysis, the cost-reimbursement variable proved to be an insignificant factor in determining cost per admission, even though the proportion of hospital expenses covered by cost-reimbursement plans was taken into account. However, after adjusting for changes in utilization and rising wage rates, Davis found hospital average cost to be higher after Medicare than before. She concluded, therefore, that one could not dismiss the possibility of a linkage between Medicare and rising hospital costs, even if there was no evidence of a direct relationship between increased costs and cost-reimbursement per se (Davis, 1973a).

M. Feldstein identified that linkage as the demand-pull theory of inflation. For Feldstein, increases in labor inputs and nonlabor inputs explain how costs have changed, not why. The "why" is embodied in shifts in the factors influencing consumer demand for hospital care—greater faith in the curative power of medicine, higher prices for other goods and services, rising personal income and, most important, growing insurance coverage (1971). Through government or employer contributions and periodic premiums of modest size, insurance increases the amount of money available for health services and, as a result, the demand for such services (Klarman, 1969b). Likewise, it is alleged that, by lowering the net price or out-of-pocket cost of care at the time of treatment, insurance encourages a greater demand for services than would be the case if quantity and price were clearly associated (M. Feldstein, 1973; Klarman, 1969b).

While there are no statistics on faith in medical technology or the prices of substitute goods or services not consumed, support for the demand-pull theory can be found in the trend data on income and insurance. The median income of both families and unrelated individuals has increased steadily. In like manner, according to estimates of the Health Insurance Association of America, the number of persons with private health insurance for hospital care rose from 12 million in 1940 to 179 million in 1977. It should be noted as well that, in 1977, 23.8 million persons over 65 were enrolled for hospital insurance under Medicare, while approximately 24 million eligible poor received payment under Medicaid (Health Insurance Institute, 1979).

A data foundation also exists for theorizing about effects of low net price on service utilization. From 1950 to 1978, out-of-pocket payments decreased from 59% to 21% of private expenditures for hospital care (Gibson, derived from Table 8). Thus, in 1950, when the average cost of a day of care was about $16, out-of-pocket payments were approximately $9. In 1978, such payments totaled only $40, or 21% of $194, that year's average cost per day (American Hospital Association, 1979). M. Feldstein (1973) argued that even this small dollar difference overstates the real rise in net costs to the consumer, since the devaluation of the dollar has not been taken into account. Davis, in turn, highlighted the potential for hospital cost increases embodied in such relatively stable out-of-pocket payments. If a hospital could charge $100 a day and maintain desired occupancy in the absence of hospitalization insurance, it could charge $500 a day if insurance coverage reduced the net price to 20% of hospital charges (Davis, 1972b).

A number of studies support this positive relationship between hospital usage and insurance coverage. Weisbrod and Fiesler, for example, linked a broadening of insurance benefits to both admissions and the use of ancillary services (1961). Studying third-party payment and length of stay for 22 disease categories in Iowa hospitals, Joseph (1972) found a statistically significant relationship in seven categories representing less serious illnesses or conditions, indicating that economic forces do influence hospital usage when physical state permits. Rosenthal utilized data aggregated at the state level for the years 1950 and 1960 and demonstrated a negative relationship between price and hospital admissions, patient-days, and length of stay, and a positive relationship between insurance coverage and the three variables (1964).

P. Feldstein's empirical research on the factors of demand showed that hospital insurance coverage is positively and significantly related to both patient-days and hospital expenditures (1964). Over 25 years ago, Anderson and Feldman concluded, after a nationwide survey, that, at every income level, insured individuals use more of every kind of health service (1956). Working with data on 2,367 families across the United States,

Anderson and Benham reported a dramatic increase in demand for medical services following the extension of insurance benefits to low-income groups (1970). Newhouse and Phelps focus upon marginal price. Their results, drawn from data gathered in a household survey in 1963, indicated that choice of hospital, as measured by room and board charges, is highly sensitive to coinsurance rates (1974). Finally, Friedman documented an increase in service intensity following the advent of Medicare. From aggregated data, he showed a rising trend in charges per case, a function of length of stay and increased use of resources per patient-day. From a review of the Massachusetts Tumor Registry, he reported a doubling of the number of new cases of breast cancer treated by both surgery and radiation between 1965 and 1967 (Friedman, 1974). In brief, the research supporting an association between third-party payment and hospital use and expenditures is considerable.

There is, then, a basis for subscribing to the demand-pull theory of cost inflation. Rising incomes and the growth of third-party payment have made a greater number of dollars available for a service believed to be valued more and more for its curative powers. In addition, insurance has increased the possibility of unnecessary hospital usage attributable to both patient and provider behavior or misbehavior. From the patient's standpoint, it is the added precaution taken, the extra day spent in the hospital. From the physician's standpoint, it may be the additional test and more, for the physician is the gatekeeper to hospital care.

Putting all of this information together, the "demand-pull" and "scientific progress" theories seem to be the most useful in explaining that proportion of increased hospital costs and, in turn, increased health care costs that cannot be explained by general inflation. To the extent that "scientific progress" is poorly planned, duplicative, or of questionable utility, and to the extent that new purchasing power is created with minimal attention to cost-control and in a manner that tends to favor utilization of one part of the delivery system (hospitals), the "waste" and "cost-reimbursement" theories are applicable.

The complexity of the problem suggests that any recommendation for containing cost inflation must be multifaceted. The aftermath of the Economic Stabilization Program proves the evanescence of cost-containment achieved through directly imposed wage and price controls (Worthington, 1975a). Ways must be found to encourage improved and lasting performance by the private market sector. Certainly, the evidence is sufficient to warrant attention to restructuring hospital insurance. Research, if not action, is indicated on plans that provide greater protection against the large bill and less against the small, that incorporate cost-sharing by patients, and that set limits on payments to providers. Attention should also be directed to the regionalization of expensive tertiary care facilities and services and to basic changes in the method of health care delivery, changes that promote cost-containment. Effecting a shift away from present reliance upon hospital services, away from almost total dependence upon the physician when medical care is indicated, and toward less costly, equally effective modes of care may well be termed a necessary step.

Conclusion

Money fuels the health care delivery system, but the routes dollars take from consumer to providers can be labyrinthine. Some dollars go directly, some via the government, some through insurance companies. Most health care providers are paid by salary, but some, the higher-income ones for the most part, are paid on a piecework basis. Some institutions get paid on the basis of what they charge, some on the basis of calculated costs per item of service, and some get an annual budget to privide a set of services.

In the United States, in the mid-1970s, a health insurance system that emphasized coverage for hospital care, as well as the practice of having most physicians working both in and out of hospitals, with hospital care generally being more lucrative, "tilted" the system in the direction of utilization and overutilization of the most expensive component of the system. Technological change, a significant factor in rising health care costs, has been poorly planned and evaluated, with decisions often being made on the basis of each provider being there with the most rather than on a cost-benefit analysis. However, as expenditures rise, and as an increasing proportion goes through government hands, the government's interest in cost control rises. Thus we now turn our attention to various aspects of the role of government in the health care delivery system. It is well known that he who pays the piper calls the tune.

References

Abel-Smith, B. "Value for Money in Health Services." *Social Security Bulletin, 37,* 17, July 1974.

"Amendments to Australia's National Health Act." *Social Security Bulletin, 34,* 28, December 1971.

American Hospital Association. *Hospitals, Guide Issue, 40,* August 1, 1966.

——————. *Hospital Statistics, 1979.* Chicago: American Hospital Association, 1979.

American Medical Association. "Medical Education in the United States, 1978– 1979." *Journal of the American Medical Association, 243,* March 7, 1980.

Andersen, R., and Anderson, O. *A Decade of Health Services: Social Survey Trends in Use and Expenditure.* Chicago: University of Chicago Press, 1967.

Anderson, O. *The Uneasy Equilibrium.* New Haven, Connecticut: College and University Press, 1968.

Anderson, O. W., and Feldman, J. J. *Family Medical Costs and Voluntary Health Insurance: A Nationwide Survey.* New York: Blakiston, 1956.

Anderson, R., and Benham, L. "Factors Affecting the Relationship Between Family Income and Medical Care Consumption." In Klarman, H. E., Ed., *Empirical Studies in Health Economics*. Baltimore: Johns Hopkins Press, 1970.

Bauer, K. G. *Containing Costs of Health Services through Incentive Reimbursement*. Cambridge, Massachusetts: Harvard Center for Community Health and Medical Care, 1973.

Bluestone, E. M. "Home Care: An Extra-Mural Hospital Function." *Survey Midmonthly, 84*, 99, 133, April 1948. Reprinted in Committee on Medical Care Teaching of the Association of Teachers of Preventive Medicine, Eds., *Readings in Medical Care*. Chapel Hill: University of North Carolina Press, 1958.

Bunker, C. S. "A Study to Determine the Impact of Unionization and the Threat Thereof on New York City's Voluntary Non-Profit Hospitals." Ph.D. dissertation, George Washington University, 1968.

Bureau of the Census. *Statistical Abstract of the United States, 1978*. Washington, D.C.: U.S. Department of Commerce, USGPO, 1978.

——————. *Statistical Abstract of the United States, 1979*. Washington, D.C.: U.S. Department of Commerce, USGPO, 1979.

Carroll, M. S., and Arnett, R. H., III. "Private Health Insurance Plans in 1977: Coverage, Enrollment and Financial Experience." *Health Care Financing Review, 1*, 3, Fall 1979.

Coe, R. M., et al. "Impact of Medicare on the Organization of Community Health Resources." *Milbank Memorial Fund Quarterly, 52*, 231, 1974.

Committee on the Costs of Medical Care. *Medical Care for the American People*. Chicago: University of Chicago Press, 1932. Reprinted, Washington, D.C.: USDHEW, 1970.

Congressional Research Service. *Workmen's Compensation: Role of the Federal Government*. Issue Brief Number IB75054. Washington, D.C.: Library of Congress, 1976.

Davis, K. "Community Hospital Expenses and Revenues: Pre-Medicare Inflation." *Social Security Bulletin, 35*, 3, October 1972a.

——————. "Rising Hospital Costs: Possible Causes and Cures." *Bulletin of the New York Academy of Medicine, 48*, 1354, December 1972b.

——————. "Theories of Hospital Inflation: Some Empirical Evidence." *Journal of Human Resources, 8*, 181, Spring 1973a.

——————. "Hospital Costs and the Medicare Program." *Social Security Bulletin, 36*, 18, August 1973b.

——————, and Foster, R. *Community Hospitals: Inflation in the Pre-Medicare Period*. Research Report No. 41. Washington, D.C.: Social Security Administration, 1972.

Densen, P., et al. *Prepaid Medical Care and Hospital Utilization*. Monograph No. 3. Chicago: American Hospital Association, 1958.

Dowling, W. L. "Prospective Reimbursement of Hospitals." *Inquiry, 11*, 163, 1974.

——————. "Hospital Rate-Setting Programs: How, and How Well, Do They Work?" *Topics in Health Care Financing, 6*, 15, 1979.

Drake, D. F. "Will Rate Regulation in the Hospital Industry Be Effective? A Provider Inquiry." *Topics in Health Care Financing*, 6, 25, 1979.

Dyckman, Z. Y. *A Study of Physician's Fees*. Washington, D.C.: Council on Wage and Price Stability, USGPO, March 1978.

Elkin, R. D. "Recognition and Negotiation Under Taft-Hartley." *Hospital Progress*, 55, 50, December 1974.

Encyclopaedia Britannica. "Insurance." Chicago: Encyclopaedia Britannica, 1970.

Falk, I. S., et al. *The Costs of Medical Care*. New York: Arno Press, 1972.

Feldstein, M. S. *Economic Analysis for Health Service Efficiency*. Amsterdam, Holland: North-Holland Publicity Co., 1967.

—————. *The Rising Costs of Hospital Care*. Washington, D.C.: Information Resources Press, 1971.

—————. "The Medical Economy." *Scientific American*, 229, 151, September 1973.

Feldstein, P. J. "The Demand for Medical Care." In American Medical Association, *Report of the Commission on the Cost of Medical Care*, Vol. 1, General Report. Chicago: American Medical Association, 1964.

Freeland, M. S., et al. "National Hospital Input Price Index." *Health Care Financing Review*, 1, 37, Summer 1979.

Friedman, B. "A Test of Alternative Demand—Shift Responses to the Medicare Program." In Perlman, M., Ed., *The Economics of Health and Medical Care*. New York: Wiley, 1974.

Fuchs, V. R., Ed. *Essays in the Economics of Health and Medical Care*. New York: Columbia University Press, 1972.

Fuchs, V. R. *Who Shall Live?* New York: Basic Books, 1974.

Fuchs, V. R., and Kramer, M. J. "Determinants of Expenditures for Physicians' Services in the United States 1948–1968." Washington, D.C.: USDHEW Pub. No., (HSM) 73–3013, USGPO, 1973.

Gibson, R. M. "National Health Expenditures, 1978." *Health Care Financing Review*, 1, 1, Summer 1979.

Gibson, R. M., and Fisher, C. R. "National Health Expenditures, Fiscal Year 1977." *Social Security Bulletin*, 41, 3, July 1978.

Gibson, R. M., and Fisher, C. R. "Age Differences in Health Care Spending, Fiscal Year 1977." *Social Security Bulletin*, 42, 3, 1979.

Glaser, W. A. *Paying the Doctor*. Baltimore: Johns Hopkins University Press, 1970.

Goldberg, J. H. "Working for a Paycheck: One MD's Paean . . . Is Another Man's Pain." *Hospital Physician*, 7, 68, 1971.

Goldberg, L. G., and Greenberg, W. *The Health Maintenance Organization and Its Effects on Competition: Staff Report to the Federal Trade Commission*. Washington, D.C.: (Mimeographed) July 1977.

Goldstein, H. "Health and Medicine." In Schuckster, G., and Dale, E., Jr., Eds., *The Economist Looks at Society*. Lexington, Massachusetts: Xerox Publishing Co., 1973.

Harvard Law Review. "The Role of Prepaid Group Practice in Relieving the Medical Care Crisis." 84, 948, 1971.

Haveman, R. H., and Knopf, K. A. *The Market System*. New York: Wiley, 1970.

Hayt, E. "The Practice of Medicine by Hospitals." *Hospital Management, 100*, 30, 1965.

Health Insurance Institute. *Source Book of Health Insurance Data, 1974–75*. New York, 1975.

————. *Source Book of Health Insurance Data, 1978–79*. New York, 1979.

Jeffers, J. R., and Siebert, C. D. "Measurement of Hospital Costs Variation: Case Mix, Service Intensity and Input Productivity Factors." *Health Services Research, 9*, 293, Winter 1974.

Jonas, S. "Japan Strains under Complex Health System." *Hospitals, J.A.H.A.*, September 1, 1975, p. 56.

————. "Fee-for-Service Private Practice Medicine: Problems and Contradictions." *Consumer Health Perspectives, 6*, No. 4, August 1979, p. 1.

————. "Fee-for-Service Private Practice Medicine: The End Is in Sight." *Consumer Health Perspectives, 7*, No. 2, April 1980.

Joseph, H. "Hospital Insurance and Moral Hazard." *Journal of Human Resources, 7*, 152, Spring 1972.

Klarman, H. E. "The Increased Cost of Hospital Care." In Mushkin, S. J., Ed., *The Economics of Health and Medical Care*. Ann Arbor: University of Michigan, 1964.

Klarman, H. E. *The Economics of Health*. New York: Columbia University Press, 1965.

————. "Approaches to Moderating the Increases in Medical Care Costs." *Medical Care, 7*, 175, May–June 1969a.

————. "Reimbursing the Hospital—The Difference the Third Party Makes." *Journal of Risk and Insurance, 36*, 553, December 1969b.

————. "What Kind of Health Insurance Should the United States Choose?" In Morrale, J. C., Ed., *The U. S. Medical Care Industry: The Economist's Point of View*. Ann Arbor: University of Michigan, 1974.

Korcok, M. "Medicine in Canada." Parts 1 and 2. *American Medical News*, March 20, 1972.

Kramer, C., and Roemer, R. *Health Manpower and the Organization of Health Services*. Los Angeles: University of California, Manpower Research Center, Institute of Industrial Relations, 1972.

Krizay, J., and Wilson, A. *The Patient as Consumer*. Lexington, Massachusetts: Heath, 1974.

Law, S. A. *Blue Cross: What Went Wrong?* New Haven, Connecticut: Yale University Press, 1974.

Lee, S. "Teaching Hospitals: Alone or Together." *Bulletin of the New York Academy of Medicine, 48*, 1467, December 1972.

Lium, R. "Choice, Fees, and Quality." *Harvard Medical Alumni Bulletin, 4*, 1971.

Lytton, H. D. "Recent Productivity Trends in the Federal Government: An Exploratory Study. *Review of Economics and Statistics, 41*, 341, November 1959.

McCarthy, C. M. "Incentive Reimbursement as an Impetus to Cost Containment." *Inquiry, 12*, 320, December 1975.

Mueller, M. S. "Private Health Insurance in 1973: A Review of Coverage, Enrollment and Financial Experience." *Social Security Bulletin, 38,* 21, February 1975.

Mueller, M. S., and Gibson, R. M. "National Health Expenditures, Fiscal Year 1975." *Social Security Bulletin, 39,* 3, February 1976.

Mueller, M. S., and Piro, P. A. "Private Health Insurance in 1974: A Review of Coverage, Enrollment and Financial Experience." *Social Security Bulletin, 39,* 3, March 1976.

Mushkin, S. J. "Toward a Definition of Health Economics." *Public Health Reports, 73,* 785, 1958.

New York Times. "Doctors Strong, Patients Weak, Costs Up." April 26, 1976.

Newhouse, J. P. "Toward a Theory of Nonprofit Institutions: An Economic Model of a Hospital." *American Economic Review, 60,* 64, March 1970.

Newhouse, J. P., and Phelps, C. E. "Price and Income Elasticities for Medical Care Services." In Perlman, M., Ed., *The Economics of Health and Medical Care.* New York: Wiley, 1974.

Pauly, M. V., and Drake, D. F. "Effect of Third-Party Methods of Reimbursement on Hospital Performance." In Klarman, H. E., Ed., *Empirical Studies in Health Economics.* Baltimore: Johns Hopkins Press, 1970.

Price, D. N. "Workers' Compensation Program in the 1970s." *Social Security Bulletin, 42,* No. 5, p. 3, 1979a.

————. "Workers' Compensation: Coverage, Payments, and Costs, 1977." *Social Security Bulletin, 42,* No. 10. p. 18, 1979b.

Ricketts, H. T. "Forty Years of Full-Time Medicine at the University of Chicago." *Journal of the American Medical Association, 208,* 2069, 1969.

Roemer, M. I. "On Paying the Doctor and the Implications of Different Methods." *Journal of Health and Human Behavior, 3,* 4, Spring 1962.

————. "An Ideal Health Care System for America." *Transaction, 8,* 31, 1971.

Rosenthal, G. D. *The Demand for General Hospital Facilities.* American Hospital Association Hospital Monograph Series No. 14. Chicago: American Hospital Association, 1964.

Russel, L., et al. *Federal Health Spending, 1969–74.* Washington, D.C.: National Planning Association, 1974.

Sade, R. M. "Medical Care as a Right: A Refutation." *New England Journal of Medicine, 285,* 1288, 1971.

Salmon, J. W. "The Maintenance Organization Strategy: A Corporate Takeover of Health Services Delivery." *International Journal of Health Services, 5,* 609, 1975.

Samuelson, P. A. *Economics,* 9th ed. New York: McGraw-Hill, 1973.

Shinefield, H. R., and Smillie, J. G. "Prepaid Group Practice and Health Care." *Advances in Pediatrics, 20,* 205, 1973.

Sigmond, R. M. "The Notion of Hospital Incentives." *Hospital Progress, 50,* 63, January 1969.

Somers, H., and Somers, A. R. *Doctors, Patients and Health Insurance.* Washington, D.C.: The Brookings Institution, 1961.

Strickland, S. *U. S. Health Care: What's Wrong and What's Right?* New York: Universe Books, 1972.

U.S. Council on Wage and Price Stability. *The Complex Puzzle of Rising Health Care Costs: Can the Private Sector Fit It Together?* Washington, D.C.: Executive Office of the President, December 1976.

USDHEW. *Towards a Comprehensive Health Policy for the 1970's: A White Paper.* Washington, D.C.: USGPO, 1971.

──────. *Health United States, 1978.* USDHEW Pub. No. (PHS) 78–1232, Hyattsville, Maryland: USGPO, 1978.

U.S. Department of Labor. *State Workers' Compensation Laws in Effect on January 1, 1980 Compared with the 19 Essential Recommendations of the National Commission on State Workmen's Compensation Laws.* Washington, D.C.: December 27, 1979.

U.S. National Commission on State Workmen's Compensation Laws. *Report.* Washington, D.C.: USGPO, 1973.

Waldman, S. *The Effect of Changing Technology on Hospital Costs.* Social Security Administration, Office of Research and Statistics, Note No. 4. Washington, D.C.: The Office, February 28, 1972.

Wasyluka, R. G. "New Blood for Tired Hospitals." *Harvard Business Review, 48,* 66, October 1970.

Weisbrod, B. A., and Fiesler, R. J. "Hospitalization Insurance and Hospital Utilization." *American Economic Review, 51,* 126, 1961.

Williams, G. "Kaiser: What Is It? How Does It Work? Why Does It Work?" *Modern Hospital, 116,* 67, February 1971.

Wolkstein, I. "Incentive Reimbursement Plans Offer a Variety of Approaches to Cost Control." *Hospitals, J.A.H.A.,* June 16, 1969.

Worthington, N. "National Health Expenditures, 1929–74." *Social Security Bulletin, 38,* 2, February 1975.a.

──────. "Expenditures for Hospital Care and Physicians' Services: Factors Affecting Annual Charges." *Social Security Bulletin, 38,* 3, November 1975b.

11

Government in the Health Care Delivery System

Steven Jonas and David Banta

Introduction

Thus far we have examined four principal elements of the United States health care delivery system: the people whom it serves, the personnel it employs, the organizational structures and facilities through which care is provided, and the fiscal mechanisms that enable the system to operate. There is a fifth crucial element of any health care delivery system: government. In our earlier discussions, we have seen some ways in which various components of the government and the health care delivery system interrelate; now we will look more directly at government operations in administration, legislation, regulation, adjudication, planning, quality control, and the development of national health insurance. We will also discuss some activities of the private sector in those areas.

In the United States, the government operates neither the health care delivery system nor, as of 1981, the financing system in its entirety; in fact, our government is less involved in health care than the governments of most other industrialized countries. Among the many reasons for this difference, perhaps the most important is the strength of the private sector and its opposition to "government control and interference," except in select areas, such as care of the sick poor, care of the mentally ill, and infectious disease control. Restricted as the government's role is, however, on an absolute scale it looms rather large. This role has developed and expanded gradually over a long period of time.

In the 1940s, the Committee on Medicine and the Changing Order of the New York Academy of Medicine sponsored a series of monographs on the health care delivery system. One—*Medical Services by Government: Local, State and Federal,* by one of the first medical sociologists, Bernhard J. Stern (1946)—had a preface by W. G. Smillie, one of the noted authorities on public health of the day. Many of the observations are strikingly relevant to our present situation.

In the preface, Smillie said (Stern):

Our forefathers certainly had no concept of responsibility of the Federal
Government, nor of the state government, for health protection of the
people. This was solely a local governmental responsibility. When Benjamin
Franklin wrote "Health is Wealth" in the Farmers' Almanac, he was saying
that health was a commodity to be bought, to be sold, to be conserved, or to
be wasted. But he considered that health conservation was the responsibility
of the individual, not of government. The local community was responsible
only for the protection of its citizens against the hazards of community life.
Thus government responsibility for health protection consisted of (a) promotion of sanitation and (b) communicable disease control. The Federal Constitution, as well as the Constitutions of most of the states, contains no
reference or intimation of a federal or state function in medical care.

The care of the sick poor was a local community responsibility from
earliest pioneer days. This activity was assumed first by voluntary philanthropy; later, it was transferred, and became an official governmental obligation. . . . (p. xiii)

Professor Stern continued that line of thought in his introduction:

Government action in the field has traditionally been limited to the care of
the indigent and has been dominated in its scope and administration by the
restraining influences of the parochial poor laws. Gradually, and especially
after the passage of the Social Security Act and during [World War II],
government medical care has increasingly been furnished to some nonindigent groups. New patterns of government medical care are being formulated and the role of local, state, and federal governments in the field is
changing. . . . Government agencies, after protracted delays and faltering
beginnings, are making significant strides in the development of effective
administrative procedures and in the provision of skilled and experienced
personnel. The attitudes of the medical profession and of the public toward
government medical programs will determine whether these resources are
to be used progressively to distribute more medical care of higher quality to
the American people. (pp. 4–5)

Government at all jurisdictional levels in the United States is involved
in the health care delivery system to a much greater degree now than in
1946. The kind of involvement has changed too, with such initiatives as
Medicare and Medicaid, planning acts, new regulatory powers, and support of biomedical research and health professions education. But certain
characteristics have remained unchanged, and they are most significant.
To quote Smillie again (Stern):

. . . Practically all governmental procedures in medical care stem from the
original local community responsibility for the care of the sick poor, and

many of our great municipal hospitals, clinics, and health services of today still bear the stigma of pauperism. Two separate types of governmental medicine developed through the years: official public health services, a health department function which attempted to prevent disease, and medical care of the sick poor, which was provided by departments of welfare. Though these frequently impinged and overlapped, they seldom were interrelated, and almost never were fused. (p. xiv)

The pauper stigma, that "poor equals bad" and that poverty is the fault of the poor, is still attached to much government activity in direct care delivery. It is rooted in the Protestant ethic, which held people directly accountable for their state in life. The legal implementation of the Protestant ethic goes back at least as far as the Elizabethan Poor Laws. Today our society may accept sociological explanations as to why some people are well-off and others are destitute; but attitudes toward the proper role of government in health care are still colored by old values and prejudices.

The Constitutional Basis of Government Authority in Health

To understand how the government operates in the health care delivery system, it is essential to understand the structure of the government itself.* A basic principle of the United States Constitution is the sharing of sovereign power between the federal and state governments. The Constitution represents an agreement by the states to delegate some of their powers to the federal government; the states reserve certain inherent powers, among which is police power, the basis of the states' role in health (Mustard, pp. 17–21). As Grad points out:

> The state's police power, i.e., the power "to enact and enforce laws to protect and promote the health, safety, morals, order, peace, comfort, and general welfare of the people" is an attribute of a sovereign government—a sovereign government in this context, being a government with power that derives from its very nature as a government, i.e., with plenary and inherent (rather than delegated) power. Thus, the fifty states are separate repositories of police power, while the national government, which, in its origins, is a government of delegated power, does not possess the police power, at least not in its usual broad sense. (p. 5)

Another basis of the states' authority in health is the Tenth Amendment of the United States Constitution, which states: "The powers not delegated to the United States by the Constitution, nor prohibited by it to the states, are

*The *Public Health Law Manual* by Frank P. Grad (1975) is a valuable guide to the legal basis of government activity in health care and to the many legal procedures involved in the enforcement of public health law.

reserved to the states respectively, or to the people."

Among the states' other inherent powers are those of delegation of authority. The states have used it to create the third tier of the governmental system, local government, and most states have delegated some of their powers in health matters to local governments.

The powers of the federal government in health are not specifically mentioned in the Constitution; they derive from the powers to tax and spend in order to provide for the general welfare, and to regulate interstate and foreign commerce. These powers are stipulated in Article I, Section 8 of the Constitution (Grad, p. 8).

The separation of powers, the clear constitutional division of the federal government into the executive, legislative, and judicial branches, is the second basic principle of the Constitution. Under separation of powers, each branch of the federal government is independent and has its own powers limited by the Constitution through the system of "checks and balances." The tripartite form, with checks and balances, is followed fairly closely by state governments. At the local level, the boundaries between branches sometimes become blurred: in suburban and rural areas, for example, the chief local executive officer may preside over the local legislative body. Nevertheless, in most jurisdictions, separation of powers is found as a major principle of government.

The Functions of Government in the United States Health Care Delivery System

The bulk of this chapter deals with the operations of the three jurisdictional levels of government—federal, state, and local—in the delivery of personal health services. However, there are other governmental functions in health, some of which are considered in other chapters. We will briefly review them and indicate in which chapters more detailed discussions may be found.

Licensing, particularly of physicians, is a basic government function in health care. Licensing of individuals determines who may and may not deliver what kinds of health services, and in theory, establishes minimum standards. Licensing of institutions also sets minimum standards and to some extent investigates the characteristics of owners and providers. Licensing is carried out primarily by the states, and all three branches of government are involved: the legislatures enact the statutes, the executive branches administer them, and the courts interpret and enforce them.

The licensing system, which is discussed in detail in Chapter 14, gives physicians tight control over the central product of the system: medical services. By exercising this control, physicians largely determine the structure of the health care delivery system—how it is organized, the types and functions of the institutions, and the powers of personnel. The states hold this power, which may be the single most important one in determining the character of the United States' health care delivery system.

Legislatures. In addition to enacting the legal framework within which the health care delivery system functions, legislatures may impose certain requirements for planning and development of the system (see Chapter 13) and for quality measurement and control (see Chapter 14). If the government is to participate in health care financing (see Chapters 10 and 15), or directly deliver services (see this chapter and Chapters 6, 7, 8, and 9), or support research efforts, those programs must first be established by legislative acts. Chapter 12 describes legislative functioning in health care at the federal level in some detail.

The judiciary. The judicial branches in the three levels of government have important powers, but since they cannot apprehend transgressors, or prosecute them, or carry out punishment on their own, they must work in concert with the law enforcement arms of the executive branches. Together they form the civil and criminal justice systems.

The civil and criminal justice systems support the work of the other components of the government in adjudicating disputes related to health care, and in protecting the rights of individuals under the due process and equal protection clauses of the Constitution. Most importantly, although a legislature creates a licensing law for physicians, and an executive branch administers it, the criminal justice system enforces it, if necessary by sending to jail a person who "practices medicine without a license."

Legislatures are passing an increasing number of laws attempting to regulate one or another part of the health care delivery system. Executive branches then interpret those laws and write regulations for their administration. Often one or another provider group, objecting that the new legislation inhibits its prerogatives, turns to the civil justice system for relief. Through litigation, providers avail themselves of the functions of one branch of the government to deal with what they feel are unconstitutional, illegal, or unwarranted intrusions into their work by one or more other branches.

Finally, malpractice litigation is one method by which dissatisfied customers attempt to get some kind of satisfaction from providers whom the consumers feel have wronged them in some fashion. The civil justice system is the arena in which malpractice litigation is carried out (see Chapter 14).

The executive—an overview. In speaking of "government in health care," we usually mean the executive branch that administers programs, not the legislature that creates them, or the courts that adjudicate disputes arising from them. In the remainder of the chapter, the term "government" will refer to the "executive branch of government." We will use the shorter term because it is common parlance, and much less cumbersome.

Personal health services provided by the federal government for the most part are for categories of persons: merchant seamen, American Indians, veterans, members of the uniformed services and their families, and so on. Personal health services provided by state governments for the most part are for categories of disease: mental illness and tuberculosis. Local government personal health services generally are for the lower socioeconomic class and the medically indigent. There are some overlaps: the federal government cares for those afflicted with leprosy and narcotics addiction, and operates St. Elizabeth's Hospital, a mental institution in the District of Columbia; governments at all levels provide care for prisoners; but by and large the distinction holds.

For community health services, government at all levels is the major provider in such areas as pure water supply and sanitary sewage disposal; food and drug inspection and regulation; communicable disease control; vital statistics and public health laboratory work.* However, there are certain activities that are shared with the private sector. In public health education the voluntary agencies—for example, the American Cancer Society and the American Heart Association—are very important. Private refuse collectors are important in solid waste disposal. Private organizations are very active in environmental protection. Private institutions of course play a vital role in health sciences education and research.

Government is an important factor in the delivery of combined health services, those which have both personal and community aspects—for example, immunization and treatment of venereal disease and tuberculosis.

Government participates in the financing system in three ways. First, there is spending for governmental delivery of services, personal, community, and combined. This can be direct—as in the federal government's care to veterans in hospitals that it owns and operates—or indirect, as in the federal government's "grant-in-aid" program to state governments to provide care in state tuberculosis hospitals. Likewise, state and federal governments spend directly to collect vital statistics, and give money to local governments to assist them in so doing. Governments also give money by grants and contracts to nongovernmental agencies (and in certain cases, other governmental agencies), for specific projects such as a program

---

*A great deal of valuable detail on government activities in community health services is contained in *Public Health: Administration and Practice* by John J. Hanlon and George E. Pickett, (St. Louis: C. V. Mosby, 1979).

in biomedical research, support of health facilities construction, and support for the development of Health Maintenance Organizations. Third, governments pay providers on an item-of-service basis for the delivery of care to third parties, e.g., under Medicare and Medicaid.

Agencies and Health Care Delivery

Many federal agencies are involved in the delivery of personal and community health services. About one-sixth of the population, aside from beneficiaries of Medicare and Medicaid, are eligible to receive at least some personal health services from or through the federal government. Table 11.1 shows which agencies have health-related activities, by category of activity, and how much was expected to be spent in each category in fiscal 1979. Note that the federal role is for the most part indirect. It has many programs for financial assistance—formula grants and categorical grants, not to mention revenue-sharing. It gives assistance to individuals and families, states and localities, and educational and other institutions. Through Medicare and Medicaid, it is a major third-party payor for personal health services. Although the government is weak in the health care system of the United States, relative to those of other countries, public funds accounted for over 40% of national health expenditures.

Federal health policy in our pluralistic system results from an interplay among five major participants: the President, the Congress, the federal bureaucracy, state and local government, and interest groups. Some of the interplay will be described in Chapter 12. As is to be expected, the U. S. Department of Health and Human Services (USDHHS) is the most important federal department in health care activity. For Medicare and Medicaid, which are administered by the Health Care Financing Administration (HCFA) and account for the bulk of USDHHS expenditures, it is primarily a third-party payor and secondarily a regulator (see Chapters 10 and 15). The Health Services Administration and Alcohol, Drug Abuse and Mental Health Administration provide significant indirect support for a variety of health services through the grant and contract mechanism. USDHHS, through the National Institutes of Health and other agencies, is the largest federal supporter of biomedical research. It is also a significant factor in health sciences education and health facilities construction, health care planning, and prevention.

Two other federal agencies with large direct expenditures for health care are the Veterans' Administration and the Department of Defense. They pay primarily for care in their own facilities, but are also involved in research, education, construction, and paying for care for beneficiaries in other institutions. Other federal agencies with significant health-related

Table 11.1

Estimated Outlays for Medical and Health-Related Activities by Agency, 1979
(In millions of dollars)

Agency	Indirect federal hospital and medical services	Direct federal hospital and medical services	Health research	Training and education	Construction	Health planning activities	Consumer and occupational health and safety	Total
Department of Health, Education, and Welfare (total)	44,108	606	2,895	785	397	303	276	49,370
Health Services Administration	1,070	527	15	45	109	18	1	1,785
Health Resources Administration	—	—	—	337	166	179	—	682
Alcohol, Drug Abuse, and Mental Health Administration	624	72	199	111	36	17	—	1,058
Center for Disease Control	166	—	58	8	—	—	4	235
National Institutes of Health	—	—	2,532	203	81	—	—	2,816
Food and Drug Administration	—	—	26	—	5	—	266	298
Assistant Secretary for Health	—	8	32	1	1	82	5	130
Health Care Financing Administration	41,973	—	18	—	—	7	—	41,991
Other HEW	273	—	16	80	—	8	—	376
Department of Defense	670	2,697	132	337	258	8	50	4,152
Veterans' Administration	362	4,436	113	334	394	28	—	5,667

								Total
Department of Housing and Urban Development	33	—	—	—	63	1	29	126
Department of Agriculture	2	—	97	—	24	5	349	477
Environmental Protection Agency	—	—	84	—	—	—	—	84
National Aeronautics and Space Administration	—	—	51	—	2	—	6	59
Department of Energy	—	—	199	—	8	1	—	208
Department of Labor	—	—	4	27	—	2	233	265
Department of State	20	—	4	9	3	—	36	72
National Science Foundation	—	—	63	—	—	—	—	63
Department of Interior	11	—	47	—	5	16	3	66
Department of Transportation	1	28	6	—	16	9	14	78
Department of Justice	86	38	1	—	2	5	15	62
Other Agencies	—	1	54	58	93	23	168	483
Agency contributions to employee health funds	2,145	—	—	—	—	—	1	2,146
Total outlays for health, 1979	47,436	7,809	3,750	1,553	1,262	384	1,180	63,374

Source: Special Analysis, Budget of the United States Government, Fiscal Year 1977, Washington, D.C.: Government Printing Office, 1979, p. 261.

expenditures include the Department of Agriculture (meat and poultry inspection; Food Stamps); the Environmental Protection Agency; and the Department of Labor (the Occupational Safety and Health Act.)

The Department of Health and Human Services*

In 1979, the Department of Health, Education and Welfare, the predecessor in health and welfare matters of the USDHHS, administered at least 200 programs through 13 operating agencies and 10 regional offices; more than 100 of the programs were health programs or were health-related. They were administered through two of the major administrative divisions of the department: the Public Health Service, which has six major agencies plus the Office of the Assistant Secretary for Health, which administers the USPHS; and the Health Care Financing Administration. The operating agencies and the number of personnel employed by each at the end of 1979 were as follows:

Public Health Service	
Office of the Assistant Secretary for Health	1,872
National Institutes of Health	11,131
Food and Drug Administration	7,705
Center for Disease Control	3,833
Health Resources Administration	1,187
Health Services Administration	18,839
Alcohol, Drug Abuse and Mental Health Administration	5,816
Health Care Financing Administration	4,560
Total	54,943

The Assistant Secretary for Health, who is also the Surgeon General of the Public Health Service, has a role of potential conflict; he has an empire to protect, but is also supposed to give impartial staff advice on health matters to the Secretary, including on Medicare and Medicaid. A major reorganization of the DHEW in 1977 removed the Medicare Program from the Social Security Administration and the Medicaid Program from the Social and Rehabilitation Service and combined them under the Health Care Financing Administration (HCFA). It is not under the Assistant Secretary's control, but rather has its own Administrator. Another 1977 reorganization moved the National Center for Health Statistics and the National Center for Health Services Research from the Health Resources Administration to the Office of the Assistant Secretary for Health (OASH), under a Deputy Assistant Secretary for Health. In 1978, the new National

*The most comprehensive description of the USDHHS is still Rufus E. Miles, Jr.'s, *The Department of Health, Education and Welfare* (New York: Praeger Publishers, 1974).

Center for Health Care Technology was created by statute and was also placed in OASH under the same Deputy Assistant Secretary as Health Statistics and Health Services Research. The USDHHS itself was created by Congress in 1979 when it passed legislation developed by the administration following a campaign promise of President Carter to create a separate Department of Education.

Public Health Service

The Public Health Service is directed by the Assistant Secretary for Health. The Public Health Service has a long and proud history, dating back to the 1798 Act creating the Marine Hospital Service (Schmeckebier, Chapter 1; Mustard, pp. 23–81; Stern, pp. 145–154; Wilson and Neuhauser, pp. 105–115, 147–170). In 1878, foreign quarantine activities were added by Congressional act, leading to the development of a quasi-military personnel system (the "commissioned corps") in 1889, a group that was largely made up of career medical people. The Public Health Service continued to gain responsibilities gradually, and grew rapidly in the area of communicable disease control during World War II. Since World War II, its responsibilities have grown greatly, with the passage of the Hospital Survey and Construction Act of 1946 (Hill-Burton Act), the rapid growth of the National Institutes of Health, the creation of the Communicable Disease Center in Atlanta (later the Center for Disease Control), and the development of drug abuse control, mental retardation and mental health centers, and comprehensive health planning. The Public Health Service, however, has suffered a relative decline in recent years for several reasons.

With the passage of Medicare and Medicaid legislation in 1965, the health financing programs began to predominate among federal health activities, and then to compete actively with PHS programs for financial support. Several reorganizations in rapid succession hurt morale. During the 1960s the Budget Bureau (later the Office of Management and Budget) embarked on a crusade to close the PHS hospitals, which damaged Service morale greatly, and also attempted to abolish the commissioned corps (Miles, pp. 192–200). Further, the unclear role of the Assistant Secretary of Health—and his lack of a top policy-analysis staff—have hampered active health leadership from the Public Health Service. In 1968, the functions of the Surgeon General of the PHS were given to the Assistant Secretary for Health (Miles, p. 73). Many observers feel that the Public Health Service, as a result of the changing nature of government health responsibilities, has largely lost its once great vibrancy and morale. From 1977 to 1979, USDHEW Secretary Joseph Califano continued to downplay the importance and autonomy of the PHS. However, with the succession of Patricia Roberts Harris to the Secretaryship in 1979, and the simultaneous release of *Healthy People: The Surgeon General's Report on Health Promotion and*

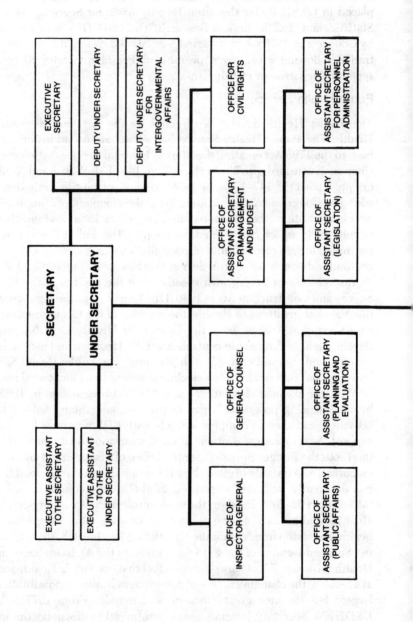

SECRETARY

UNDER SECRETARY

EXECUTIVE SECRETARY

DEPUTY UNDER SECRETARY

DEPUTY UNDER SECRETARY FOR INTERGOVERNMENTAL AFFAIRS

EXECUTIVE ASSISTANT TO THE SECRETARY

EXECUTIVE ASSISTANT TO THE UNDER SECRETARY

OFFICE OF INSPECTOR GENERAL

OFFICE OF GENERAL COUNSEL

OFFICE OF ASSISTANT SECRETARY FOR MANAGEMENT AND BUDGET

OFFICE FOR CIVIL RIGHTS

OFFICE OF ASSISTANT SECRETARY (PUBLIC AFFAIRS)

OFFICE OF ASSISTANT SECRETARY (PLANNING AND EVALUATION)

OFFICE OF ASSISTANT SECRETARY (LEGISLATION)

OFFICE OF ASSISTANT SECRETARY FOR PERSONNEL ADMINISTRATION

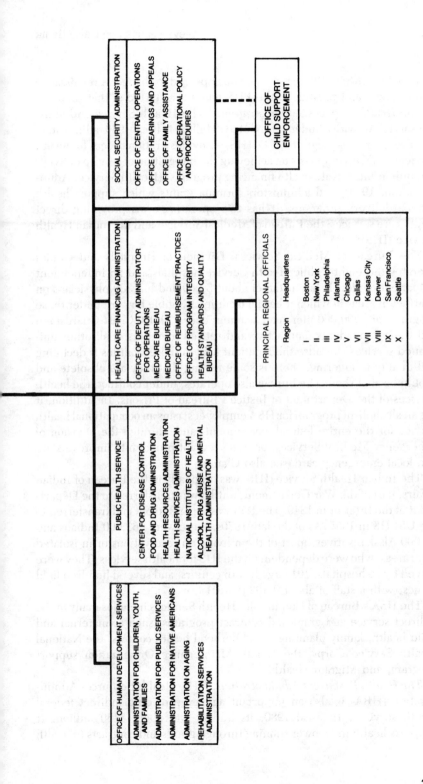

Figure 11.1 Organization Chart of the Department of Health and Human Services

Disease Prevention (1979), the situation appeared to change. A renaissance of the power and prestige of the PHS may have started at that time.

   The Health Services Administration.   The Health Services Administration (HSA), with a budget of about $1.3 billion in fiscal 1980, administers the direct services programs of DHHS, "provides a rational focus for health services . . . with emphasis on achieving the integration of service delivery and public and private health financing programs" (Health Services Administration, 1974), and administers formula grants which support health service delivery programs. It has two operating arms providing direct health care services: the Bureau of Medical Services and the Indian Health Service (IHS).

   The Bureau of Medical Services' Division of Hospitals and Clinics operates the eight Public Health Service hospitals and 26 independent outpatient clinics. It has a staff of about 5,000 and has 330 physicians on contract in areas in which it has no facilities. Eligible for care under these programs are 200,000 merchant seamen, over 130,000 Coast Guardsmen and their dependents, and active and retired members of all other uniformed services. Because the inpatient load in those facilities is declining and quality is suffering, there is some feeling that they are obsolete and should be abolished. The Bureau also operates, under contract, the health services of the Department of Justice's Bureau of Prisons. In addition, it has an alcoholism program for HSA employees; runs an occupational health service for the entire federal government, and, through the Division of Emergency Medical Services, operates a grant program to improve state and local emergency care (see also Chapter 6).

   The Indian Health Service (IHS) was originally in the Bureau of Indian Affairs, part of the War Department, until it was transferred to the Department of the Interior in 1849. The IHS was separated out and transferred to the USPHS in 1955. As of the late 1970s, there were 663,000 Indians and 71,000 Alaska Natives, most of them living on reservations or in isolated rural areas, who were dependent on the IHS for health services. They were served by 49 hospitals, 101 large health centers, and several hundred field clinics, with a staff of about 9,400 (USPHS, p. 87).

   The HSA's Bureau of Community Health Services includes many of the indirect service and grant and contract programs, such as maternal and child health, family planning, neighborhood health centers, the National Health Service Corps, the Health Maintenance Organization support program, and Migrant Health.

   The Health Resources Administration.   The Health Resources Administration (HRA) is also an important agency providing indirect federal health services. In fiscal 1980, its budget was about $450 million. It supports health manpower training through grants and contracts to health professions schools; provides leadership and support for the development of comprehensive health planning; and supports activities concerned with health facility development. Its mission is "to identify health care resource problems and maintain or strengthen the distribution, supply, utilization, quality, and cost-effectiveness of these resources to improve the health care system and individual health status" (Health Resources Administration). The functional divisions of HRA are the Bureau of Health Professions, the Bureau of Health Planning, and the Bureau of Health Facilities.

The Center for Disease Control. The Center for Disease Control (CDC) had a budget of about $280 million in FY 1980. It functions primarily to prevent and control communicable disease, to direct foreign and interstate quarantine operations, to improve the performance of clinical laboratories, and to develop the standards necessary to insure safe and healthful working conditions for all working people. It maintains excellent reference laboratories and carries out training programs. It also awards project grants to state and local health agencies to support immunization, particularly for children, and has health education responsibilities.

The Food and Drug Administration. The Food and Drug Administration, with a budget of about $320 million in FY 1980, functions to protect the public against hazards of various products and to assure potency and effectiveness of such products as drugs. FDA has six divisions, each covering a major type of product: the Bureau of Foods, the Bureau of Drugs, the Bureau of Veterinary Medicine, the Bureau of Radiological Health, the Bureau of Biologics, and the Bureau of Medical Devices. It also includes a National Center for Toxicological Research.

The Bureau of Drugs, which has responsibility under the Kefauver-Harris Amendments of 1962 for assuring the efficacy of all drugs, is perhaps the most controversial FDA agency. Some have contended that potentially useful drugs are being kept off the market by a lengthy and expensive approval process. Others feel that such premarket approval is essential to protect the public. Congress, through its consideration of bills to strengthen FDA, and its passage in 1976 of legislation to bring medical devices under similar controls, has shown its belief in the necessity of such assurances of efficacy and safety.

In the late 1970s, several legislative proposals that would substantially reform the drug review, approval, and control process were before the Congress. The Carter Administration's proposal contained provisions that would: increase consumer protection; increase consumer information and protect patient rights; encourage drug innovation; make additional drugs available; promote competition and cost savings through the use of generic drugs; increase FDA openness and public accountability; improve FDA enforcement; and encourage research and training. Considerable con-

troversy was raised by these proposals and by others emanating from the
Congress itself. The pharmaceutical industry and consumer organizations
were involved in lobbying on all sides of the issue.

The National Institutes of Health. The National Institutes of Health
(NIH), with a budget of about $3.4 billion in FY 1980, is responsible for
supporting and carrying out health research through its 11 institutes.
Although a number of other federal agencies support health research, the
NIH alone accounts for about two-thirds of the federal investment in health
research. NIH has its own (intramural) research program on its campus in
Bethesda, Maryland, and supports research at many other institutions
around the country through (extramural) grants and contracts. NIH also
fosters research by supporting training, resource development, and construction.

NIH has been subject to a number of investigations and has been
consistently found to be a high-quality research institution (House of
Representatives; President's Biomedical Research Panel). However, the
reports have also raised certain concerns. It was probably this problem that
stimulated Secretary Califano to initiate an activity to develop goals for
biomedical research in the United States (*DHEW Health Research Principles*). The principles that resulted stressed the importance of basic or
fundamental research.

The *Research Principles* also stressed the importance of mission-
oriented research. One form of targeted research that has become publicly
visible in the past several years is the evaluation of medical practices or
technologies. Driven by the rising costs of medical care, a number of
analyses examined the benefits of medical technology. The main finding
was that technologies are often introduced and used widely without clear
scientific evidence that they are beneficial to the health of the people
(Office of Technology Assessment; Banta and Behney). Although NIH
supports a reasonably large number of clinical trials, it has not been
mandated to do so. Examination of this situation led Congress in late 1978
to pass legislation establishing a new agency, the National Center for
Health Care Technology (NCHCT). Its main goal was to "better equip [the
PHS] to assess, systematically, the potential of technological applications
in medicine and to promote those which offer advances in health care"
(Richmond, p. 2).

The NCHCT is part of the Office of Health Research, Statistics, and
Technology, also established in 1979 in the office of the Assistant Secretary
for Health. It includes as well the National Center for Health Services
Research (NCHSR) and the National Center for Health Statistics (NCHS).
The principal responsibility of the NCHS is to carry out one of the historically oldest public health functions, the counting and analysis of statistics
on morbid and fatal events and their relationships in populations. The

NCHS collects and publishes a wide range of health and illness data, gathered in a number of ongoing studies by itself and by many other federal, state, and local government agencies, in a broad range of publications. The NCHS also conducts research in statistical and survey methodology. NCHSR is the primary federal agency responsible for research to improve the provision and quality of health services. NCHSR sponsors research in many private agencies and has its own intramural research program as well. In 1979, it identified nine priority issues for intensive study: (1) technology assessment; (2) health insurance; (3) cost containment; (4) planning and regulation; (5) quality of care; (6) health care and the disadvantaged; (7) health manpower; (8) emergency medical services and ambulatory care; and (9) long-term care (Richmond).

The Alcohol, Drug Abuse and Mental Health Administration. The Alcohol, Drug Abuse and Mental Health Administration (ADAMHA), with a budget of over $9.7 billion in FY 1980, is divided into three parts: the National Institute on Alcohol Abuse and Alcoholism, the National Institute on Drug Abuse, and the National Institute of Mental Health (NIMH).

Each division of ADAMHA supports treatment, rehabilitation, prevention, and research activities in its area of interest. The National Institute on Drug Abuse has given special emphasis to assuring treatment facilities for heroin addicts; the National Institute on Alcohol Abuse and Alcoholism supports treatment and prevention demonstration programs; the National Institute of Mental Health administers an intramural research program on the grounds of NIH and also controls a large nationwide program of community mental health centers.

ADAMHA is controversial because each of its divisions supports both service and research programs. Many feel that service programs will inevitably erode support for research and doubt that such an agency can support first-class research. A 1976 report from the President's Biomedical Research Panel recommended that ADAMHA's research activities be increased.

The Veterans' Administration

The Veterans' Administration (VA) is an independent agency of the federal government reporting directly to the President. The VA operates the largest centrally directed hospital and clinic system in the United States: in the late 1970s, about 30 million veterans, 14% of the population, were eligible to receive at least a portion of their medical care in a VA medical facility.

The origins of the VA medical services can be traced to a 1776 report of a committee of the Continental Congress established "to consider what provision ought to be made for such as are wounded or disabled in the land or sea service, and report a plan for that purpose" (*Journals of the Con-*

tinental Congress, vol. 5, p. 469). The committee had recommended the establishment of a pension system for disabled veterans. (Precedent for such a system can be traced back to an act of the English Parliament in its 1592–93 session that provided relief for veterans of the 1588 war with Spain.) By the time of the American Revolution, every colony had some program to assist disabled veterans (House Committee Print No. 4, p. 29). The federal government took over the responsibilities in 1789.

Following the American Civil War, the federal government established the "National Military and Naval Home" to care for Union Army veterans with service-connected disabilities causing "economic distress." Later, the facilities were made available to all veterans, and "for economic distress" not necessarily related to military service. There were 11 homes throughout the country, primarily for residence, with medical care a secondary consideration.

After World War I, the Public Health Service hospital system was assigned the responsibility of caring for the large influx of disabled veterans. The system was expanded greatly by the addition of certain military hospitals and the construction of new ones—by June 1920, there were 11,639 beds in 52 hospitals. In 1922, the veterans' hospitals were transferred to the Veterans' Bureau, which became the Veterans' Administration in 1930.

In fiscal 1978, the VA was operating 172 medical centers with 90,154 hospital beds: 43,749 medical (including about 11,000 extended care beds); 18,878 surgical; and 27,527 psychiatric (Cleland, pp. 9–10). There were 47 satellite or independent clinics. Nursing home care units were operated by 91 of the centers and 15 operated domiciliaries. There were about 190,000 full-time equivalents in staff, including 11,000 physicians, 1,100 dentists, and 27,000 nurses. There was a VA hospital in every state except Alaska and Hawaii, where veterans are hospitalized in civilian facilities under contract, and Puerto Rico. The VA's annual health care budget was $5.2 billion; 2.5 million veterans made over 15 million outpatient visits and provided over 1.2 million admissions to VA hospitals.

There are four overlapping groups of veterans eligible to receive VA medical care: (1) veterans with service-connected disabilities; (2) recipients of VA pensions; (3) veterans 65 years and older; and (4) "medically indigent" veterans (Veterans' Administration, 1979, p. 5). The means test is self-administered and there are no financial investigations. Over 50% of discharges from VA hospitals in FY 1978 were for patients who had no service-connected disability and drew no VA pension (Cleland, p. 26). A veteran is anyone who served 90 days or more in an armed service, but he/she must have received an honorable or general discharge in order to be automatically eligible. Thus, for eligibility there is a "moral means test" based on discharge status.

Medical staffing in the majority of VA hospitals is provided under a unique arrangement. Following World War II, press reports of abysmal medical care in VA hospitals led to the establishment of affiliation agreements with medical schools under which graduate (and eventually undergraduate) education would be carried out in them, with the VA paying the salaries of the house staff and certain faculty members. These activities are supervised by "Deans' Committees."

The government thus divided its responsibility and authority over its paid VA staff with medical schools and faculty that had neither received government grants or salaries for VA purposes, nor were assigned any accountability for their actions to the government or to the taxpayers; the VA remained ultimately responsible for the quality of services. Neither the schools nor the individual medical personnel were in the employ of the government; nonetheless, the Deans' Committees since 1946 have controlled the expenditure of many millions of dollars each year for VA residents, interns, full-time and part-time staff, consultants, and attendants, usually from medical school faculties. The committees have, in addition, influenced the annual expenditure of millions of dollars for medical supplies and equipment that, in their judgment, are needed for education, research, and patient care (Lewis, pp. 156–62). Until June 1973, the agreements had been quite informal and were largely verbal understandings. However, these arrangements generally worked well, and many feel they have been the salvation of the VA system. In 1973, the VA Central Office decided that a little more formality was in order and directed that letters of understanding—quite simple in language and very liberal in policy—be completed. By the late 1970s, 136 VA hospitals had medical school affiliation agreements.

In 1966, federal legislation opened up the VA hospitals for affiliation with other types of health sciences educational institutions. By 1978, VA hospitals had educational agreements with 58 dental schools, 130 graduate departments of psychology, 153 nursing schools, 108 rehabilitation medicine schools (primarily physical, occupational, and speech therapy), 148 social work schools, and several hundred other allied health units in universities, colleges, and technical institutions.

In 1977, the National Academy of Sciences (1977) reported on a Congressionally mandated *Study of Health Care for American Veterans*. The study was in depth, the report large, and the recommendations many. The most controversial one was that "VA policies and programs should be designed to permit the VA system ultimately to be phased in to the general delivery of health services in communities across the country" (National Academy of Sciences, p. 279), assuming that medical care services for veterans would continue to be paid for under existing policies, or under a to-be-enacted national health insurance program. The VA's response was swift and predictable (Veterans' Administration, 1977). In a massive document, the VA rejected out of hand the proposal that its hospital system be gradually dismantled as a separate entity and be incorporated into the nation's general medical care system. The special, veteran-centered system was to be maintained as a national resource and obligation. By 1980, no starts had been made to implement any of the major NAS recommendations. The two documents together provide a fascinating insight into this unique health care delivery subsystem, however.

Department of Defense

There are about 9 million people in the United States who receive all or most of the health care under the auspices of the Department of Defense, or DOD, about 4% of the population (Rice, p. 80). According to the Army Surgeon General, speaking in 1978, military medicine's four principal objectives are as follows (Comptroller General):

- To maintain physically and mentally fit servicemen and trained health manpower to support combat, contingency, and mobilization plans;
- To provide care and treatment capabilities in a theater of operations and in the United States for combat casualties;
- To provide health services for dependents of soldiers, retired career servicemen and their dependents, and dependents and survivors of deceased career servicemen; and
- To provide a major incentive for soldiers, including health professionals, to select military service as a career. (p. 1)

According to a House Armed Services Committee Report, in addition to active-duty servicemen, their dependents and surviving dependents of servicemen killed on active duty are *entitled* to care. Career retirees and their dependents *may* be given care at a military facility, if the capacity exists. However, many of the latter category of person feel that they too are *entitled* to care. This difference of perception created problems for the military medicine system in the late 1970s (Comptroller General, pp. 2–5). It is an aspect of the larger contradiction faced by the DOD medical services: being constantly prepared for war on the one hand while trying to operate a huge conventional health care delivery system on the other (Rice, p. 81).

As of 1979, DOD operated 170 hospitals, of which 129 were in the Continental United States (CONUS). Although the total peacetime bed capacity was 37,609, only 20,650 beds (17,636 in CONUS) were operating, with occupancy rates varying from 49% to 97%. There were 302 freestanding clinics and dispensaries and 19 drug and alcohol rehabilitation centers. There were about 95,000 military and 39,000 civilian personnel to staff these facilities, including 11,000 physicians and 10,000 nurses (Rice, p. 81). These facilities and people provided over 900,000 hospital admissions and 46 million outpatient visits (Comptroller General, p. 1).

The Civilian Health and Medical Program of the Uniformed Services (CHAMPUS) is an important medical care resource for non-uniformed beneficiaries. CHAMPUS is a reimbursement system that pays for the costs of care in the private sector for dependents of active-duty members, career retirees and their dependents, and surviving dependents of members killed while on active duty. Theoretically, all persons potentially eligible under CHAMPUS must first seek care from a military medical facility and be unable to obtain it, for one reason or another (Comptroller General, p. 4).

A serious problem faced by DOD at the end of the 1970s, resulting in part from the perceived rights of retiree families and survivors' dependents for care, and leading to an increased use of CHAMPUS, was a chronic and severe shortage of physicians in an all-volunteer army. This problem has persisted despite various attempts to solve it. First, the inequities in income differential between military physicians and those in private practice have been reduced somewhat (but apparently not enough); second, there are educational scholarship support programs that obligate physician graduates to a given term of service; and third, the roles of other medical care providers are being redefined to extend the capabilities of those physicians in service (Cowan, 1975, 1976). All of the services have traditionally relied on medics, particularly in the field, but they are now increasingly turning toward formally trained physicians' assistants and clinical nurse practitioners. Moreover, trained administrators are replacing physician-executives. Finally, in the Uniformed Service University of the Health Sciences, the DOD is training its own physicians, as well as other health care providers (*Medical World News;* Boffey). Nevertheless, a great deal of dissatisfaction remains among DOD physicians (Comptroller General, pp. 44–49).

An unusual aspect of military medical departments is that they are charged not only with providing a full range of direct health services but also with providing for the environmental health of their communities. This combination of administrative responsibilities for personal and community preventive and treatment services is rarely found in the U.S. health care delivery system.

Other Federal Departments

As noted in Table 11.1, a number of other federal government departments engage in health-related activities not involving the delivery of personal health services. The United States Department of Agriculture (USDA) has major responsibilities for human, animal, and plant health (Office of the

Secretary of Agriculture). Most of its health-related money is spent on research and preventive activities. Focusing on improved crop and animal production, in 1979 the USDA dealt with hog cholera, African swine fever, contagious equine metritis, fruit flies, and boll weevils. The USDA is also active in various aspects of human nutrition. It operates a National School Lunch Program and the Food Stamp Program, which helps poor people to buy food. It establishes recommended daily allowances for nutrients. In 1980, in cooperation with the USDHEW, it issued overall dietary guidelines as part of a program to establish a national nutrition policy (USDA). It supervises food safety regulations in cooperation with the FDA, and grades meats and other foods for consumers. It also has programs in nutrition education and research.

The Department of Housing and Urban Development invests most of its health-related expenditure in construction, especially of rural hospitals and neighborhood clinics; its Federal Housing Authority (FHA) provides mortgage insurance for hospitals, group practice facilities, and long-term care facilities.

The Department of Labor invests most of its health-related expenditure in preventive activities in the workplace, through its Occupational Safety and Health Administration (OSHA). OSHA uses criteria developed by the National Institute of Occupational Safety and Health (NIOSH), part of the CDC, to set national standards for occupational safety and health (*President's Report on Occupational Safety and Health, 1979;* U.S. Department of Labor, 1977, 1979a, 1979b). The major responsibilities of OSHA are to develop workplace health and safety standards, to enforce and gain compliance with the standards, to engage in education and training, to guarantee workers' rights, and to aid business in meeting OSHA requirements. In the late 1970s, OSHA was concentrating on focusing resources on high-risk industries and workplace hazards, rather than on trivia, improving its aid to employers for meeting standards, educating workers in occupational safety and health, and simplifying regulations and eliminating unnecessary rules.

The Environmental Protection Agency (EPA) is an independent (nondepartmental) federal government agency that has major responsibilities for air and water quality and pollution control, solid waste disposal control, pesticide regulation, radiation hazard control, noise abatement, and toxic substances (U.S. Environmental Protection Agency, 1979a, 1979b). The Environmental Protection Agency conducts research on air pollution control technology and the effects of air pollution on humans, develops criteria and promulgates national standards for pollutants, and enforces compliance with these standards.*

*For further information on the health-related activities of OSHA and EPA, see Chapter 17 of *Public Health and Preventive Medicine*, John Last, Ed., New York: Appleton-Century-Crofts, 1980.

Fragmentation and Reorganization of Health Programs

As a candidate in 1976, President Carter campaigned vigorously for the need to reorganize the federal bureaucracy. And indeed, it has been pointed out (Roemer et al.) that:

> A bewildering array of programs, services, and agencies confronts the individual seeking health care in the United States. Listings of federal assistance programs have revealed hundreds of separate health programs at the federal level of government alone, within the Department of Health, Education and Welfare and other departments. (p. 2)

This multiplicity of programs leads to fragmented responsibility and provision of services, as well as to overlapping within geographic areas and political jurisdictions. The result is a lack of coherent policy. Roemer et al. note that these programs have been developed for various reasons:

> The complexity of the health service system in the United States is the result of the accretion of programs and agencies over the years as new needs in health services have been recognized, of the specialized and categorical character of these services, of the sheer numbers of individuals and organizations that provide health care, and of the lack of a rational pattern for fitting the many parts into an effective whole. (p. 11)

These programs, then, are generally addressed to real needs, and in many cases the programs' problems stem less from organizational disorder than from lack of money to do the whole job. The separation of DOD health programs from categorical HHS programs, for example, is not necessarily a problem. On the other hand, a serious organizational problem does exist in HHS: the separation of the financing programs, Medicare and Medicaid, from the resources development and health planning activities found in the Public Health Service. As will be discussed in Chapter 12, this split reflects the organization structure of the Congress, and is difficult to attack for that reason.

There are many possible solutions to these problems, which relate not only to the complexity of the federal government's role in health care delivery and the nature of the "pluralistic" system of medical care, but more broadly to the complexity of the structure and role of government. "Reorganization" is one commonly proposed solution. The theory of scientific management is often cited. The Congressional Research Service notes (Moe): "Every major study of the executive branch has reflected, to some degree, the influence of these administrative values." As Seidman says: "Reorganization is deemed synonymous with reform and reform with progress. Periodic reorganizations are prescribed if for no other purpose than to purify the bureaucratic blood and to prevent stagnation" (p. 3).

One goal of reorganization favored by special-interest groups is to raise the bureaucratic level of the office supervising the program in which they are interested. Seidman notes: "Rare indeed is the Commission or Presidential task force with the self-restraint to forgo proposing an organizational answer to the problems it cannot solve" (p. 4). For example, in 1976, the Diabetes Commission suggested placing diabetes activities under a National Diabetes Advisory Board in the Office of the Assistant Secretary for Health (National Commission on Diabetes). In 1977, as mentioned earlier, several research centers were moved into the Office of the Assistant Secretary for Health, as had been proposed by those interested in those programs for years.

Although understandable, this effort can only add to the "tangled net of programs." It is difficult to apply organizational theory to the executive branch for just this reason. The structure inevitably "reflects the values, conflicts, and competing forces to be found in a pluralistic society" (Seidman, p. 13). "Rational organization" can mean excluding some elements of society from effective participation in the system and an equitable share of its benefits. The organization of the executive branch has an organic function that may not be perceived by even the wisest reformers. For example, some overlapping of programs in different parts of the organization may assure plurality of funding that acts against dogmatic program development. Categorical programs or specific programs, while tending to fragment the executive branch, do elicit Congressional and public support—thus the change in the name of the National Microbiological Institute to the National Institute of Allergy and Infectious Diseases (Seidman, p. 34).

Such jurisdictional problems have probably been the main force preventing reorganization. Although the President did gain new authority in 1977 to reorganize the executive branch, the goals of effective management, economy, and efficiency are often incompatible. Because truly effective reorganization is difficult to achieve, form rather than substance is often emphasized. As Seidman notes: "Frequently studies of executive branch structure degenerate into sterile box-shuffling and another version of the numbers game" (p. 12).

In outlining some of the drawbacks to reorganization, we do not argue against it per se. Reorganization is often valuable and even critical: the old organizational framework may become anachronistic, and, for political reasons, a controversial program may be buried deep in the bureaucracy, or a prestigious one brought into public view. The 1977 reorganization that placed the Medicare and Medicaid programs in one organizational structure seems to make good sense. On the other hand, it is necessary to look on reorganization skeptically. It may be the result of a naive faith in management science and a lack of trust in democracy. It may also be an attempt to avoid the real problem, which in part is a proliferation of underfunded categorical programs.

It is worth pointing out that NIH, FDA, and CDC have had considerable stability over a number of years and will probably continue in much their present form, however government programs change. It is the other agencies, which are sometimes made up of a bundle of unrelated programs, that can be expected to be subject to further reorganizations.

Regulation

"Regulation" has become an unpopular word, and deregulation a popular concept. The flood of advertisements, speeches, articles, and books continues unabated. Analyses purport to show that various regulations cost more than seems reasonable. Mobil Oil decries a "national orgy of regulation" (quoted in Green). It is undeniable that the scope of federal regulations has increased markedly within the past decade. The growth of regulation has been costly. And there are certainly problems of implementation, such as delays by regulatory agencies, duplication of reporting requirements, hastily issued and ill-conceived regulations, and conflicting regulations by different agencies (Allen). The purpose of this section is to discuss briefly an important general issue as it applies to health care.

Regulation is pervasive in the health care system (O'Donoghue: Institute of Medicine; Havighurst). Many regulations have been discussed in various chapters. For example, physicians are regulated basically through a licensing system operated by the states (see Chapter 14). Hospitals are licensed by states (see Chapter 14). Any program with a statutory base develops regulations to implement the programs. It is these regulations, which have force of law, that are referred to in the term "regulation."

The federal government administers three regulatory programs that have direct implications for medical care. They are the product regulations for drugs, devices, and biologics of the Food and Drug Administration; the regulations developed in the health planning program (see Chapter 13); and the PSRO program (see Chapter 14), our main quality-assurance mechanism.

Why do regulatory programs develop? As Hutt (1976) says:

> The rationale customarily given for government regulation . . . is that, in a complex society, individual consumers can no longer protect their own interests and the government must therefore do it for them. Implicit in this well-recognized principle is that there is something against which the public in fact does need protection. . . . The history of the increasing government regulation (of consumer products) is the history of the perceived failure of business to regulate itself in a way sufficient to satisfy the public's felt needs. Time and again, Congress has acted in response to what it believed to be a demonstrated danger.

Thus, regulation is an extension of government power into the private sector to protect the public. In effect, it is a contract between consumers and the private sector, in which consumers agree to a market economy if business avoids unnecessary injury and death and establishes minimum conditions to protect the public (Green). This formulation applies well to the three programs mentioned above.

Is this formulation consistent with public attitudes? It seems to be. A comprehensive review of public opinion polls relating to regulation concluded that although public support for regulation has slipped a bit, government regulation is widely accepted and even popular in some areas. Americans have been ambivalent toward regulation for four decades. They have said that they opposed greater regulation, but they have also expressed approval of existing regulation and said that they did not want to roll back the tide. The public does not express lack of faith in business, but expects the government to act as a watchdog to make sure that business does not inappropriately exploit its powerful position. Although the public lacks faith in government as the solution to anticipated problems, it turns to government regulation as the only answer (Lipset and Schneider).

It does seem that Congress expressed a more pervasive skepticism against regulation in the late 1970s than one might believe from these polls. Not since passage of the Medical Device Amendments of 1976 has Congress strengthened health regulatory programs. In 1979, it weakened the health planning program in some ways. The proposed Drug Reform Act of 1978 found little receptivity in Congress. Congress rejected cost-containment legislation.

The claim is that the costs of regulation are unreasonable. A review by the Library of Congress in 1978 found that estimates of the cost of regulation were sketchy, incomplete, and of doubtful validity (Allen). However, the cost question does dominate debate. Several studies examined the PSRO program and concluded that it was not cost-effective because it cost more to operate than it can be demonstrated to have saved (Congressional Budget Office; Health Services Administration, 1978). (That situation was reversed by 1979, however; see Chapter 14.) The problem with this reasoning is that regulatory programs have goals that are very difficult to quantitate. The Food and Drug Administration exists to prevent unsafe drugs from being used; the costs of using unsafe drugs can hardly be quantitated. The PSRO program has quality-assurance goals that go well beyond financial costs.

The essential point is that regulation has developed to meet real needs. While programs can be improved, and some alternatives such as financial incentives may have a place, regulation in the health care system is an essential function that is certain to continue.

State and Local Governments
Federal-State-Local Relationships

As pointed out at the beginning of this chapter, like the federal government, state and local governments have multiple functions in the health care delivery system. In considering the states' and localities' roles in health care, we shall first examine some aspects of their relationships with the federal government.

Money transfers from the federal government to state and local governments began very early in the history of the United States, but did not become significant until after World War II. As late as 1950, such transfers for all purposes totaled only $2 billion (Office of Managment and Budget, Table H–7). After 1960, the amount rose rapidly; the expected 1980 expenditure is $83 billion. That was about 24% of total state and local government expenditures (Office of Management and Budget, Table H–7).

About $33 billion of the total (40%) came from the DHEW (Office of Management and Budget, Table H–5). Health expenditures showed the most dramatic growth, rising from 4% of federal aid in 1958 to 19% in 1980. The estimated federal expenditures for health services' aid to the state and local governments was about $14.5 billion (Office of Management and Budget, Table H–3). The increase has been largely due to the Medicaid program (see Chapters 10 and 15). Income security, a separate but important health-related function that includes the federal share of unemployment and Welfare payments, and railroad retirement and other programs, accounted for more than $15 billion in federal aid to state and local governments in 1980.

Federal aid developed as "categorical" grants to support specific activities. Categorical programs are those developed to aid certain groups, such as the maternal and child health (MCH) program or the tuberculosis control program. The first such program was created by the Sheppard-Towner Act of 1921. Enacted over the bitter opposition of the AMA, it provided for grants-in-aid to the states, setting the pattern for future categorical federal programs (Stern, pp. 123–124; Mustard, pp. 73–77; Burrow, pp. 157–165).

By the late 1960s, however, there was increasing concern about uncoordinated programs, excessive federal requirements on the funds, and rigid funding arrangements that prevented local innovation and decision-making. James Haughton (1968) wrote rather vehemently:

> The worst way to finance health care is by categorical grants. Categorical grants tend to attract programs to where the money is rather than where the need is . . . rather than developing services on a broad basis so that people get

the services they need, categorical grants tend to stimulate programs that match the money that is available. (p. 773)

Reforms instituted by the Nixon Administration in the early 1970s and continued under the Carter Administration included: (1) decentralization of decision-making to federal field offices in 10 regions; (2) simplification of federal grant administrative requirements; (3) maximum possible sharing of planning and management functions with state and local governments; and (4) consolidation of overlapping federal grant programs (Office of Management and Budget, p. 229). This led to the development in 1973 of what was called "general revenue-sharing," designed principally to get away from the categorical approach, to give money to states based on a formula reflecting population and relative economic status, and then, within very broad program guidelines, to let the states—and through them the local governments—decide how to spend the money, based on their knowledge of specific community needs. However, in the Nixon approach, general revenue-sharing had other goals, in particular to slow the growth of federal aid to states (Whitman). The 1976 estimate of outlays for general revenue-sharing and other broad-based grants was $9.6 billion (Office of Management and Budget, p. 230), about 22% of the total. However, reductions in numerous grant programs were likely to lead to reduced levels of social services, especially to the poor, and to less innovative government activity in urban areas (Whitman). Thus, revenue-sharing was partially in conflict with the stated goals of the earlier reforms.

These changes attempt to redefine the appropriate role of government and the relationship between state and federal government. An overall reduction in spending implies that the public wishes to have fewer programs. A shift to state and local initiative indicates a growing awareness that not all governmental programs can be administered from Washington. It makes good sense to decentralize as many functions as possible, if the states are capable of handling them; but many experts are skeptical on this point (Seggel, pp. 110–112). Federal program administration has also been largely decentralized to regional offices, despite Congressional opposition. Indications are that these offices lack the expertise required to furnish technical assistance, a critical federal role (Martin; Seggel, pp. 112–113).

Another consideration is equity. The history of welfare programs in the United States is not reassuring in this regard. Welfare has been run through grants-in-aid to the states, but as Burns points out (p. 49), states have been required to carry some of the costs, on the assumption that this will help to assure responsible administration. Purely local program development can lead to great inequities because of unequal resources, the traditional pauper stigma, and racial prejudice. The innumerable different state benefits, exclusions, and unreasonable eligibility requirements have led to proposals to federalize welfare. Proponents point to the Supplemental Security Income (SSI) program for Social Security beneficiaries, a partial federalization of welfare. By 1975, it had relieved the states of responsibility for about $1 billion annually in expenditures for public assistance to the aged, blind, and disabled, and simultaneously abolished the inequities (Seggel, p. 71).

The Medicaid program is also plagued with inequities. Although President Ford proposed early in 1976 that more of the administrative and financial responsibility for this program should be turned back to the states, the above considerations make that unlikely. In fact, the federalization of Medicaid has been proposed in several national health insurance bills, and seems inevitable. Several NHI proposals, however, have included state administration (see Chapter 15).

Thus the debate continues. A concept of policy-direction from Washington—along with considerable financial assistance, in the federal government's role as income-transfer agent—has evolved, but the specifics of this philosophy applied to each program will have to be worked out over time. It is clear that this will remain one of the critical policy issues of American government.

The State Government's Role in Health Services

As at the federal level, many different agencies are involved in health services at the state level. In most states, two of the most important health-related functions are provided by departments other than the state health department: mental illness treatment services are usually run by an independent department, and the Medicaid program is often run by the state welfare department. In recent years, the Association of State and Territorial Health Officials (ASTHO) has taken on the task of annually surveying the activities of the nation's state health departments (1980). There is no readily available information on the totality of health functions of other state agencies.

Licensing of health manpower often resides in the education department; vocational rehabilitation in a special agency; occupational health in the labor department; school health in the local boards of education; and in some states, environmental protection programs are found in a special agency too. Most states also have a board of health, usually appointed by the Governor, which has varying administrative, policy, and advisory functions.

The National Commission on Community Health Services (1966) recommended consolidation of official health services in a single state health agency. One state that has attempted such consolidation is Massachusetts, which previously had classical public health programs plus certification of need and licensing of private health facilities in a Department of Public Health, but had the following programs in other agencies as well:

1. Rate-setting—the Office of Administration and Finance
2. Regulation of health insurance—the Commissioner of Insurance
3. Licensing and standard-setting for health personnel—Office of Consumer Affairs
4. Administration and standard-setting for the Medicaid program— Department of Public Welfare
5. Health planning activities—Office of Human Services.

These functions were reorganized into a Health Systems Regulation Administration in 1974 (Executive Office of Human Services, 1974).

In Chapter 6, in considering the role of local health departments in ambulatory care, we discussed the political struggles with the private practitioners in the 1920s that led to the departments being generally limited in functions to Haven Emerson's "Basic Six." The "Basic Six" are vital statistics, public health laboratories, communicable-disease control, environmental sanitation, maternal and child health, and public health education (Wilson and Neuhauser, p. 204). Local governments (usually not local health departments, however) were also given responsibility for providing general medical services for the poor. State governments were generally confined to the Basic Six as well (excluding general medical care for the poor), but also ran the public mental hospitals. In recent years, additional responsibilities have been given to state governments, and on occasion to large local governments, in regulation and quality-control, rate-setting, institutional licensure, planning, and acting as a third-party payor under Medicaid.

Activities of State Health Agencies. Not all states call their principal government health agency the health department. Thus ASTHO established the designation "State Health Agency" (SHA), defined as "the agency or department headed by the state or territorial health official" (Association of State and Territorial Health Officials, p. iv). The "states" in this definition include the fifty states plus the District of Columbia, American Samoa, Guam, Puerto Rico, the Trust Territory of the Pacific Islands, the Northern Mariana Islands, and the Virgin Islands. Thus there are 57 SHAs.

ASTHO has defined six program areas for SHAs. It defines a program as: "A set of identifiable services organized to solve health-related problems or to meet specific health or health-related needs, provided to or on behalf of the public, by or under the direction of an organizational entity in a State Health Agency, and for which reasonably accurate estimates of expenditures can be made" (Association of State and Territorial Health Officials, p. vii). The six areas are "personal health, environmental health, health resources, laboratory, general administration and services, and funds to local health departments not allocated to program areas" (Association of State and Territorial Health Officials, p. 9). All SHAs had personal health programs, 54 reported environmental health programs, 54 had health resources programs, 53 had laboratory programs, and 56 had general administration and services.

Regarding identifiable public health services, a significant number of SHAs report having programs, some of which are actually provided by local health departments, in the following areas:

- Maternal and child health, including prenatal and postnatal services, family planning, immunization, and well-baby care
- Communicable disease control, including immunization, tuberculosis and venereal disease control, epidemiology, and laboratory services
- Dental health, emphasizing preventive services
- Chronic-disease screening
- Environmental health, including consumer protection and sanitation, air and water quality control, waste management, occupational health and safety, and radiation control
- Health planning and resources development, regulation, and statistics.

The meaning of this fairly comprehensive list for the health of the American people ought to be evaluated at least in part in terms of the amount of money spent. In fiscal 1978, the 57 SHAs reporting spent a total of $3.3 billion, 1.7% of total national health expenditure during that year. Of the $3.3 billion 72% went for personal health programs. Included were many personal preventive services such as maternal and child health, communicable disease control, dental health, and chronic disease control. Of the $3.3 billion, 29% was spent on SHA-operated institutional treatment programs. However, $238 million (7%) went to environmental health programs; $299 million (9%) was spent on health resources programs (planning, etc.); and $131 million (4%) was paid for laboratory programs. These figures do not represent an overwhelming commitment by the states to public health services. The amount being spent on public health programs by other, non-SHA state agencies, e.g., environmental protection administrations, is not known. Of the total expenditure by SHAs, 55% came from the states themselves, 35% from the federal government, and the balance from miscellaneous sources. State expenditures of their own funds on SHA programs amounted to less than 1% of total state expenditures on all programs. About two-thirds of the federal funds came from HEW. Federal funds given to SHAs amounted to about 2.6% of all federal health-related expenditures, and about three-quarters of these federal funds went to support personal health services.

Personal health programs. Almost all SHAs reported having programs in maternal and child health, communicable disease control, chronic disease control, and dental health (Association of State and Territorial Health Officials, Table V–1). About 75% operated programs for crippled children; 45% operated mental health programs including mental retardation and substance abuse (recall that most states have a separate mental health department); about three-quarters operated other personal health services; and 44% operated patient-care institutions.

Although state public health services are in theory available to the general population, according to the ASTHO survey most programs were targeted toward persons with low incomes (Association of State and Territorial Health Officials, p. 65). Local health departments participated in the delivery of at least some of their programs, 47 SHAs reported.

Environmental health programs. In the examination of federal programs, it has already been pointed out that many agencies are active in environmental health. At the state level the picture is even more complicated. Under federal law dealing with environmental health, the governor of each state has designated a "lead environmental agency." In 19 states, it is the SHA (Association of State and Territorial Health Officials, p. 72). In the others, however, it is an environmental protection agency or a natural resources agency. Nevertheless, in some of the states in which the SHA is not the designated lead environmental agency, it still has important environmental health functions, especially in such areas as sanitation, pure water supply, and sanitary sewage disposal. Although in fiscal 1977, SHAs spent $238 million on environmental health activities, the total amount spent must be a considerably greater figure. It is unknown.

The major environmental health programs carried out by SHAs are (Association of State and Territorial Health Officials, p. 69):

- Consumer protection and sanitation: food and milk control, substance control and product safety, sanitation of health care facilities and other institutions, housing and recreational sanitation, and vector and zoonotic disease control
- Water-quality services: public and individual water supply and individual sewage disposal. (Public water pollution control services are usually provided by an agency other than the SHA.)
- Radiation control
- Occupational health and safety, accident prevention, and noise pollution control
- Solid- and hazardous-waste mangement

- Environmental health personnel training
- Environmental health planning, design, and impact studies.

Air quality control was provided by only 19 SHAs, the responsibility being lodged in other agencies in the balance of the states.

Health resources. Among the oldest of public health functions is the collection and analysis of vital and health statistics. In recent years, SHAs have expanded their activities in such areas as health planning, health resources development, and health resources regulation.

The National Health Planning and Resources Development Act of 1974 required that states establish a lead health planning agency, known as the State Health Planning and Development Agency, or SHPDA (see Chapter 13). In 35 states, the SHA houses the SHPDA (Association of State and Territorial Health Officials, p. 88). SHAs in some states make health facility construction grants and/or provide technical assistance for construction. Most SHAs are involved in one aspect or another of health manpower development, licensing, and regulation, as well as in health facility licensing, certification, and regulation. Public health laboratory services, another of the traditional public health services, are provided by 53 of the 57 SHAs.

Staffing. According to the 1978 ASTHO survey, about 125,000 full-time-equivalent people worked in SHAs. The categories most frequently reported (Association of State and Territorial Health Officials, p. 43) were registered nurses (17,800); engineers, sanitarians, and related employees (9,200); professional and technical laboratory employees (6,200); licensed practical nurses (6,300); and physicians (3,900). There were 65% of staff in personal health programs, 9% in environmental health programs, 8% in health resources programs, 5% in laboratory programs, 8% in general services, and the balance (5%) not assigned to specific program areas.

Local Government

It is even more difficult to speak authoritatively about local health departments than about state health departments. First, there is no generally agreed-to definition of a local health department. Second, there is no national roster or ongoing annual reporting system for local health departments. However, in the 1970s, Miller and his colleagues commenced a series of studies of local health departments, which have provided much useful information (Miller, 1975; Miller et al., 1977a, 1977b, 1979). Following a survey of what state health officers considered to be local health departments (LHD), Miller and his colleagues developed a definition of an LHD: "An administrative and service unit of local or state government, concerned with health, employing at least one full-time person and carrying some responsibility for the health of a jurisdiction smaller than a state" (1977a, p. 931). Because of the paucity of data, the surveyors were able to provide only a rough estimate of the number of LHDs fitting this definition. The surveyors surmised that it "probably falls between the inflated estimate of 2,073 represented by [our] address list . . . and the 1,073 reported . . . in 1966."

On the other hand, the National Public Health Program Reporting System (NPHPRS) of ASTHO, using a different definition of an LHD, came up with a much larger estimate. The NPHPRS defines an LHD as follows (Association of State and Territorial Health Officials):

> An official (governmental) public health agency which is in whole or in part responsible to a sub-state governmental entity or entities. The latter may be a city, county, city-county, federation of counties, borough, township, or any other type of sub-state governmental entity. In addition, a local health department must meet these criteria: (A) It has a staff of one or more full-time professional public health employees (e.g., public health nurse, sanitarian); (B) it delivers public health services; (C) it serves a definable geographic area; and (D) it has identifiable expenditures and/or budget in the political subdivision(s) which it serves. (p. 36)

Using this definition, 46 SHAs reported a total of 2,783 LHDs in their states in fiscal 1977, while 11 SHAs (including those of four states) reported that by the NPHPRS definition there were no LHDs in their states (Association of State and Territorial Health Officials, p. 36). No one has compared the Miller et al. and NPHPRS lists to attempt to explain the wide disparity between the numbers reported.

Miller et al. reported that there are three organizational patterns for LHDs: (1) they are operated by the SHA directly; (2) they are operated by local government entirely; and (3) they are operated jointly by local and state government (1977a). The majority of LHDs are based on single local government jurisdictions: city, county, town, etc. Mergers with other local government health agencies are a relatively recent development (Shonick and Price, 1977, 1978).

Regarding expenditures, once again, the data are limited. Miller et al. reported total LHD expenditures of $1.8 billion for fiscal 1974 (1977a). ASTHO reports another figure for fiscal 1978 (1980, p. 35). There is disagreement too on sources of funds. Miller et al. (1979) reported that 60% of LHD funding came from local government, 20% from the states, and 9% from federal sources. According to ASTHO, the figures are, respectively, 51%, 22%, and 16%, plus 11% from other sources (Association of State and Territorial Health Officials, p. 39).

According to Miller et al. (1979) the average number of employees in an

LHD is 35, one-third of whom are administrative/support personnel, one-third registered nurses, and one-fourth sanitarians. There is one physician for every 30 employees in the average LHD.

The types of functions carried out by LHDs are many. LHDs tend to be limited to the Basic Six, although some of them in recent years have become involved in the direct delivery of ambulatory services to the poor (Miller et al., 1979). Following the state and federal model, local health services are also provided by various agencies other than health departments. For example: cities and counties are likely to place their hospitals for the poor (see Chapter 7) and their mental health services (see Chapter 9) in separate agencies. Water supply, sanitary sewage and solid waste disposal, and pollution control are also likely to be in separate agencies, if they are not handled in the private sector.

According to Miller et al. (1977a), at least one-half of LHDs provide one or more of the following services: immunization, environmental surveillance, tuberculosis control, maternal and child health, school health, venereal disease control, chronic disease control, home care, family planning, ambulatory care, and health code enforcement. Thus, it is the LHDs in cooperation with SHAs and other state agencies, particularly in environmental health, which are the backbone of the system for providing public health and preventive services to the people. Nevertheless, LHD directors feel that major constraints were placed on performance and expansion of service by lack of funds and lack of staff (Miller et al., 1977a).

Conclusion

It should be quite clear that government is heavily involved in the health care delivery system in the United States. Our constitutional structure and our economic system determine and limit the nature of that involvement to a great extent. Government provides the legal underpinning for the system through the licensing laws, and regulates its workings through covering financing and quality of care. Government is a direct financier and a direct provider of service. It is preeminent in community health services and plays an important part in supporting health sciences education and research. However, the resistance to "government interference in the practice of medicine" is still very prominent among private medical practitioners, and in many laws concerning the health care delivery system—for example, the Social Security amendments establishing the Medicare program—such interference is expressly prohibited. Nonetheless, most providers recognize the reality of the situation—that government is already heavily involved in the practice of medicine—and they welcome participation in certain critical areas: licensing; care of the mentally ill, the tubercular, and the poor; and community health services.

We now face the problem of determining the precise role of government in the health system: what proportion of payment for health services will be public money, who shall plan how funds are used, who shall assure quality of care in physicians' offices, and so forth. The "tangled net of programs," with multiple jurisdictions and interests, leading to overlapping coverage for many people and lack of any coverage for others, presents a major difficulty. But a more serious problem is defining the relation between government and the private sector. What we need is not a "government takeover," but a rational division of labor between the public and private sectors; a cooperative effort aimed at benefiting the citizenry rather than aggrandizing either sector. However, it is easier to state the need for this alliance than to identify the programs and procedures that can bring it about.

In the remaining chapters we will examine how government is involved and will be involved in solving our health care problems in legislative action, planning, quality control, and national health insurance.

References

Allen, J. *Estimating the Costs of Federal Regulation: Review of Problems and Accomplishments to Date*. Washington, D.C.: Library of Congress, Congressional Research Service, 1978.

Association of State and Territorial Health Officials. *Comprehensive National Public Health Program Reporting System Report: Services, Expenditures and Programs of State and Territorial Health Agencies, Fiscal Year 1978*. Silver Springs, Maryland: ASTHO, 1980.

Banta, D., and Behney, C. "Medical Technology: Policies and Problems." *Health Care Management Review* (In Press).

Boffey, P. M. "Military Medical School: It Survives Despite All Efforts to Kill It." *Science, 190*, 860, 1975.

Burns, E. *Health Services for Tomorrow*. New York: Dunellen, 1974.

Burrow, J. G. *AMA: Voice of American Medicine*. Baltimore, Maryland: Johns Hopkins Press, 1963.

Cleland, M. *Veterans Administration: Annual Report, 1978*. Washington, D.C.: USGPO, 1978.

Comptroller General. *Military Medicine Is in Trouble: Complete Reassessment Needed*. Washington, D.C.: General Accounting Office, 1979.

Congressional Budget Office. *The Effect of PSROs on Health Care Costs: Current Findings and Future Evaluations*. Washington, D.C.: USGPO, 1979.

Cowan, J. R. "Retention Biggest Problem for DOD." *U.S. Medicine*, January 15, 1975, pp. 17–20.

————. "Volunteer Force: DOD Successful." *U.S. Medicine*, January 15, 1976, pp. 7–9.

DHEW Health Research Principles. Volume 1. Documents Relating to the Development of Draft Health Research Principles for the Department of Health, Education, and Welfare, April-December, 1978. USDHEW Pub. No. (NIH) 79–1890. Washington, D.C.: USGPO, 1978.

Executive Office of Human Services, Commonwealth of Massachusetts. *Statement of Rationale for the Health Systems Regulation Administration.* Proposed in House 6120, July 17, 1973, Boston.

——————. *Statement of Rationale for the Health Systems Regulation Administration.* July 17, 1974. Mimeograph.

Grad, F. P. *Public Health Law Manual.* Washington, D.C.: American Public Health Association, 1975.

Green, M. "The Faked Case Against Regulation." *The Washington Post,* Sunday, January 21, 1979, pp. C1, C5.

Haughton, J. G. *Hearings before the Subcommittee on Executive Reorganization of the Committee on Intergovernment Operations.* U.S. Senate, 90th Cong., 2nd Sess., July 1968.

Havighurst, C. C. *Regulating Health Facilities Construction.* Washington, D.C.: American Enterprise Institute, 1974.

Health Resources Administration. "Statement of Organization, Functions and Delegations of Authority." *Federal Register, 43,* 39423. September 5, 1978.

Health Services Administration. "Statement of Organization, Functions and Delegations of Authority." *Federal Register, 39,* 10462. March 20, 1974.

——————. *Professional Standards Review Organizations: Program Evaluation.* Report No. OPEL 77–12. Washington, D.C.: USGPO, 1978.

House Committee Print No. 4. *Medical Care of Veterans.* 90th Congress, 1st Session. Washington, D.C.: USGPO, April 1967.

House of Representatives. *Investigation of the National Institutes of Health.* Prepared by the Staff for the Use of the Committee on Interstate and Foreign Commerce and Its Subcommittee on Health and the Environment. Washington, D.C.: USGPO, 1976.

Hutt, P. "Balanced Government Regulation of Consumer Products." Presented at a Symposium on "Who Regulates the Regulator While the Regulator Regulates?" Published by the Center for Drug Development, University of Rochester Medical Center, Rochester, New York, Fall 1976.

Institute of Medicine. *Controls on Health Care.* Washington, D.C.: National Academy of Sciences, 1975.

Journals of the Continental Congress. Volume 5.

Lewis, B. J. *Veterans Administration Medical Program Relationship with Medical Schools in the United States.* House Committee Print No. 170, 91st Congress, 2nd Session. Washington, D.C.: USGPO, 1970.

Lipset, S., and Schneider, W. "The Public View of Regulation." *Public Opinion, 2,* 6, 1979.

Martin, J. *Statement of the General Accounting Office (GAO) before the Subcommittee on Health, Committee on Labor and Public Welfare, U.S. Senate, on the Implementation of the Health Maintenance Organization Act of 1973. November 21, 1975.* Washington, D.C.: USGPO, 1975.

Medical World News. "Military Medical Schools Launched." *16,* No. 17, p. 32.

Miles, R. *The Department of Health, Education and Welfare*. New York: Praeger,
    1974.
Miller, C. A. "Issues of Health Policy: Local Government and the Public's Health."
    American Journal of Public Health, 65, 1330, 1975.
Miller, C. A., et al. "A Survey of Local Public Health Departments and Their
    Directors." *American Journal of Public Health*, 67, 931, 1977a.
Miller, C. A., et al. "Statutory Authorizations for the Work of Local Health
    Departments." *American Journal of Public Health*, 67, 940, 1977b.
Miller, C. A., et al. "A Study of Local Health Departments." *Bulletin of the
    Association of Public Health Physicians*, 26, 1, January 1979.
Moe, R. *Executive Branch Reorganization: An Overview*. Washington, D.C.:
    Library of Congress, Congressional Research Service, 1977, pp. 3–4.
Mustard, H. S. *Government in Public Health*. New York: The Commonwealth
    Fund, 1945.
National Academy of Sciences. *Study of Health Care for American Veterans*.
    Washington, D.C.: USGPO, 1977.
National Commission on Community Health Services. *Health Is a Community
    Affair*. Cambridge, Massachusetts: Harvard University Press, 1966.
National Commission on Diabetes. *Report to the Congress of the United States*.
    USDHEW Pub. No. (NIH) 76–1018. Washington, D.C.: USGPO, 1975.
O'Donoghue, P. *Evidence About the Effects of Health Care Regulation*. Denver,
    Colorado: Spectrum Research, Inc., 1974.
Office of Management and Budget. *Special Analyses, Budget of the United States
    Government, Fiscal Year 1980*. Washington, D.C.: USGPO, 1979.
Office of the Secretary of Agriculture. *Annual Report, 1978*. Washington, D.C.:
    USGPO, 1979.
Office of Technology Assessment, U.S. Congress. *Assessing the Efficacy and
    Safety of Medical Technologies*. Washington, D.C.: USGPO, 1978.
President's Biomedical Research Panel. *Report Submitted to the President and the
    Congress of the United States*. USDHEW Pub. No. (OS) 76–500. Washing-
    ton, D.C.: USGPO, 1976.
President's Report on Occupational Safety and Health: 1975. Washington, D.C.:
    USGPO, 1979.
Rice, D. B. *Defense Resource Management Study: Final Report*. Washington,
    D.C.: USGPO, 1979.
Richmond, J. B. *Organizational Changes in the Public Health Service*. Washing-
    ton, D.C.: USDHEW, January 10, 1979.
Roemer, R., et al. *Planning Urban Health Services: From Jungle to System*. New
    York: Springer Publishing Co., 1975.
Schmeckebier, L. F. *The Public Health Service*. Institute for Government Re-
    search, Service Monographs of the U.S. Government, No. 10. Baltimore,
    Maryland: Johns Hopkins Press, 1923.
Seggel, R. "Social and Human Service Functions." In S. Humes and G. Graham,
    Eds., *Policy Formulator*, pp. 61–116. Fort Lauderdale, Florida: Nova Uni-
    versity Press, 1975.
Seidman, H. *Politics, Position, and Power*. New York: Oxford University Press,
    1970.

Shonick W., and Price, W. "Reorganization of Health Agencies by Local Government in American Urban Centers: What Do They Portend for Public Health?" *Health and Society*, 55, 233, 1977.

Shonick, W., and Price, W. "Organizational Milieus of Local Public Health Units: Analysis of Response to Questionnaire." *Public Health Reports*, 93, 648, 1978.

Stern, B. J. *Medical Services by Government: Local, State, and Federal*. New York: The Commonwealth Fund, 1946.

Surgeon General. *Healthy People: The Surgeon General's Report on Health Promotion and Disease Prevention*. USDHEW Pub. No. (PHS) 79–55071. Washington, D.C.: USGPO, 1979.

USDA. *Nutrition and Your Health*. Washington, D.C.: USGPO, 1980.

U.S. Code, Title 38, Chapter 17, Sec. 610.

U.S. Department of Labor. *All About OSHA*. Washington, D.C.: USGPO, 1977.

—————. *Sixty-Sixth Annual Report: Fiscal Year 1978*. Washington, D.C.: USGPO, 1979a.

—————. "Briefing Paper: Occupational Safety and Health Administration." Washington, D.C.: Photocopy, 1979b.

U.S. Environmental Protection Agency. *Legislation, Programs, and Organization*. Washington, D.C.: EPA, 1979a.

—————. *1978 Report: Better Health and Regulatory Reform*. Washington, D.C.: USGPO, 1979b.

USPHS. *Annual Report to Congress, Fiscal 1978*. Washington, D.C.: USDHEW, 1979 (duplicated).

Veterans' Administration. *Veterans' Administration's Response to the Study of Health Care for American Veterans*. Washington, D.C.: USGPO, 1977.

—————. *Federal Benefits for Veterans and Dependents*. Washington, D.C.: USGPO, 1979.

Whitman, R. D. "The Future of Revenue Sharing." *Challenge*, July–August, 1975, p. 14.

Wilson, F. A., and Neuhauser, D. *Health Services in the United States*. Cambridge, Massachusetts: Ballinger, 1976.

12

The Federal Legislative Process and Health Care

David Banta

Introduction

Most national public policies are established by legislative enactment, although some policy-making powers do lie with the executive branch and the courts (Lindblom, pp. 72–73). In the previous chapter, we described the major functions of government in the delivery of health care services. This chapter describes the role of Congress in the health care delivery system and its modus operandi in decision-making and the establishment of policy.

Policy may be defined as "any set of values, opinions, and actions which moves decision-making . . . in certain directions" (Anderson). Those who analyze policy generally think in terms of rational objectives, such as eliminating poverty or curing cancer (Rivlin). But thinking of the policy process as rational "fails to evoke or suggest the distinctively political aspects of policy-making, its apparent disorder and the consequent strikingly different ways in which policies emerge" (Lindblom, p. 4). In particular, rational planning is difficult to achieve in a democracy. Planning seeks to maximize the public good, but different groups within the society have a different concept of "public good" (Lindblom, p. 17). Moreover, rational policy-making is stymied because Congress, like the country it represents, is complex. It is chaotic and decentralized in its functioning.

The Constitutional separation of powers also complicates the policy-making process, as pointed out in Chapter 11. The goals of the Executive branch often conflict with the provincial interests of Congressmen. These conflicts are exacerbated when different political parties control the White House and the Congress. As chief administrative officer of the Executive branch, the President obviously has important policy functions. Even in the legislative arena, the President may (and usually does) propose legislation; he presents the budget; and he must approve, and may veto legislation. The President must rely heavily on the Department of Health and

352

Human Services for policy suggestions. However, the department is almost as fragmented as the Congress and will ordinarily limit itself to suggestions for marginal changes in existing programs (Brown).

Of course, governmental health policies are not determined only at the federal level, as was discussed in Chapter 11. States and localities retain considerable power in the health field and may have philosophies and plans that may conflict with federal policies. Policy is molded by a variety of societal forces beyond those of the policy-making system, such as the wealth of the nation and its social structure. The fact that major elements of the health system remain largely in private and disparate hands not only limits federal influence on the health system but makes the development of health policies difficult.

Nonetheless, the broad outlines of a national health policy for the United States are beginning to emerge (Anderson; Kennedy; McNerney; Somers; Weinerman; White). There is agreement on certain critical needs concerning the organization of medical and health care: the need to assure access to primary health care services; to plan and organize health services in a region; to foster group practice and team medicine; to train health manpower to carry out the tasks of the future; and to establish a national health insurance system. In dealing with all of these questions, the role of the government must be carefully defined. In particular, the society must grapple with the appropriate method of assuring an effective public-private mix in health services. If Edwards (1975) is correct in saying that the private health sector has failed to accept leadership responsibility, functioning instead merely as an array of special interests, a deeper penetration of government in medicine is likely.

The public is generally in favor of national health insurance (NHI), for example. A 1979 Gallup Poll showed that 67% of the public feels that there is a need for NHI, and 54% feel strongly that there is a need. Only 20% feel that there is no need for NHI. Of respondents, 43% preferred to pay for the plan through premiums, while 38% preferred increased taxation; 45% wanted private insurance company administration, while 38% preferred government. While a plurality of respondents felt that government regulation increases the costs of health care, a majority thought that the advantages of regulation outweigh the disadvantages (Health Law Newsletter). Polls have consistently shown that the public finds serious problems with the system of health care, with the costs of health care gaining the most attention (American Medical Association; Health Insurance Institute). In one poll, 71% of those questioned said they were dissatisfied with the costs of medical care (Health Insurance Institute). Such opinion is certain to have a continuing impact on Congress.

The Congress and Its Organization

The Congress has been evocatively described: "It is organized quite differently from the conventional bureaucracy, which Casual Observer professes to despise, but which he and his friends comprehend. Instead of having a single head, Congress looks like the hydra (or perhaps the Medusa) of Greek mythology. Instead of neatly delegating work downward and responsibility upward, Congress is a complex, redundant, not always predictable, and purposely unwieldy network of crisscrossing and overlapping lines of authority and information" (Polsby, 1971).

Basically, Congress has the following functions: (1) legislating, (2) overseeing government programs, (3) expressing public opinion, and (4) servicing constituents (Mayhew, p. 8). These functions, however, do not coincide with the main interests of an individual Congressman. Indeed, a Congressman's three primary goals have been said to be: (1) getting reelected, (2) achieving influence in Congress, and (3) making good public policy, perhaps in that order (Fenno, 1973). Studies have indicated that a substantial part, perhaps as much as half, of the factors determining the outcome of a Congressional election are local; for this reason, a Congressman must be attuned to his constituents. On the other hand, the average voter has a limited awareness of the voting records and general effectiveness of his representative, so the Congressman takes special note of the opinions of those active in politics, particularly if they are prominent. (It is also worth noting that different groups vote at different rates, with the poor, least-educated, and least-involved in the community voting the least [Schattschneider, p. 105]). As will be discussed later, organized groups are more effective at producing campaign contributions and volunteers for the campaign. Thus, the electoral process connects a Congressman primarily to important persons and groups of people with strong feelings on particular issues (Mayhew, pp. 40–42).

Certain ingrained structural characteristics tend to weaken Congress, while others strengthen it. Congressmen are *formally* equal to each other, which distinguishes them from members of bureaucracies. This formal equality tends to fragment the Congress, as does the committee structure. Forces acting to preserve and strengthen the institution include the political parties and certain committees, especially in the House of Representatives. The complex rules of the House control the fragmentation and moderate the power of interest groups (Mayhew, pp. 146–155). However, Congress presently tends to be more decentralized in its functioning, as a result of reforms in the early 1970s (Dodd).

The seniority system has been an important mechanism for maintaining institutional integrity. Seniority assures that those in positions of leadership have knowledge of the government, as well as knowledge of specific policy issues in such areas as health. Because of the seniority system, most leadership positions are held by members from "safe" districts. They are therefore able to use their judgment more and to resist special interest lobbying (Fenno, 1973). However, more than half of Congress has been elected since 1970. In the House, the seniority system has been greatly weakened because of abuses by some committee chairmen, and it is not clear what can take its place (Dodd; Ornstein).

The two houses of Congress operate in quite different ways. The House of Representatives, with 435 members, is a large, unwieldy body. It is the place to gain access to decision-making—the epitome of representative democracy (Jones). Each member is assigned to only one or sometimes two committees. The resulting specialization reduces conflict (Fenno, 1973). Floor debate in the House is often limited to committee members, who have traditionally been expected to concentrate their attention on the area of jurisdiction of their committee.

The Senate is less structured. Senators are fewer, more prominent socially, may be quite wealthy (Perkins), serve longer terms, and except for states with small populations, represent more people. The Senate, much more than the House, is the place of the individual, and much of the business is done by unanimous consent (Huitt, p. 91). "The essence of the Senate is that it is a great forum, an echo chamber, a publicity machine" (Polsby, p. 3). Each senator serves on many committees and subcommittees; few specialize. The Senate tends to develop policies through a process that has been called "random innovation" (Jones), and in recent years has been likely to pass legislation dealing with a new issue much more quickly than does the House.

Congressional Committees: Structure and Function

The Congressional committees are important loci of power; indeed, in the House, they have been referred to as the "backbone of the decision-making structure" (Fenno, 1973, pp. 64–65). There are 22 standing committees in the House and 15 in the Senate, as well as a number of select, special, and joint committees. At the beginning of the 96th Congress (1979), standing committees had almost 100 subcommittees in the Senate and 148 in the House (Joint Committee on Printing).* The principal committees and subcommittees with health functions are shown in Table 12.1.

Changes resulting from the Legislative Reform Acts of 1946 and 1970, as well as from alterations in the Democratic caucus, have given such pre-

---

*Congressional committees and subcommittees are listed periodically in the *Official Congressional Directory*, published by the Government Printing Office.

Table 12.1

Some Key Congressional Committees and Subcommittees with Health Functions, 1980

Committee and Subcommittee	Area of Health Activity
Senate:	
Committee on Labor and Human Resources	
Subcommittee on Health and Scientific Research	Most health legislation, jurisdiction over the Public Health Service Act (most programs in DHHS)
Committee on Finance	Taxes, Social Security
Subcommittee on Health	Medicare, Medicaid, PSROs
Committee on Appropriations	
Subcommittee on Labor, Health and Human Services	Allocation of tax funds in the budget — DHSS health programs, except Medicare and Medicaid
Committee on Budget	
No subcommittees	Budget resolutions — overall priority-setting
House of Representatives:	
Committee on Interstate and Foreign Commerce	
Subcommittee on Health and Environment	Most health programs in DHSS, including Medicaid and Part B of Medicare
Committee on Ways and Means	Taxes, Social Security
Subcommittee on Health	Medicare, Part A
Subcommittee on Labor, Health, and Human Services	Allocation of tax funds in the budget — DHSS health programs, except Medicare and Medicaid
Committee on Budget	
Subcommittee (Task Force) on Human and Community Resources	Budget resolutions — overall priority-setting

rogatives as budgets and staff to subcommittee chairmen (*Congressional Quarterly*, 1979a, pp. 3–12). Subcommittees have also become more important because of the complexity of the issues. Since the mid-1970s, both houses have limited the number of chairmanships that members can hold (*Congressional Quarterly*, 1979a, p. 9; Mayhew, pp. 96–97). Naturally, this has diffused power (Fox and Hammond, pp. 158–162.)

Role of Staff

Congressmen's claims to expertise derive from their own knowledge *plus* that of their staffs, the staff having much more policy input than is generally recognized. Congressional staff is divided into office staff, which works directly for a Congressman or senator, primarily on constituent problems and requests, and committee staff, which identifies problems, provides facts and questions, and carries out the day-to-day work of the committee, such as writing reports. In practice, the line between these two types of staff can be very fuzzy. Both types have expanded rapidly with the increasing complexity of the federal government, becoming quite large (Fox and Hammond; Seidman). For example, by 1975 there were 26 professionals, including four physicians, on the staffs of the four Senate and House authorizing committees and two appropriations subcommittees that write the great majority of federal health legislation (Iglehart). Total office and committee staff more than doubled, to 17,000, from 1970 to 1979 (Salisbury and Shepsle).

The role of staff differs considerably in the two houses. Since representatives are much better versed on the technical issues, their staff has a limited role. In the Senate, where members tend to spread themselves thin, committee staff especially have considerably more autonomy. Few senators are interested enough in health to spend a great deal of their time on it, so the task of creating and constructing legislation is delegated almost entirely to staff. Of course, staff works within limits defined by each senator.

In addition to the two types of staff described, Congress has technical resources available, although these are miniscule in comparison to those of the Executive branch. The Congressional Research Service of the Library of Congress has several health experts, as do the Office of Technology Assessment and the Congressional Budget Office. The Office of the Legislative Counsel has experts in health law. And the General Accounting Office, part of the Legislative branch, employs about 200 people to carry out program evaluations in the health field and is the primary tool for carrying out Congressional "oversight" of Executive branch programs (Rourke).

The Legislative Process

During each two-year Congressional term, approximately 25,000 legislative proposals are introduced by members of the House and Senate, with as many as 2,000 in health or health-related fields (American Hospital Association). Any member of either house can submit a bill for consideration by his house on any subject. These bills can be written by the member, staff, lobbyists, members of the Executive branch, constituents, or anyone else designated by the member.

During the mid-1960s, perhaps 90% of health legislation originated with the Executive branch, and was actively pushed by members of the Administration. Until the late 1960s, Congress responded to the proposals of the Executive branch, and demonstrated little inclination to initiate substantive policy-oriented legislation. Legislation establishing Medicare, Medicaid, and Comprehensive Health Planning was essentially fashioned by the Executive. However, the Nixon/Ford Presidency (1969–1977) saw considerable conflict between the White House and the Congress, and Congress began to attempt to establish independent positions. With more activist chairmen of the several health subcommittees, plus increased staff, some proposals originated in the Congress. For example, the bill to establish a National Center for Health Care Technology, passed in 1978, originated in the Senate Labor and Human Resources Committee.

Most legislative work is spent renewing expiring authorities, except on the appropriations committees. Authorization measures establish programs and provide for spending goals, while appropriations, which require separate votes, specify exactly how much money is to be made available for a particular authorized program. Almost all authorizing legislation is written with a time limit, usually two or three years. The renewal process gives Congress a chance to review programs, collect testimony, and consider changes. For example, health manpower legislation has been substantively altered each time it has been considered, beginning in 1960. The 1968 Act involved little more than an attempt to insure financial viability of health professions schools. The 1971 Act, in addition to providing per capita support for students, included requirements for the schools—for example, that they expand enrollment and institute special programs in such areas as primary care. The legislation passed in 1976 required further changes in medical school policies in return for the "capitation" payments. The renewal process also affords Congress an opportunity to carry out "oversight" on federally funded programs. The legislative process on these renewals is essentially identical to that for new legislation. That process requires consideration of the bill by subcommittee and committee, passage by both houses, a conference to reconcile the differences between the two bills, and Presidential signature.

After introduction, each bill, whether for a new program or a renewal, is assigned to the standing committee that has jurisdiction over the subject area of the bill.* Most bills dealing with health programs are assigned in the House to the Committee on Interstate and Foreign Commerce and in the

---

*The legislative process has been clearly described in detail in *How Our Laws Are Made* (Washington, D.C.: House of Representatives, USGPO, 1971), and in Jewell and Patterson's *The Legislative Process in the United States* (New York: Random House, 1966).

Senate to the Committee on Labor and Human Resources, both of which have health subcommittees (see Table 12.1). However, the bulk of federal health spending is in the Medicare and Medicaid programs (see Chapter 10), which fall under the jurisdiction of the Committee on Finance in the Senate. In the House, Medicaid falls under the jurisdiction of Interstate and Foreign Commerce, as does Part B of Medicare.

Jurisdictional disputes are common. An important one in 1979 centered on the question of which of the two main authorizing committees in the Senate would control national health insurance legislation, the Committee on Finance or the Committee on Labor and Human Resources (Senator Kennedy or Senator Long). Such disputes often block potentially valuable legislation, as occurred with a Senate proposal to use the leverage of Medicare and Medicaid funds to force changes in medical residency training programs.

Lack of space prevents our describing in detail each of the committees involved in health policy. The committees have their own personalities, which tend to be stable over time (Fenno, 1973). For example, Labor and Human Resources has been a very liberal committee for more than 10 years.

In addition to the four authorizing committees (Labor and Human Resources and Finance in the Senate; Commerce and Ways and Means in the House), a number of others have jurisdiction over some health programs or health-related programs. Particularly important ones controlling the authorization of health care expenditures are the Armed Services and Veterans' Affairs Committees. As noted in Chapter 11, the Department of Defense and the Veterans' Administration operate large health care programs.

After a bill is referred to the appropriate committee or subcommittee, if the leaders consider it important, public hearings will be held. Interested organizations and individuals, including Executive branch officials, will be invited to express their opinions. Of the bills presented to Congress, approximately 10% receive hearings (Fenno, 1965). After hearings, a subcommittee "mark-up" session will be held, during which the bill is rewritten by the members, taking into account testimony heard in hearings. This mark-up may take months in the House, where Congressmen are very involved in the details of legislation, but in the Senate the process generally takes less time. The bill will also be considered by the full committee, which may also hold hearings. Then, if it is favorably endorsed by the committee, it is reported to the floor of the respective house. During the process, a great deal of informal coalition-building occurs.

In the health area, floor votes are generally predictable. Members are likely to defer to the judgment of the committee unless there is great controversy, ideological conflict, or a split committee (Fenno, 1965). With a few recent exceptions, notably national health insurance and health manpower legislation, health has not been a controversial area; Congressmen know that their constituents favor an expansion of the government role. Nonetheless, important committee decisions are more often questioned on the floor than used to be the case.

Often, problem areas will be the subject of similar, but not identical, bills passed by each house. In that case, what is called a "conference committee" will be necessary to reconcile the areas of difference. If agreement is reached, the Conference Committee Report, essentially a revision of the bill passed in each house into a mutually acceptable version, must be resubmitted to both houses for approval. If no agreement can be reached, the bill "dies in conference," as did health manpower legislation in December 1980.

The final bill may well bear the "marks of executive uncertainty and obfuscation, extensive congressional reworking to build a majority coalition, and considerable interest group accommodation" (Brown).

The Budgetary Process

As previously mentioned, authorization and appropriation functions are separated in the Congress. Authorization does not assure a program a place in the budget. The authorization committees are by far the most publicly visible, but the budget process is obviously crucial, as a "policy" is generally meaningless without monetary support.

During the late 1960s, a number of signs indicated breakdown of the budget process. The Congress was unable to complete its budgetary process by July 1, the beginning of the fiscal year at that time, leading to a number of "continuing appropriations." The gaps between authorizations and appropriations became larger and larger. Congress became unable to monitor actual spending because of increases in spending outside the regular appropriations process and "uncontrollables," entitlement programs such as Medicare that do not require appropriation. Finally, President Nixon claimed the right to refuse to expend funds appropriated by Congress, a process called "impoundment" (Kotler). All of these factors led Congress to pass the Congressional Budget and Impoundment Control Act of 1974, which entirely overhauled the budget process. Table 12.2 lays out the major milestones in the new process.

The budget process begins in the Executive branch each spring, when agency programs are evaluated and budgetary projections are made by the Office of Management and Budget (OMB).* After discussions with the

---

*The entire budget process is well-described in Office of Management and Budget's "The Budget Process," in *The Budget of the United States Government, Fiscal Year 1980,* (Washington, D.C.: USGPO, 1979).

Table 12.2

Schedule of Presidential and Congressional Action on the Budget

On or before	Action to be completed
November 10	President submits current services budget.
15th day after Congress meets	President submits his budget.
March 15	Committees and joint committees submit reports to budget committees.
April 1	Congressional Budget Office submits report to budget committee.
April 15	Budget committees report first concurrent resolution on the budget to their houses.
May 15	Committees report bills and resolutions authorizing new budget authority.
May 15	Congress completes action on first concurrent resolution on the budget.
7th day after Labor Day	Congress completes action on bills and resolutions providing new budget authority and new spending authority.
September 15	Congress completes action on second required concurrent resolution on the budget.
September 25	Congress completes action on reconciliation bills or resolution, or both, implementing second required concurrent resolution.
October 1	Fiscal year begins.

Source: N. Kotler, "The Politics of the New Congressional Budget Process: Or, Can Reformers Use It to Undo the System of Privilege." In M. Raskin, Ed., *The Federal Budget and Social Reconstruction* Washington, D.C.; Institute for Policy Studies, 1978.

President, general policy directions and planning ceilings are given to the agencies. Each department and agency has produced its own budget proposals, beginning at the program level, as well as estimates of the amount required to continue programs in the upcoming fiscal year without changes. The budget proposals from the agencies are aggregated and modified, with many discussions through the levels of each department and with OMB staff, to arrive at the President's final budget. Under the Budget Act, the current services estimates are required to be sent to Congress by November 10, but because of difficulties in producing the information by that date, the Congress has allowed them to be submitted with the President's budget in January.

Congressional review of the budget proposals begins in the House Appropriations Committee. However, under the procedures established by the Budget Act, the Congress considers budget totals before it completes action on the budget. Each standing committee submits reports on budget estimates to the House and Senate Budget Committees by March 15. The Congressional Budget Office submits a fiscal policy report by April 1. Then Congress adopts the first concurrent budget resolution, containing targets of total receipts and outlays.

The House Appropriations Committee and its subcommittees considers the President's budget line by line through a process of hearings and mark-ups to passage by the full House. It is then forwarded to the Senate, where a similar process is followed. In case of disagreement between the two houses, a conference committee meets to resolve the issues, and the resulting report must be approved by both houses.

After action has been completed on all appropriations bills, the Congress adopts the second concurrent budget resolution containing budget ceilings. This resolution can revise the levels set earlier in the year and can direct the appropriations committees to change their bills. After the Congress completes action on the final amended appropriations bills, it may not consider legislation that would breach levels set in the second resolution.

The Budget Act is still new, but it appears to be enhancing Congressional control over the budget. The former diffusion of power largely benefited the wealthy, organized, powerful special interests (Kotler). Budget committees can withstand lobbies better, because they are not controlled by one group. The process is less fragmented, but it remains incremental, with small changes being made in the budgets of existing programs. The Act has fostered a questioning of program effectiveness and has democratized the budget process within the Congress. However, it has stirred the resentment of entrenched committees and may not survive for that reason (Kotler). An important implication of the resulting process is that House budget resolutions represent a majority party budget (Democratic in recent years), so that the parties have been strengthened. Clear budget choices can now be made (Ellwood and Thurber).*

The "Cozy Triumvirates"

The legislative process does not operate in a vacuum. Influencing the process are the "cozy triumvirates," a term used to denote a coalition

*The politics of the budget process have been studied by Wildavsky, *The Politics of the Budgetary Process* (Boston: Little, Brown, 1974). Budget priorities are described each year in Office of Management and Budget, *The Budget of the United States Government,* and are analyzed by a report from the Brookings Institution (J. Pechman, Ed., *Setting National Priorities, The 1980 Budget.* Washington, D.C., 1979).

between an outside pressure or interest group, professionals working on a particular program in the Administration, and a like-minded group in Congress. The clearest example in the health area is biomedical research, where researchers and concerned lay people make alliances with staff at the National Institutes of Health and staff and members of Congress to assure growth of certain research areas. Coalitions have formed around such areas as cancer, lung diseases, environmental health problems, Sickle cell disease, and diabetes. These coalitions do not consider broader questions, such as overall health programs or budget limitations: they lobby specifically for expansion of one particular program.

To initiate such an alliance, agency bureaucrats take their proposals directly to the Congress, usually secretly. In the early 1970s, the Administration tried very hard to stamp out this practice, with some success. Interest groups are an inevitable part of the democratic process, as concerned constituents and physicians cannot be prevented from contacting a Congressman. On the other hand, the President does need some control over the Executive bureaucracy if he is to lead. Any rational planner would be opposed to this inefficient pulling and tugging; however, Lindblom (1968) has argued that what he calls "muddling through" is quite natural in a democracy, especially in dealing with social programs. Maddox (1971) points out that the process of muddling through yields some important advantages: (1) making politically feasible decisions, (2) avoiding or minimizing major mistakes, and (3) allowing for maximum participation. Several case studies have described how this process works for specific issues (Marmor; Redman; Rettig; Spingarn; Strickland).

Role of Lobbyists

Many interest groups set up their own offices to "lobby" the Congress and the Executive branch; sometimes they hire a professional lobbying firm. In the health area, the best-known of the many lobbying groups are the American Medical Association (AMA), the Association of American Medical Colleges, (see The New Physician), the American Hospital Association, and the American Federation of Labor/Congress of Industrial Organizations.

A legitimate difference exists between "special interest" groups and "public interest" groups. A special interest is shared by a few members of society, whereas a public interest is shared by a substantial number of citizens of the community or nation (Schattschneider, pp. 23–25). In practice, this distinction is often difficult to make, for special-interest groups universally use the language of public interest. For example the AMA's public concern for the quality of medical care is little different from the argument of organized business that profits are the best guarantee of the public good. A characteristic shared by both types of interest groups is their elitist bias; they are led by and responsive to the educated and the affluent, making for a de facto exclusion of the poor and powerless from participation in the system.

Lobbying activity is targeted toward Congress. Groups monitor government activity that might affect them, initiate government action to promote their interests, and block action that would be to their detriment. Lobby groups are important to political figures, especially legislators, for a number of reasons: (1) they provide information; (2) they can assist with political strategy; (3) they provide ideas and innovative proposals; (4) lobbyists are often trusted friends; (5) they can provide campaign or electoral assistance (Ornstein and Elder). There are also sanctions that lobby groups can apply, such as trying to block committee assignment for a particular individual or working for the election of opponents.

Aside from the diffusion of power in the Congress, along with the resulting openness and expanded staff, both of which enhance lobbying by organized groups, the development of political action committees (PACs) is the most important development in recent years. With limitations on corporate and union contributions, as well as on individual support, large campaign contributions must come from voluntary gifts to the PACs. There were 1,938 PACs in operation in the 1978 Congressional campaign (*Congressional Quarterly*, 1979b, p. 73). The AMA PAC was number one in contributions, with $1.9 million. Other health-related groups defending the status quo were also large, such as the American Dental Political Action Committee. Conservative groups such as these did well in the 1980 elections.

This expanded activity by formal groups has a number of negative consequences: increased legislative activity along with an increased dependence on formal groups for information results; the Congressional process has become further fragmented. Throughout the society, individuals tend to select a subgroup to identify with, rather than broader social issues. It is not too much to say that the cohesion of the entire society is threatened by this development (Ornstein and Elder, pp. 228–229).

Implementation

After legislation is passed, it must be implemented, and the first step is generally the development of what are called "regulations," which describe how the law is to be administered (Altman and Sapolsky; American Hospital Association). During the early stages of regulation-writing, personnel in the designated agency generally consult with the groups involved, including Congressional members and staff, officials of state and local governments, and lobbyists. In effect, this is a legislative process with all the forces contending, but it is a hidden process compared to the rather open Congressional operations. Draft regulations are published in a daily official publication called the *Federal Register*, with invitations to all interested parties to comment. Final regulations are then published, usually 90 days after the appearance of the draft regulations. They have the force of law. (For additional discussion of the regulatory process, see pp. 337–338.)

Oversight

If Congress is to legislate effectively, it must know which programs work and which do not. It learns this through the process of legislative "oversight." It can investigate programs by different means, including hearings and studies by its own staff or its support agencies. However, Congress does not carry out oversight effectively (Ogul, p. 5). One of the key reasons is that authorizing committees are not sufficiently critical of programs they oversee because of the "cozy triumvirates" (Dodd). Future reorganizations of the Congress may be expected to pay more attention to this important activity (Ogul, p. 197).

Outlook and Discussion

Congress has serious problems meeting modern challenges. The decentralization, fragmentation, and specialization in Congress all militate against an integrated perspective. The diffusion of power within both houses, the increase in staff, and the growth in special-interest groups have all weakened Congress. Reforms have weakened the committee structure for some good reasons, but no integrative force has yet developed to take its place. One possibility is the resurgence of political parties (Broder). Another is the development of Congressional leadership that can take advantage of the young, motivated members who now make up the Congress, especially the House of Representatives (Ornstein).

However, our form of government requires a strong Congress to prevent Executive branch abuses. It seems likely that a cycle of centralization of power in the Congress will occur (Dodd). In order for that to happen, the support of the public for the Congress is necessary. The health of the democrataic system depends on citizen involvement and respect for governmental processes. Without an informed citizenry, this cannot be expected, and the continued evolution of Congress will be slowed or prevented.

References

Altman, D., and Sapolsky H. "Writing the Regulations for Health." *Policy Sciences*, 7, 417, 1976.
American Hospital Association. "A Summary of Federal Legislative Process and

the Process of Federal Program and Regulation Development." *Washington Developments*, 3, 1974 (Supplement).

American Medical Association. *Health Care Issues: Physician and Public Attitudes*. Compiled from studies conducted by the Gallup Organization, Inc. Chicago, Illinois, 1978.

Anderson, O. "Influence of Social and Economic Research on Public Policy in the Health Field, a Review." *Milbank Memorial Fund Quarterly*, 44, 11, 1966 (Part 2).

Broder, D. "Let 100 Single-Issue Groups Bloom." *The Washington Post*, January 7, 1979, p. C1.

Brown, L. "The Formulation of Federal Health Care Policy." *Bulletin of the New York Academy of Medicine*, 54, 45, 1978.

Congressional Quarterly. "Inside Congress." Washington, D.C., 1979a.

Congressional Quarterly. "The Washington Lobby." Washington, D.C., 1979b.

Dodd, L. "Congress and the Quest for Power." In Dodd, L., and Oppenheimer, B., Eds., *Congress Reconsidered*. New York: Praeger Publishers, 1977.

Edwards, C. "The Federal Involvement in Health: A Personal View of Current Problems and Future Needs." *New England Journal of Medicine*, 292, 559, 1975.

Ellwood, J., and Thurber, J. "The New Congressional Budget Process: The Hows and Whys of House-Senate Differences." In Dodd, L., and Oppenheimer, B., Eds., *Congress Reconsidered*. New York: Praeger Publishers, 1977.

Fenno, R. "The Internal Distribution of Influence: The House." In Truman, D., Ed., *The Congress and America's Future*. Englewood Cliffs, New Jersey: Prentice-Hall, 1965.

——————. *Congressmen in Committees*. Boston: Little, Brown, 1973.

Fox, H., and Hammond, S. *Congressional Staffs, The Invisible Force in American Lawmaking*. New York: The Free Press, 1977.

Health Insurance Institute. *Health and Health Insurance: The Public's View*. Washington, D.C., 1979, p. 14.

Health Law Newsletter. "Americans Want NHI." *105*, January 1980, p. 1.

House of Representatives. *How Our Laws Are Made*. Washington, D.C.: USGPO, 1971.

Huitt, R. "The Internal Distribution of Influence: The Senate." In Truman, D., Ed., *The Congress and America's Future*. Englewood Cliffs, New Jersey: Prentice-Hall, 1965.

Iglehart, J. "Health Report: Congress Expands Capacity to Contest Executive Policy." *National Journal Reports*, 7, 730, 1975.

Jewell, M., and Patterson, S. *The Legislative Process in the United States*. New York: Random House, 1966.

Joint Committee on Printing. *1979 Official Congressional Directory*. Washington, D.C.: USGPO, 1979.

Jones, C. "Will Reform Change Congress?" In Dodd, L., and Oppenheimer, B., Eds., *Congress Reconsidered*. New York: Praeger Publishers, 1977.

Kennedy, E. "The Congress and National Health Policy." *American Journal of Public Health*, 68, 241, 1978.

Kotler, N. "The Politics of the New Congressional Budget Process: Or, Can Reformers Use It to Undo the System of Privilege." In Raskin, M., Ed., *The Federal Budget and Social Reconstruction*. Washington, D.C.: Institute for Policy Studies, 1978.

Lindblom, C. *The Policy-Making Process*. Englewood Cliffs, New Jersey: Prentice-Hall, 1968.

McNerney, W. "Health Care Financing and Delivery in the Decade Ahead." *Journal of the American Medical Association*, 222, 1150, 1972.

Maddox, G. "Muddling Through: Planning for Health Care in England." *Medical Care*, 9, 459, 1971.

Marmor, T. *The Politics of Medicare*. Chicago: Aldine, 1970.

Mayhew, D. *Congress: The Electoral Connection*. New Haven, Connecticut: Yale University Press, 1974.

New Physician, The. Special Issue. "The AAMC: Medicine's New Superpower." October 1974.

Office of Management and Budget. "The Budget Process." In *The Budget of the United States Government, Fiscal Year 1980*. Washington, D.C.: USGPO, 1979.

Ogul, M. *Congress Oversees the Bureaucracy*. Pittsburgh: University of Pittsburgh Press, 1976.

Ornstein, N. "Is Congress Too Good for Us?" *The Washington Post*, November 18, 1979, p. C5.

Ornstein, N., and Elder, S. *Interest Groups, Lobbying and Policymaking*. Washington, D.C.: Congressional Quarterly Press, 1978.

Pechman, J., Ed. *Setting National Priorities, The 1980 Budget*. Washington, D.C.: The Brookings Institution, 1979.

Perkins, J. "Danforth, Heinz Richest in Senate?" *The Washington Star*, May 20, 1978, p. 2.

Polsby, N. "Strengthening Congress in National Policymaking." In Polsby, N., Ed., *Congressional Behavior*. New York: Random House, 1971.

Redman, E. *The Dance of Legislation*. New York: Simon and Schuster, 1973.

Rettig, R. *Cancer Crusade*. Princeton, New Jersey: Princeton University Press, 1977.

Rivlin, A. *Social Policy: Alternate Strategies for the Federal Government*. Washington, D.C.: The Brookings Institution, 1974.

Rourke, J. "The GAO: An Evolving Role." *Public Administration Review*, 453, 1978.

Salisbury, R., and Shepsle, K. "Understanding the Role and Impact of Congressional Staff: A Research Agenda." *Staff*, Issue 2, p. 1 ff, March 1979.

Schattschneider, E. *The Semi-Sovereign People*. Hinsdale, Illinois: The Dryden Press, 1960.

Seidman, H. *Politics, Position and Power: The Dynamics of Federal Organization*. New York: Oxford University Press, 1970.

Somers, A. "Some Basic Determinants of Medical Care and Health Policy." *Milbank Memorial Fund Quarterly*, 46, 13, 1968.

Spingarn, N. *Heartbeat: The Politics of Health Research*. Washington, D.C.: Robert B. Luce, Inc., 1976.

Strickland, S. *Politics, Science, and Dread Disease*. Cambridge, Massachusetts: Harvard University Press, 1972.

Weinerman, E. "Anchor Points Underlying the Planning for Tomorrow's Health Care." *Bulletin of the New York Academy of Medicine, 41*, 1213, 1965.

White, K. "Organization and Delivery of Personal Health Services: Public Policy Issues." *Milbank Memorial Fund Quarterly, 46*, 225, 1968.

Wildavsky, A. *The Politics of the Budgetary Process*. Boston: Little, Brown, 1974.

13

Planning for Health Services

Carol McCarthy and Steven Jonas

In this chapter, we turn to a consideration of health services planning, an activity for which government has historically borne a major responsibility. After discussing the basic principles and problems of health services planning, we examine the historical antecedents of government activity in the field, and then discuss the major planning efforts that the federal and state governments have undertaken since World War II.

Principles and Problems of Health Care Planning
Basic Concepts

Herman Hilleboe, M. D., one of the fathers of the modern approach to health services planning, described planning as follows (1967):

> Planning is an orderly process, put in writing, of: 1. defining the extent and characteristics of community health problems and identifying unmet needs, 2. assessing available and potential resources, 3. establishing priority goals (by matching needs and resources and considering alternatives and their consequences), 4. formulating the necessary administrative action to achieve program goals, and 5. relating results to goals by continuing evaluative studies.

According to Gottlieb, health services planning must keep in mind certain assumptions, which have been summarized as follows: (1) resources are scarce; thus ways must be found to secure optimum value from allocations devoted to health; (2) health care serves social purposes and should, therefore, be valued above activity undertaken in pursuit of economic or other social ends; (3) an effective health care system is rooted in responsiveness to consumer needs and requires public accountability. Rosenfeld sums up these thoughts well: "The aim of planning must be the achievement of optimum use of available resources for the betterment of human welfare."

Health services planning can take place on multiple levels. The macro level is concerned with health services systems or major pieces thereof: the nation, a region, or one or more states. The micro level is concerned with one of the following: an institution, such as a hospital or a health mainte-nance organization; a single, categorical health service being provided to a geographic area, such as family planning or chronic disease detection; or a health care provider's private office. Spiegel and Hyman, in *Basic Health Planning Methods,* a very useful textbook and guide for the field of health services planning, describe six common types of health services planning, all of which can take place at both the macro and micro levels:

1. Problem-solving planning: Identifying and resolving a specific problem, using the scientific method.
2. Program planning: Setting a course of action to deal with a circum-scribed problem, usually one that has already been described else-where.
3. Coordination of efforts and activities planning: Aiming to increase the availability, efficiency, productivity, and effectiveness of var-ious activities and programs.
4. Planning for resource allocation: Choosing among various alterna-tives defined in earlier stages of the planning process in order to achieve the optimal outcome, given limited resources.
5. Creation of a plan: Developing a blueprint for action, including recommendations and supporting data.
6. Design of standard operating procedures: Creating sets of standards of practice and/or criteria for operation and evaluation. (p. 11)

Any particular planning process consists of one or more of these types of planning.

Regardless of the type of planning being undertaken, it is of vital importance to the success of the process that its desired goals and objec-tives be clearly stated, understood, and agreed to by all parties concerned. The most frequent cause of failure in planning is neglecting to establish clear, agreed-upon goals and objectives, either as the first step or at least before the program planning phase (step 4 in the Hilleboe formulation) is begun.

Goals and Objectives

Goals are broad, usually long-range statements of ideal desired outcomes, e.g., "All Americans shall have equal access to health care of high quality." Objectives refer to specific targets of action, usually to be reached within a named time period, that are considered to be attainable; the degree of attainment achieved within the specified time is considered to be measurable, e.g., "Within ten years there shall be one primary care practitioner for every 1,000 Americans." Only by clearly defining goals and objectives can one know in which direction one is headed. When goals and objectives are not clearly stated, and this does happen with depressing frequency in health services planning in the United States, the following pitfalls are usually encountered:

1. There is no way to evaluate the effectiveness of the planning process, because what was being planned *for* was never defined.
2. Reams of data may be collected, much of it useless, or few data are collected and decisions are made in their absence, because without goals and objectives, data needs cannot be defined.
3. Planning for *functions* can be confused with and sometimes superseded by planning for a *building*. A great deal of present health services planning does result in a new or remodeled building. Failure to define goals and objectives often leads to planning for the building alone, employing available land and available money, rather than intended use, as basic design criteria. This approach, of course, reverses Frank Lloyd Wright's architectural dictum: "Form should follow function." Instead of asking, toward the end of the planning process, "What space do we need for these needs?" one says, "What needs do we meet with this space?"

There are a number of reasons why goals and objectives are sometimes ignored in the planning process. First, the larger the group of affected persons, the more difficult it is to define goals and objectives that all parties can agree to. It is sometimes easier to skip the stage than to go through the political process necessary to hammer out goals and objectives. Second, some of the parties involved may have goals and objectives in mind that they feel would not be accepted under close scrutiny, or be justified by data collection and analysis, or be economically feasible. If such persons are in positions of power from which they can implement programs without going through the goal-and-objective stage of planning, they will often do so. Third, the glitter of the *techniques* of planning, the collection and analysis of data, the designing of administrative structures and staffing patterns, the development of budgets, and above all, the laying out of space, can easily outshine the fundamental, unglamorous, much more difficult job of determining "Why are we doing this?"

In setting goals and objectives, it is important to remember that there is no such thing as "value-free planning" (Fein). Every planner and participant in the planning process is influenced by his or her "ideological baggage." It is one's "ideological baggage" or *Weltanschauung* that influences, indeed, determines, one's value judgments and ordering of social priorities. Recall Rosenfeld's statement (above) on the aim of planning: "[It] must be the achievement of *optimum use* of *available resources* for *the betterment of human welfare*." (Our italics added.) The definition of just what constitutes "optimum use," "available resources," and "the betterment of human welfare" will vary from person to person and will, even in the presence of scientifically gathered data, be strongly influenced by each person's social values and priorities.

The workings of the health care delivery system have outcomes relating to the needs of the people it serves for health and sickness services. They also have outcomes relating to the needs of the people who work in it. Often, the needs of those who work in the health care delivery system are the same as those of the people being served, related to improving the population's health status and combating disease, but occasionally they are not. Provider needs can be of a different order: power, profits, institutional preservation and growth, career advancement, intellectual stimulation and development, and political gain. When they exist side by side, the two sets of goals do not necessarily lead to plans that are rational.

One can state goals and objectives *for* the planning process, and goals and objectives *of* the planning process. The former are technical entities: what kind of product (a report, an analysis, a functional program, a building design) is to be achieved, by when. The latter are substantive, and are produced by the planning process itself.

It should be apparent that one cannot write a *complete* set of goals and objectives before beginning a planning process. If one could do the former, one would not need to do the latter. In fact, at the beginning it is more likely that one will be able to write goals than that one will be able to write objectives. But as data are gathered, and no planning process can take place without data-gathering, then specific objectives can be defined. As the planning process proceeds, it may be found appropriate or necessary to add to or modify previously written goals and objectives. This "feedback loop" mechanism is one of the principal engines of the planning process.

The Health Services Planning Process

The basic concepts of health services planning are straightforward. However, the fragmented health care delivery system in the United States affects the nature of the technical planning process. In brief, the science rather than the art of planning consists of collecting and using data. The data needed depend on the existing level of health knowledge and planning knowledge, on the particular health care delivery system at issue, and on characteristics of the larger social framework. Since the planning process is a continuous, cyclical whole (Sigmond), all categories of data are relevant throughout, although one may be more heavily relied upon at a particular stage than another.

Planning for health services requires knowledge of: (1) the population to be served, (2) its health status, and (3) existing health care resources and their utilization. Without such information, one cannot determine whether the demand for medical services is greater than, equal to, or less than the quantity of services health professionals estimate are required. (This quantity is known as "need.") The difference between demand and need estimates must be taken into account in rational planning (Jeffers et al.).

Measuring health status.   The first step is to measure health and illness levels in the population to be served, whether it be the population of the nation as a whole, of a defined community, or of users of a particular existing service that is a candidate for redesign. Then the total health service needs of the population can be estimated.

Demographic data on populations to be served (Chapman and Coulson; Rienke and Baker; Spiegel and Hyman, Chapter 2; Susser and Watson) are discussed in Chapter 3. A population's health status is assessed through measures of mortality and morbidity or combinations of the two. Traditionally, mortality has been the primary indicator—infant, perinatal, maternal, and other age-adjusted death rates. Mortality indices, however, are less than optimal measures of health. Their interpretation is confounded by multiple causes of death, poor reporting systems (Guralnick), and the shift from acute to chronic diseases as the major killers of our time. Furthermore, death is an opposite of health. Therefore, it is only an indirect measure of health status.

Measures of morbidity (the presence of a disease condition or active pathology) and disability (restricted performance of normal roles) present similar problems, as well as others. There are a limited number of reportable diseases, and selective reporting leads to inaccurate data (Blum; D. F. Sullivan). In addition, the definition and classification of morbidity states entail difficulties. The same clinically defined disease appears with different complaints in different ethnic populations (Zola). A cross-culturally valid index for each disease is needed, one that will encompass physical, emotional, and social causal factors; incidence (the number of new cases in a specified time period); prevalence (the number of extant cases in a specified time period); duration; and severity.

In the National Health Survey, outlined in Chapter 3, disability is measured in terms of the number of days of restricted activity in the six months preceding the study interview. Data are gathered from a random sample of civilian, noninstitutional households. In the survey conducted by the Social Security Administration, respondents are classified along a con-

tinuum based on the extent of their work limitations. Although the resultant "functional limitations index" provides a greater degree of specificity
about disability (Haber), highly sensitive measures of acute and chronic
disability are still unavailable.

A variety of other health status indicators have been used to attempt to
define the health of a population adequately (Balinsky and Berger; Berg;
Goldsmith). Among them are: activity counts (USDHEW, 1969); the Q
value developed by the Indian Health Service (J. E. Miller); an index of
physical, mental, and social health devised by the Human Population
Laboratory in Berkeley, California (Meltzer and Hochstim); and diverse
mathematical models (National Center for Health Statistics). Bush and
others (Bush et al.; Fanshel and Bush) have done a great deal of work in this
area. Bush et al. have developed an index which consists of two dimensions, a function level and a prognosis (Spiegel and Hyman, pp. 37–44). It
seems quite promising.

Describing existing resources.   The next step is to undertake an inven-
tory and evaluation of existing services (Spiegel and Hyman, Chapter 3).
Resources are of three kinds: human, physical, and financial. The number,
age, sex, education, specialization, type of practice, productivity, and
geographic location of available manpower must be determined, along with
the output of operating and approved training programs. Sites of care must
be inventoried as to number, type, distribution, and characteristics such as
size, type, volume, and quality of services offered, physical condition,
approvals, policies, financial solvency, and referral patterns. For each
facility, patient characteristics must be noted and utilization measures
compiled—the number of patient visits, average daily census, percent
occupancy, length of stay. (The two vantage points from which utilization
can be measured are discussed in Chapter 3.) Financial data concerning
the number and types of insurance mechanisms, government-supported
programs, median family income, and sources of philanthropy must be
obtained.

In comparing the health service needs of the population with the level of
need that can be met by the existing resources, if the population's needs
are greater than the needs that the existing resources are capable of
meeting, the population's "unmet need" has been defined. Available resources constitute the supply side of the planning equation; sociodemographic factors, health status measures, and professional assessments of
undetected problems, the demand/need side. By using the mathematical
tools and subjective estimates at his or her command, the planner weighs
one against the other and both against established standards to identify
problems requiring attention (Spiegel and Hyman, Chapter 4). The next
stage of the planning process is concerned with creating a program to meet

unmet needs. At this point, the original goals must be reconsidered in light of the data obtained and analyzed. Goals may remain unchanged or they may be redefined, reduced, or enlarged. Objectives can now be written with a great deal of specificity. As is the development of goals and objectives at the beginning of the planning process, the redevelopment and enhancement of goals and objectives before program planning begins is critical to a successful outcome. Realistic goals and objectives are rooted in sound priority-setting (Spiegel and Hyman, Chapter 5); sound priorities depend on the vulnerability of a health or health care problem to attack. To the extent feasible, the health planner quantifies vulnerability so that priorities are defensible (Ahumada et al.). In program planning, he or she is careful not to neglect time-series graphs and curve-fitting techniques (Bright), as well as cost-benefit analysis (Prest and Turvey). All three planning tools take into account the time span between planning and implementation and the "objective" merits of viable program alternatives.

Finally, without planning data, there is no baseline against which the impact of implemented programs can be measured. Information is needed on the extent to which anticipated changes in health status occur, at what cost, and with what positive or negative spillover. Indeed, baseline data provide the foundation for systems of continuous feedback, systems that must be in place if inappropriate goals or inadequate work activities are to be identified and corrected.

Program planning. In planning a program to meet unmet needs, the following must be provided for: description of services to be offered; personnel requirements and staffing patterns; policy-setting and administrative structure and mechanisms; financing systems to raise, budget, and pay out the funds needed for program operation; physical space; and a means for program evaluation and ongoing forward planning. As mentioned above, in order to have the best chance of creating a service that will truly meet community needs, program planning should always precede physical space planning.

If at all possible, proposed programs should be tested by one means or another before implementation. It is rarely possible in the real world to run a purely scientific, prospective experiment of a planned program before it is fully implemented. However, it is often possible to undertake a retrospective evaluation of other, similar, previously implemented programs. This can be done through the literature, by private mail and telephone surveys, and by direct observation. This kind of analysis, not always done in the real world, can prove to be very useful. Pitfalls can be skirted, "reinvention of the wheel" can be avoided, and successful planning and implementation strategies can be adapted to use.

Evaluation. Once implemented, programs must be evaluated

(Spiegel and Hyman, Chapter 7). Taylor (1972) indicates the need for a two-pronged approach: evaluation for administrative purposes (Are targets being met within specified time frames and in accordance with standards set?) and evaluation for plan revision (Are original goals appropriate? Are the necessary resources being developed as anticipated?). Five levels of evaluation have been outlined. (Blum):

1. Activity. Is the program operative?
2. Criteria. Is the program operating according to standards (of quality, access, etc.)?
3. Cost. Are program costs in line with those agreed upon? Can unit cost be improved?
4. Effectiveness. How well is the program achieving the desired output?
5. Outcome validity. To what extent has the program realized the ultimate goal for which it was designed?

Avoiding biased measures of outcome is a primary concern. Indeed, the literature on laboratory and field experiments is replete with cautions against evaluator contamination. Program designers are advised against evaluating their own programs, evaluation designers against implementing their own designs. Morehouse notes that evaluations can fail in two ways: for methodological reasons and for failure to produce "acceptable" findings—that is, those consistent with the policymaker's commitment to program success. A planning imperative thus becomes clear. The shifting power structure in health must be given attention (Elling) and a coalition of support for thorough and factual program evaluation, regardless of political repercussions, must be formed.

Early History of Regional and Comprehensive Health Planning in the United States*

The use of the health planning techniques outlined above, as well as efforts at regional health planning (planning across several political jurisdictions) and comprehensive health planning (planning for more than one disease category, population, or facet of the health care delivery system), are relatively recent. Diverse forces have affected our health delivery system over the past 50 years. Planning has been stimulated by advances in health care technology and the lag between the development and general avail-

*A useful overview of regional health planning in the United States is provided by Ernest W. Saward (Ed.) and his colleagues in *The Regionalization of Personal Health Services*, New York: PRODIST, 1976.

ability of such advances; by more widespread education and a concomitant rise in consumer health care expectations; by the arrival of organized third-party payors and unionized health care workers; by urbanization and increased health hazards; by suburban sprawl and resultant accessibility problems; by a shortage of medical manpower; and by skyrocketing health care costs.

Recognition of the need for regional and comprehensive health care planning can be traced back to the establishment in 1927 of the Committee on the Costs of Medical Care, to which we have referred elsewhere. To review, the 42-man committee had been formed in response to the desire of leading physicians, public health personnel, and economists for sound studies on the economic and social aspects of health services. Supported by $1 million from six foundations, the committee and its staff studied the incidence of disease and disability in the United States; health care facilities open to the general public and those organized to serve particular population groups; family expenditures for health care; and income earned by providers of care (Anderson). Citing the rising costs of diagnosis and treatment and the inequitable distribution of health services across the nation, the final report of the majority of the committee, published in 1932, recommended support for group medical practice and group prepayment for health care services, or health insurance. The strong reactions elicited by that report stimulated a series of changes in health care financing and delivery. Equally important from the vantage point of regional and comprehensive health planning was the committee's call for the coordination of primary and specialty services within defined geographic areas (Committee on the Costs of Medical Care, 1932).

At first the call was picked up locally. Efforts were few in number, however, and generally limited to exploring the feasibility of a "regionalized" or three-tiered system of institutionalized care. Regionalization in this context denoted integrated networks, with primary care delivered through rural or outlying hospitals and clinics; secondary (more specialized, consultant care) at district or "intermediate" hospitals; and tertiary (highly specialized, technologically based care) at medical centers (Mountin et al.). In rural New England, for example, the Bingham Associates Fund worked to coordinate medical services for area residents. To that end, program linkages were established between the Pratt Clinic, New England Center Hospital, and Tufts Medical School (Gartland). In Michigan, the Hospital Survey Commission explored that state's bed needs in the context of regionalization (Commission on Hospital Care, 1946).

Only in 1944, when the American Hospital Association's (AHA) Committee on Postwar Planning took up the standard, was regionalized planning for health services promoted on a nationwide basis. A Commission on

Hospital Care was established by the AHA and local, district, and state councils formed to work in conjunction with "the official state planning agency." The outcome was a recommendation to coordinate the regionalization of hospital services, equipment, and personnel. The Commission on Hospital Care (1947) was explicit in its report:

> The haphazard development of hospital services of the past should not be extended to the future. The public must be made aware of, must assume its responsibility for the development and support of adequate hospital care on a communitywide basis. The expansion and development of individual institutions must be in accord with an overall planned program for the community. Direct benefits will accrue to both hospitals and public through organized effort in the intelligent planning of hospital care. (p. xi)

Legislation for Areawide Planning
The Hill-Burton Act

The first attempt by the federal government to translate a generalized health planning concept into action came in 1946 with the passage of the Hospital Survey and Construction Act, better known as the Hill-Burton program, after its sponsors, Senator Hill of Alabama and Congressman Burton of Michigan. The stated intent of the act was to improve the hospital bed-to-population ratio in rural areas and to upgrade facilities and standards. Federal grant assistance was authorized to the states for surveying their needs and developing state plans for hospital facilities based on those surveys. With plans in existence and minimum standards for hospitals incorporated in state licensing laws, federal funds were to be made available on a matching basis (up to one-third federal) to construct and equip public and voluntary nonprofit general, mental, tuberculosis, and chronic disease hospitals and public health centers (Public Law 79–725).

The Hill-Burton mandate for a state health facilities plan and the requirement that a single state agency assume responsibility for plan development and program implementation were important. (The word "survey" in "Hospital Survey and Construction Act" was added only after the work of the Commission on Hospital Care and the "regional plan" or three-tiered concept of the Public Health Service were discussed in hearings on the bill.) For the first time, a determination of need was to form the basis of priorities for action, and such priorities were to be explicitly stated. Centering the responsibility for such action in a single authority was also new. However, the law's emphasis on construction alone, rather than construction and coordination of facilities, supports the interpretation that the single agency requirement was adopted primarily for orderly management of funds.

Between 1949 and 1970, the Hill-Burton program was amended to provide additional grants, loans, and loan guarantees to improve geographic bed distribution. Moreover, from 1956, the United States Public Health Service received appropriations under the law for research and demonstrations relating to the development, utilization, and coordination of hospital services, facilities, and resources.

From the planning standpoint, however, the most significant additions to the Hill-Burton program came in 1964 with the Hospital and Medical Facilities Amendments. Along with $1.34 billion for the construction, modernization, and replacement of health care facilities, project grants were made available to develop comprehensive plans for health and health-related facilities on a regional, metropolitan, or other basis. Furthermore, the arbitrary bed-to-population ratio utilized in determining priorities for grant and loan requests was abandoned. A new formula, incorporating known hospital utilization data, projected population estimates, and a desirable standard of occupancy (80%) was instituted as a more sensitive measure of area hospital needs.

The legislation that continued the Hill-Burton program into the 1970s maintained the grant program and provided both guaranteed and direct loans for construction, modernization, or replacement purposes. In addition to hospitals, neighborhood health centers and emergency room facilities were made eligible for funding, a major departure from the original law. With regard to areawide planning, the continuing legislation stipulated that, in order to be approved, projects must comply with plans established by state or areawide planning agencies, creations of the Comprehensive Health Planning Act of 1966, described below.

Thus, the Hill-Burton legislation was a landmark program in two ways. It provided the stimulus and the means for a much-needed building and reconstruction program. In 1944, the American Hospital Association's Committee on Governmental Aid for Postwar Reconstruction had estimated a deficiency of 180,000 beds in the United States delivery system (Bugbee). By June of 1970, projects approved under the Hill-Burton program included construction of 334,438 hospital beds, 93,749 long-term care beds, 1,032 outpatient facilities, 520 rehabilitation facilities, 1,258 public health centers, and 41 state health laboratories (USDHEW, 1970). Moreover, efforts were concentrated in those areas where shortages were most acute. The program also introduced new approaches to facilities planning and development. Each of the 53 states and possessions, for example, had established plans and methods for establishing priorities. Documentation of need, however general, was no longer a totally untried concept. Finally, through the "strings" attached to grants, loans, and loan guarantees, the Hill-Burton initiative also promoted progress toward the equal-access goal of health planning. Institutions receiving Hill-Burton funds were required to assure the same service availability to Medicaid and Medicare patients that was accorded private-pay patients.

From the standpoint of the planning principles outlined earlier, however, the Hill-Burton program was not an unqualified success. It was a regional rather than comprehensive approach to remedying health delivery system inadequacies. Its overwhelming emphasis on bed scarcity indicates the absence of a comprehensive goal-setting process rooted in identified community needs. In fact, Hill-Burton program planning involved minimal interaction between provider and consumer and between Hill-Burton and other planning activities (Gottlieb).

Nor did Hill-Burton planning procedures encompass the total hospital field. Because of the law's emphasis on underserved rural areas and "conforming beds" (those adhering to specified standards of designs, equipment, and structure), and its exclusion of proprietary institutions, only 25% of the nation's hospital beds were involved in the program (Hilleboe et al.). Promoters of hospital projects that were denied Hill-Burton support could raise funds elsewhere. In brief, Congress and supporters of the bill—the AMA and AHA, in particular—were amenable to federal dollar support but not to federal control over the essentially voluntary hospital system. Finally, the Hill-Burton program did not achieve the same results in physician redistribution that it did in bed redistribution (Clark and Koontz).

Regional Medical Programs

Just as the Hill-Burton Act provided for planning on the structural level (bricks and mortar), Public Law 89–239—which established Regional Medical Programs (RMPs)—facilitated functional planning (i.e., planning new or improved working arrangements for health care delivery). The law, passed in 1965, was an outgrowth of three of the major recommendations of a Presidential commission headed by Dr. Michael DeBakey (Russell). President Johnson had appointed the commission to develop a "realistic battle plan leading to the ultimate conquest of three diseases—heart disease, cancer, and stroke" (President's Commission on Heart Disease, Cancer and Stroke, p. ii).

The original draft version of Public Law 89–239 strongly echoed the intention of commission members. A nationwide series of "regional medical complexes" were to be established, one each for heart disease, cancer, and stroke. Each complex was to include a research center, a medical center, and diagnostic and treatment "stations" within a defined geographic area.

However, as a result of organized opposition during the legislative process by the American Association of General Practice and the American

Medical Association, the "regional complexes" concept was replaced by "regional medical programs." Through voluntary efforts at joint problem-solving, these programs were to make the latest scientific advances in the "killer diseases" available at the grassroots level without interfering with "the patterns or methods of financing of patient care or professional practice" (Public Law 89–239; Jonas, 1967).

On the basis of applications received, the country was divided into 56 regional medical program regions. Within each region, a public or nonprofit institution, agency, or corporation was designated grantee or fiscal agent. Overall program guidance was the responsibility of the RMP's Regional Advisory Group (RAG), a voluntary body comprising local providers, representatives of public organizations, and consumers (Creditor and Nelson). Core staffs, paid through grant funds, were to provide the technical assistance required to forge planned linkages among the various elements of the health delivery system (Komaroff). Staff and RAG set regional priorities and objectives, developed programmatic approaches, reviewed local applications for grant monies, submitted selected projects to a 20-member National Advisory Council of nonfederal reviewers in Washington, and guided and evaluated operational projects.

In many instances, RMP efforts resulted in institutions and agencies working together to increase available resources and improve utilization. Indeed, the Public Accountability Reporting Group, spokesman for the 53 RMPs in existence in 1973, cites the following accomplishments for that year: approximately 27,000 providers took part in RMP medical-audit programs designed to promote quality-assurance; 9 million Americans received health care services directly from RMP-funded activities; an estimated 12 million derived benefits from the 150,000 health professionals using new skills acquired through RMP-supported training programs (Public Accountability Reporting Group).

Some of these accomplishments are traceable to the expansion of RMP's original categorical mandate (W. R. Miller, 1972). Public Law 91–515, passed in 1970, called for RMP efforts for all major diseases and conditions, and for prevention and rehabilitation as well as diagnosis and treatment. Attention to the delivery of primary care and to improving manpower utilization were promoted. Closer ties to comprehensive planning were assured by requiring that areawide planning agencies review and comment on RMP grant requests.

In sum, despite numerous phase-out orders and Presidential impoundment of appropriated funds in 1972 (Ward), individual RMPs made possible the regionalization of certain services and the introduction of innovative approaches directed at reforms in the organization and delivery of care. On the other hand, RMPs have been criticized for the "anticomprehensiveness" of their regionalization efforts (Bodenheimer) and for concentrating on developing cooperative relations among interested providers instead of on reorganizing the delivery system (Bodenheimer; Creditor).

Comprehensive Health Planning Agencies

In addition to the Regional Medical Programs, the 89th Congress signed into law another outgrowth of DeBakey Commission recommendations, Public Health Service Act Amendments of 1966, Public Law 89–749, on comprehensive health planning. Along with Public Law 90–174, passed the next year, these amendments created what was called the "Partnership for Health Program." Section 314(a) of P. L. 89–749 outlines the objectives of the program:

> The Congress declares that fulfillment of our national purpose depends on *promoting and assuring the highest level of health attainable for every person, in an environment which contributes positively to healthful individual and family living;* that attainment of this goal depends on an effective partnership, involving close intergovernmental collaboration, official and voluntary efforts, and participation of individuals and organizations; that Federal financial assistance must be directed to support the marshalling of all health resources—national, state and local—to assure comprehensive health services of high quality for every person, but *without interference with existing patterns of private professional practice of medicine, dentistry, and related healing arts. [Authors' emphasis]*

The program was to be a distinct departure from categorical approaches to health planning, which are directed at specific diseases, population groups, or types of health services. However, the single largest segment of the U.S. health care delivery system, private practice, was to be left untouched, just as it had been under RMP.

Public Law 89–749 provided for a two-tier planning system. There were "A" and "B" agencies, named for the section of the law in which they were described. The state, or A agency, assisted by an advisory council in which consumers of health care were in the majority, was given a supportive or coordinating role. The A agencies were not charged with developing detailed plans; rather, they were to review and integrate into a state plan the efforts of local, regional, and other state health planning groups dealing with health services, manpower, and facilities (Office of Comprehensive Health Planning; Hilleboe and Schaefer).

In the regional or B agency, areawide plans were to be formulated along with developmental projects to meet identified community needs. Both plans and projects were forwarded to the A agency for approval. Unlike the A agency, the B agency, whether public or nonprofit, was required to secure 25% to 50% in local matching funds to cover the costs of operations

(Jacobs and Froh; Stebbins and Williams). Like the state agencies, areawide agencies operated with the assistance of advisory councils made up of representatives of health interests, the majority of whom were consumers. In addition, the 1967 amendments to P. L. 89–749, which extended the act into the 1970s and made additional federal funding available, also required local government representation in the areawide planning process to provide a stronger impetus to plan implementation.

In 1973, under a mandate from the Secretary of Health, Education and Welfare, the Division of Comprehensive Health Planning in Washington, D.C., undertook a nationwide assessment of both A and B agencies (1974). Their interim analysis, compiled in early 1974, indicated that most of the 48 CHPs reporting were still organizing themselves for planning and securing support for their agency as the health planning body in the community. Ardell reports similar conclusions following the review of all assessment reports (1974). He attributes CHP's failure to four factors: insufficient financial resources; less-than-adequate training of staff and volunteers; an uncertain legislative mandate and minimal enforcement powers; and blurred lines of responsibility regarding other federally funded programs.

Others have suggested that the time consumed by CHP in the general review and comment process worked against the fulfillment of the planning mandate. By 1973, A and B agencies were reviewing projects submitted for funding under at least 13 different federal programs, state mental retardation proposals, and capital expenditures for health care facilities reimbursed under Medicare, Medicaid, and the Maternal and Child Health programs (Block, McGibony, and Associates; Roseman).

Poor management of the political aspect of the planning process has also been cited as a reason for CHP's failure (Creditor), along with the need to achieve a consensus for action among advisory council members. According to Roseman (1972), providers dominated the councils through their "superior knowledge," despite the 51% consumer membership requirement. Providers espoused a policy of avoiding conflict in formulating goals and succeeded in making talk rather than action the hallmark of areawide operations. In addition, the requirement for local matching monies resulted in endless hours devoted to fund-raising and promoted inactivity because of conflict of interest.

Steven Sieverts (1976) saw the failure of the CHP system as being rooted in a fundamental misunderstanding of how health systems planning really works in the United States:

I have long believed that the flawed predictions in the late '60s about CHP's power over health facilities arose from a basic misconception of the institutional decision-making dynamics in the health system. It was somehow assumed that if one labeled as "planning" a process that involved debate and development of positions by a broad base of well-intentioned and concerned people, there inevitably would be a controlling impact on how the health system developed. Of course, that didn't happen.

On the other hand, in certain CHP areas, there were positive results from the work, which laid the foundation for possible successes under the HSA system that was to follow (West and Stevens).

Certification of Need

At the same time that RMP and CHP legislation was being developed at the federal level, the states began initiating laws requiring hospitals to demonstrate community need before they could begin constructing new facilities or undertaking major renovation of hospital bed areas and services. Certificate-of-need (CON) laws began with New York's 1964 Metcalf-McClosky Act and 1965 Folsom Act (Curran). Essentially, certificate-of-need programs establish criteria of public need for health care institutions and programs against which requests for changes in plant and, in certain states, program offerings of individual health care institutions are reviewed, approved, or disapproved (Dorsey; Havighurst, 1974). In 1968, with the support of the American Hospital Association, a nationwide drive to institute certificate-of-need laws began. By mid-1975, 23 states had certificate-of-need legislation covering at least some health facilities (Bicknell and Walsh, 1975).

State certification of need is a cousin of the federal capital expenditures review program carried out by CHP agencies and later by Health Systems Agencies (discussed below) under Section 1122 of the 1972 Social Security Act Amendments. The amendments tied reimbursement by Medicare, Medicaid, and the Maternal and Child Health programs for depreciation, interest, or return on equity capital for a capital expenditure to state and areawide planning agency approval of the project (Cohen). Indeed, in nine states, the passage of certificate-of-need laws was a defense against federal control implicit in participation in the 1122 program (USDHEW, 1976).

Wholly state-defined and state-initiated CON programs came to an end, however, in 1974 with the passage of P. L. 93–641, the National Health Planning and Resources Development Act (discussed in detail below). This new law required all states to institute CON programs in accord with federal regulations or lose federal dollar support for state health planning efforts as well as grant dollars made available under the Public Health Service Act and alcohol and drug addiction entitlements. The money at stake was large enough to occasion a doubling of the number of CON programs underway. By the fall of 1978, 41 states had passed certificate-of-need legislation. When all states have done so, Section 1122 reviews will be phased out of existence (Foley).

While similar in concept to Section 1122 review, CON, under P. L. 93-641, carries much heavier sanctions for the institution that proceeds without project approval. In addition to federal and state denial of reimbursement for interest, depreciation, and return on equity capital, many states will revoke the institution's operating license, impose civil penalties on its administration, or issue an injunction against continued facility operation. Nor can a project sponsor expect that compliance with fire, safety, licensure, or accreditation standards will guarantee CON approval for a project. Approval can follow only if the project is deemed to be a needed addition to or alteration of the health care delivery system, and if the expenditure involved is consistent with the state's health plan. Reversal of a CON decision can be accomplished only at an administrative hearing or in court (Kurt Salmon Associates, Inc.).

Like all regulatory mechanisms, certification of need has its limitations (Havighurst, 1973; Simler). Klarman points to the impossibility of establishing any quantitative criterion of need acceptable to a number of technical experts. Without that criterion, what firm basis is there for a CON decision? P. R. Sullivan et al. conclude that certification of need in Massachusetts is "too slow, too ineffective and too costly" (1979). Others have found that CON fails to control unwarranted health care and institutional growth (Hellinger; Rothenberg) or hospital cost increases (Salkever and Bice, 1978). In 1977, Salkever and Bice said: "[CON] legislation has diverted rather than checked hospital capital investments and has therefore had negligible impact on patient costs." Their study period, however, was 1968-1972. It may well be that since that time CON regulatory efforts, with more experience, are becoming more effective (*COTH Report*, 1978). In any case, CON does have its defenders (Bicknell and Walsh, 1975, 1976). It is also very much a fact of life under the HSA system. What is unfortunate is that certification of need is a negative rather than a positive health planning tool. It allows a health planning agency to prevent particular changes proposed by institutional health care providers that do not accord with established health plans. It does not increase the agency's ability to implement desired changes that have not been proposed and that require public and political support.

National Health Planning and Resources Development Act of 1974

Late in 1974, the 93rd Congress passed the National Health Planning and Resources Development Act, Public Law 93-641. Under the law, single state and areawide health planning agencies were created to perform the functions of Hill-Burton programs, Regional Medical Programs, and Comprehensive Health Planning Organizations (Coopers and Lybrand; Lively; Rubel, 1976; Werlin et al.; Whiting). By ending the fragmented approach to health planning, Congress apparently hoped to realize more than the minimal progress recorded until that time toward health care delivery and utilization goals. Certainly, the lawmakers also wished to increase external pressures directed at containing the persistent rise in health care expenditures evident since World War II (Klarman).

The provisions of P. L. 93–641 were embodied in new Titles XV and XVI of the Public Health Services Act. Part A of Title XV was a first in the annals of federal health care legislation. It required the Secretary of DHEW to issue national health planning goals based on the health priorities made explicit in the law. Previously, health planning had been characterized by mandates for rational planning without reference to any goals (Daniel). To assist the Secretary in setting goals, the act established a National Council on Health Planning and Development, with rather vague, nondirective, advisory powers.

Part B of Title XV created the units that were the core of the whole program: the Health Systems Agencies, or HSAs (Peterson). State governors were to designate health planning areas within their states, subject to the approval of the Secretary of DHEW. Designated areas, each with a federally funded HSA, were based on population (generally 500,000 to 1 million residents), the availability of health resources (at least one highly specialized health services center), and coordination with standard Metropolitan Statistical Areas, Professional Standards Review Organization boundaries, and existing regional and state planning areas. The last three of these requirements indicated a sensitivity to the difficulty of collecting data for health planning. They represented an attempt to advance planning efforts under P. L. 93–641 by coordinating them with ongoing data retrieval activities.

HSAs could be public or private nonprofit entities, but not educational entities, thus excluding the medical schools that had dominated RMP operations. (Nevertheless, health sciences centers seem to be playing an active role in HSA activities [Rubel, 1978].) Each HSA, under Section 1513 of P. L. 93–641, was charged with:

1. Gathering and analyzing suitable data;
2. Establishing (long-range) health systems plans or HSPs, and (short-range) annual implementation plans, or AIPs;
3. Providing technical and/or financial assistance to those seeking to implement provisions of the plans;
4. Coordinating activities with PSROs and other appropriate planning and regulating entities;

5. Reviewing and approving or disapproving applications for federal funds for health programs within the area;
6. Assisting states in the performance of capital expenditures reviews (certification of need);
7. Assisting states in reviewing institutional health services with respect to the appropriateness of such services;
8. Annually recommending to states projects for the modernization, construction, and conversion of medical facilities in the area.

Except for powers relating to plan development and disbursement of federal funds, the emphasis is on "assist," "recommend," "gather," and "coordinate." Nevertheless, the HSA is to carry out these tasks for critical purposes: (1) improving the health of residents of [the] health service area, (2) increasing the accessibility, . . . acceptability, continuity, and quality of . . . health services . . . (3) restrain[ing] increases in . . . cost . . . and (4) prevent[ing] . . . unnecessary duplication of health resources" (P. L. 93–641, Section 1513 (a)).

An incongruity exists in P. L. 93–641 between broad goals and limited powers (Shapiro and Russell; Wildavsky; Jonas, 1975). This gap has been characteristic of almost all health services planning legislation in the United States. Thus, in the long run, the most significant aspects of this law may turn out to be the health services data-gathering requirement (Section 1513 (b) (1)). The requirements for establishing health status measures, utilization data, health care resources data, and measures of the relations between health and health care on a national basis could be as significant as the establishment of uniform vital statistics reporting was earlier in the century. Klarman highlights, in particular, the merging of these traditional planning data with financial data on expenditures, cost, charges, and sources of payment.

P. L. 93–641 also created two planning bodies at the state level (P. L. 93–641, Part C). The first, called the State Health Planning and Development Agency (SHPDA), is an agency of the state government designated by the governor, with the approval of the Secretary of DHEW, and supported by federal grant monies. The SHPDA uses input from the areawide Health Systems Agencies to create a statewide health plan. It also reviews institutional services in the state and operates a certificate-of-need program.

The second state-level planning body is the Statewide Health Coordinating Council (SHCC). The council, aided by the SHPDA, reviews and coordinates Health Systems Agencies plans, reviews their budgets, and reviews state applications for federal funds under the Public Health Service Act, the Community Mental Health Centers Act, and the Alcoholism

Control Act of 1970. Each HSA is represented on the council. At least 50% of the council's members are consumers.

DHEW provides technical assistance to HSAs and SHPDAs in defining the minimum data needed to determine health status, health resources, and service utilization, and in planning methodologies, policies, and standards. DHEW is also empowered to establish systems for uniform cost-accounting, utilization determination, and rate-setting in hospitals, nursing homes, and other institutional settings (P. L. 93–641, Section 1533).

Title XV repeated many planning strategies from earlier legislation, but it also broke new ground. As in CHP, the governing boards of area HSAs and State Health Planning and Development Agencies have consumer majorities. The boards of the HSAs and the SHCC also include elected and appointed public officials and providers of care. Both the presence of public officials and the clear definition of the population to be served were viewed as mechanisms for increasing public accountability (Daniel). As in the case of Regional Medical Programs, broad provider representation was built into the system to encourage cooperation, accommodation, and the implementation of plans.

The most noteworthy departure from prior legislation is the establishment under P. L. 93–641 of close relations between the federal government and areas within states. In grants review, HSAs were empowered to review and *approve or disapprove* requests for funds under the Public Health Service Act and other acts. The review and comment procedures associated with CHP operations—that is, local area recommendations but state disposition—are retained only in the areas of certificate of need, Medicare and Medicaid capital controls, and decisions on the appropriateness of institutional health services. Conflicts between the state agency and HSAs over area matters are subject to resolution by the Secretary of DHEW. The relationship between the SHCC and the SHPDA provides further indication of the power of the HSA in relation to the state agency. The SHCC is empowered to "prepare and review and revise" at least annually a state health plan (a reconciliation of HSA plans in the state) and approve or disapprove state applications for funds under the Public Health Service Act and other acts. The HSAs of each state collectively hold a majority of the seats on the SHCC.

Title XVI of P. L. 93–641, Parts A through E, effected minor revisions in the old Hill-Burton program, and related construction activities more closely to the comprehensive health planning process. Part F authorized developmental grants for further implementation of approved HSA Annual Implementation Plans. The American Association for Comprehensive Health Planning had argued for including developmental activities in the law. Undoubtedly, they had the RMP experience in mind when they argued that with such monies, they could convince providers to take on mandates to alter the delivery system, mandates for which other funds were not available (Daniel).

By the end of 1978, the structural components of P. L. 93–641 were in place: 213 health planning areas had been designated and more than 200 HSAs were producing HSPs and AIPs; all 56 SHPDAs were funded and operational; most SHCCs had been organized. The National Council on Health Planning and Development was functioning. The first set of National Guidelines for Health Planning were issued in March 1978 (Foley; USDHEW, 1978), and modified somewhat in April 1979 (Kurt Salmon Associates, Inc.) The guidelines set service standards to be met by various components of the health care delivery system. They cover the following:

- Maximum general hospital bed/population ratios;
- Minimum general hospital bed occupancy rates;
- Minimum obstetrical unit service rates;
- Minimum neonatal special care unit service rates;
- Minimum number of beds and occupancy rate in pediatric units;
- Minimum number of operations to be performed by open-heart surgery units;
- Minimum number of procedures to be performed by cardiac catheterization units;
- Minimum population to be served by larger radiotherapy units;
- Minimum number of procedures to be performed by computed axial tomography (CAT) scanner units;
- Minimum standards for End-Stage Renal Disease Services.

Emphasis is placed on the need for regional planning of many of these services. All Health Systems Plans developed after December 31, 1978, must be consistent with the requirements of the guidelines. They attempt to introduce greater rationality and economy into the construction, installation, and utilization of the most commonly used health facilities and equipment.

In 1979, DHEW released draft guidelines covering the types and characteristics of health services that should be the goals of the planning process, as well as very specific health status goals to be achieved by the health care delivery system (USDHEW, 1979). The health services goals call for expansion of primary care services, prepayment, group practices, surgical second-opinion programs and multi-institutional shared service arrangements; improvements in access to care, quality of care and management procedures, and mental health and dental health services; adequate technology assessment; regionalization; and energy conservation. Health status goals cover the expansion of disease prevention and health promotion services, including the integration of preventive medicine into primary care, improvement of prenatal and family planning services, expansion of immunization programs, development of accident prevention programs, fluoridation of water supplies, nutrition education, and cigarette smoking control. The health status goals set out certain specific health status outcomes in terms of the reduction of various age-specific and disease-specific death rates; the reduction of average annual days of restricted activity for older persons; the reduction of alcoholism and drug abuse rates; and the improvement of the tooth retention rate. This specification of types of health services to be emphasized and of health status measures to be achieved marks an important step forward in the health planning system, away from concentrating solely on numbers of beds, pieces of equipment, and utilization rates. The emphasis on prevention is particularly noteworthy.

Late in 1978, the General Accounting Office of the U.S. Congress released a study of the first four years of activity under the HSA system (Comptroller General). Noting that it was too early to tell whether the goals of the National Health Planning and Resources Development Act of 1974 were being achieved, the GAO leveled its major criticisms at details of administration and implementation, not at matters of principle. Thus, concerns were raised over the slowness of HEW in publishing regulations and guidelines, problems in collecting and coordinating data, inability to recruit appropriate staff, confusion over the roles of the HSA and the SHPDA in states having only one HSA area, problems with the technical assistance program established under the act, and difficulties in creating knowledgeable and effective Boards. DHEW concurred in most of the recommendations and outlined actions taken or planned to meet them.

Some of the problems raised by the GAO, and others not mentioned in the report, required legislative remedy. Late in 1979, after lengthy debate, an extension of the National Health Planning and Resources Development Act through FY 1982 was passed by Congress (P. L. 96–79; *Health Resources News*). Among the major changes made were the following:

1. Competition among health care institutions is to become a national health priority and a criterion for project reviews;
2. HSAs are to collect and publish data on rates charged by hospitals for the 25 most frequently used services;
3. CON coverage is extended to all major medical equipment used for hospital inpatients, regardless of its location;
4. Under most circumstances, HMOs are not subject to CON review;

5. Under CON, "batching," or simultaneous review of similar pro-
    posed construction projects, is required at least twice a year;
6. Dollars are made available to assist in the voluntary discon-
    tinuance or conversion of unneeded hospital facilities;
7. SHPDAs and HSAs may be granted full designation status for up
    to 36 months, rather than 12 months;
8. Fully designated state and local agencies that are not functioning
    appropriately can be returned to conditional status;
9. The health planning cycle may be a triennial rather than an annual
    process, to allow more time for implementation;
10. The selection process has been changed to assure that HSA boards
    are not self-perpetuating;
11. The conditions and criteria that HSAs can use in project review are
    clearly defined and limited;
12. The membership of the National Council on Health Planning and
    Development has been increased from 15 to 20 and is to include
    representatives of the hospital industry and the medically under-
    served.

As of 1980, it was still too early to determine if the HSA approach to
health planning would be able to achieve the goals set forth in the original
act. The performance assessments on hand were largely self-assessments.
For example, a 1979 report by the American Health Planning Association
indicated that HSAs nationally were saving about $1.8 billion a year in
capital investment initiatives denied, or about $8.00 in proposed spending
denied for every $1.00 spent in planning costs (*COTH Report*, 1979).
Similarly, in late 1979, the Bureau of Health Planning of HEW's Human
Resources Administration, which administers the HSA program, took a
look at its own work and was pleased with what it saw. Studying the work of
some of the best HSAs in the country, the bureau determined that it was
indeed possible to reduce and/or prevent excess hospital bed capacity;
improve health services availability and access; move toward the creation
of a regional hospital system; and redress the imbalance between inpatient
and ambulatory services. The challenge, as the Bureau of Health Planning
saw it, lay in expanding this work and extending it to all HSAs. Perhaps a
less involved observer would more temperately conclude that in 1980
there were some hopeful signs of planning progress.

Conclusion

Assessing how far the United States has traveled along the health planning
road is difficult. Certainly, the absence of any requirement in P. L. 93–641
to avoid interfering with established patterns of medical practice is a step

forward, as is the stipulation that areawide planning agencies review the "appropriateness" of existing health services and be given federal grant approval powers. Continuing support for the developmental function, establishing specific requirements for a planning-financial data base, and drawing areawide planning boundaries that encourage data-system sharing are also positive steps.

Such surface changes can be easily catalogued; foreseeing the impact of underlying changes is more difficult, however. One may question, for example, whether the health care consumer can be best served by placing the functions of planning, development, and regulation of health services under a single agency's jurisdiction. Experience with federal regulatory commissions has, more often than not, indicated the dangers of eliminating competition and the cross-checking of claims that retard self-aggrandizement (Huntington; Havighurst, 1973). It is not clear whether combining the three functions will reduce the degree to which self-interests are advanced and will overcome the coordination problems long inherent in our pluralistic health care system. Perhaps even greater powers or changes outside the health planning realm are required. Congressional figures behind the passage of the 1974 Health Planning and Resources Development Act saw it as a prerequisite to national health insurance. Perhaps the reverse is true: perhaps a comprehensive and flexible national health insurance scheme must be established before health planning directed at making our health care system work rationally can be accomplished. If reimbursement problems no longer plague providers, it may be possible to establish a set of values that encourages mutual adjustment for the common good. Unfortunately, there are many possibilities, but few certainties.

References

Ahumada, J., et al. *Health Planning: Problems of Concept and Method.* Washington, D.C.: Pan American Health Organization, Scientific Publication No. 111, 1965.

Anderson, O. W. "Influence of Social and Economic Research on Public Policy in the Health Field—A Review." *Milbank Memorial Fund Quarterly, 44* (Suppl.), 11, 1966.

Ardell, D. B. "The Demise of CHP and the Future of Planning." *Inquiry, 11,* 233, 1974.

Balinsky, W., and Berger, R. "A Review of the Research on General Health Status Indexes." *Medical Care, 13,* 283, 1975.

Berg, R. L. *Health Status Indexes.* Chicago: Hospital Research and Educational Trust, 1973.

Bicknell, W. J., and Walsh, D.C. "Certification of Need: the Massachusetts Experience." *New England Journal of Medicine, 20,* 1052, 1975.

Bicknell, W. J., and Walsh, D. C. "Critical Experiences in Organizing and Administering a State Certification of Need Program." *Public Health Reports, 91,* 29, 1976.

Block, McGibony and Associates, Inc. "A Discussion of Health Issues." *Special Report,* 1973.

Blum, H. L. *Planning for Health: Development and Application of Social Change Theory.* New York: Human Sciences Press, 1974.

Bodenheimer, T. S. "Regional Medical Programs: No Road to Regionalization." *Medical Care Review, 26,* 1125, 1969.

Bright, J., Ed. *Technological Forecasting in Government and Industry.* Englewood Cliffs, New Jersey: Prentice-Hall, 1968.

Bugbee, G. "The Hill-Burton Construction Bill." *Journal of the American Medical Association, 127,* 657, 1945.

Bureau of Health Planning. *Health Planning in Action: Achieving Equal Access to Quality Health Care at a Reasonable Cost.* Hyattsville, Maryland: USDHEW Pub. No. (HRA) 79–14030, 1979.

Bush, J. W., et al. *Social Indicators for Health Planning and Policy Analysis.* Springfield, Virginia: National Technical Information Service, 1974.

Chapman, J., and Coulson, A. "Community Diagnosis: An Analysis of Indicators of Health and Disease in a Metropolitan Area." *International Journal of Epidemiology, 1,* 75, 1972.

Clark, L. J., and Koontz, T. L. "Analysis of the Impact of the Hill-Burton Program on the Distribution of the Supply of General Hospital Beds and Physicians in the United States 1950–1970." Paper delivered at Annual Meeting of American Public Health Association, 1973, San Francisco.

Cohen, H. S. "Regulating Health Care Facilities: the Certificate-of-Need Process Re-examined." *Inquiry, 10,* 3, 1973.

Commission on Hospital Care. *Hospital Resources and Needs, The Report of the Michigan Hospital Survey.* Battle Creek, Michigan: Kellogg Foundation, 1946.

————. *Hospital Care in the United States.* New York: The Commonwealth Fund, 1947.

Committee on the Costs of Medical Care. *Medical Care for the American People.* Chicago: University of Chicago Press, 1932. Reprinted: Washington, D.C., USDHEW, 1970.

Comptroller General. *Status of the Implementation of the National Health Planning and Resources Development Act of 1974.* Washington, D.C.: USGPO, November 2, 1978.

Coopers and Lybrand. *Health Care in Transition.* New York, 1975.

COTH Report. "Planning Agencies Have Blocked $154 Million in Hospital Spending." Washington, D.C.: Association of American Medical Colleges, October–November 1978, p. 12.

————. "Study Attributes $1.8 Billion in Capital Savings to HSAs." Washington, D.C.: Association of American Medical Colleges, January 1979.

Creditor, M. C. "A Modest Proposal: Let CHP and RMP Run the System." *Modern Hospital, 119*, 101, 1972.

Creditor, M. C., and Nelson, D. "Regional Medical Programs and Office Management and Budget—Parallel Philosophies." *New England Journal of Medicine, 289*, 239, 1975.

Curran, W. J. "A National Survey and Analysis of State Certificate of Need Laws for Health Facilities." In Havighurst, C. C., Ed., *Regulating Health Facilities Construction*. Chapter 3. Washington, D.C.: American Institute for Public Policy Research, 1974.

Daniel, S. L. "Issues Raised by Pending Comprehensive Health Planning Legislation." *Health Politics, 4*, 3, 1974.

Division of Comprehensive Health Planning, Health Resources Administration. "Interim Analysis of Results of CHP Agency Assessments," CHP Program Letter 74–14, May 29, 1974 (E. J. Rubel, Director of the Division). Rockville, Maryland, 20852.

Dorsey, J. L. "Certification of Need Laws." *Archives of Surgery, 106*, 765, 1973.

Elling, R. H. "The Shifting Power Structure on Health." *Milbank Memorial Fund Quarterly, 46* (Suppl.), 119, 1968.

Fanshel, S., and Bush, J. W. "A Health Status Index and Its Applications to Health Service Outcomes." *Operations Research, 18*, 1021, 1970.

Fein, R. "Priorities and Decision Making in Health Planning." *Israel Journal of Medical Sciences, 10*, 67, 1974.

Foley, H. A. "Assuring the Nation's Health Resources." *Public Health Reports, 93*, 627, 1978.

Gartland, J. E. *An Experiment in Medicine: A History of the First 20 Years of the Pratt Clinic and the New England Center Hospital of Boston.* Cambridge, Massachusetts: Riverside Press, 1960.

Goldsmith, S. B. "The Status of Health Status Indicators." *Health Services Reports, 87*, 212, 1972.

Gottlieb, S. "A Brief History of Health Planning in the United States." In Havighurst, C. C., Ed., *Regulating Health Facilities Construction*. Chapter 1. Washington, D.C.: American Institute for Public Policy Research, 1974.

Guralnick, L. "Some Problems in the Use of Multiple Causes of Death." *Journal of Chronic Diseases, 19*, 979, 1966.

Haber, L. "Identifying the Disabled: Concepts and Methods in Measurement of Disability." *Social Security Bulletin, 30*, 17, 1967.

Havighurst, C. C. "Regulation of Health Facilities and Services." *Virginia Law Review, 59*, 1143, 1973.

————. "Regulation in the Health Care System." *Hospitals, 48*, 65, 1974.

Health Resources News, 6, November 1979.

Hellinger, F. J. "The Effect of Certificate-of-Need Legislation on Hospital Investment." *Inquiry, 13*, 187, 1976.

Hilleboe, H. E. "Health Planning on a Community Basis." Ann Arbor, Michigan: Delta Omega Lecture, School of Public Health, University of Michigan, July 31, 1967. (Mimeographed)

Hilleboe, H. E., and Schaefer, M. "Administrative Requirements for Comprehensive Health Planning at the State Level." *American Journal of Public Health,* 58, 1039, 1968.

Hilleboe, H. E., et al. *Approaches to National Health Planning,* Public Health Papers #46. Geneva, Switzerland: World Health Organization, 1972.

Huntington, S. P. "The Marasmus of the ICC: The Commission, the Railroads and the Public Interest." *Yale Law Journal, 61,* 467, 1952.

Jacobs, A. R., and Froh, R. B. "Significance of Public Law 89–749." *New England Journal of Medicine, 279,* 1314, 1968.

Jeffers, J., et al. "On the Demand vs. Need for Medical Services and the Concept of 'Shortage.'" *American Journal of Public Health, 61,* 46, 1971.

Jonas, S. "Heart Disease, Cancer and Stroke—Regional Medical Programs." *Journal of the National Medical Association, 59,* 7, 1967.

——————." '74 Planning Act Is Dubbed 'Sleeper'; The Prospective from the Campus." *The Nation's Health, 5,* June 1975.

Klarman, H. E. "Health Planning: Progress, Prospects, and Issues." *Milbank Memorial Fund Quarterly: Health and Society, 56,* 78, 1978.

Komaroff, Anthony L. "Regional Medical Programs in Search of a Mission." *New England Journal of Medicine, 284,* 750, 1971.

Kurt Salmon Associates, Inc. "Certificate of Need Review—Health Planning or Russian Roulette?" *Perspectives for Health Care Management,* January 1980.

Lively, C. A. "P. L. 93–641: A Recipe for Action." *Hospitals, J.A.H.A.,* 52, 65, 1978.

Meltzer, J. W., and Hochstim, J. R. "Reliability and Validity of Survey Data on Physical Health." *Public Health Reports,* 85, 1075, 1970.

Miller, J. E. "An Indicator to Aid Management in Assigning Program Priorities." *Public Health Reports,* 85, 721, 1970.

Miller, W. R. "A Five-Year Perspective of NRMP." *Minnesota Medicine,* 55, 9, 1972.

Morehouse, T. A. "Program Evaluation: Social Research versus Public Policy." *Public Administration Review, 32,* 868, 1972.

Mountin, J. W., et al. *Health Service Areas: Requirements for General Hospitals and Health Centers.* Public Health Service Pub. No. 292. Washington, D.C.: USDHEW, 1945.

National Center for Health Statistics. *An Index of Health: Mathematical Models.* U.S. Public Health Service Pub. No. 1000. Washington, D. C.: USGPO, 1965.

Office of Comprehensive Health Planning, USDHEW, Public Health Service. *Information and Policies on Grants to States for Comprehensive Health Planning.* Washington, D.C.: USGPO, 1967.

Peterson, R. L. "The Designation of Health Service Areas." *Public Health Reports, 91,* 9, 1976.

Prest, A. R., and Turvey, R. "Cost-Benefit Analysis: A Survey." *The Economic Journal, 75,* 683, 1965.

President's Commission on Heart Disease, Cancer and Stroke. *A National Program to Conquer Heart Disease, Cancer and Stroke.* Washington, D.C.: USGPO, 1964.

Public Acountability Reporting Group. *Regional Medical Programs Benefiting People and Implementing Local Health Services.* Boise, Idaho: Public Accountability Reporting Group, 1974.

Public Law 79–725. *Hospital Survey and Construction Act.* August 13, 1946.

Public Law 89–239. Amendment to the Public Health Service Act. Title IX— *Education, Research, Training and Demonstration in the Fields of Heart Disease, Cancer, Stroke and Related Diseases.* October 6, 1965.

Public Law 89–749. *Comprehensive Health Planning and Public Service Amendments of 1966,* November 3, 1966.

Public Law 93–641. *National Health Planning and Resources Development Act.* January 4, 1975.

Public Law 96–79. *Health Planning and Resources Development Amendments of 1979.* October 4, 1979.

Rienke, W. A., and Baker, T. D. "Measuring Effects of Demographic Variables on Health Service Utilization." *Health Service Research,* 2, 61, 1967.

Roseman, C. "Problems and Prospects for Comprehensive Health Planning." *American Journal of Public Health,* 62, 16, 1972.

Rosenfeld, L. S. "Problems in Planning Community Health Services." *Bulletin of the New York Academy of Medicine,* 44, 164, 1968.

Rothenberg, E. *Regulation and Expansion of Health Facilities: The Certificate of Need Experience in New York State.* New York: Praeger, 1976.

Rubel, E. J. "Implementing the National Health Planning and Resources Development Act of 1974." *Public Health Reports,* 91, 3, 1976.

——————."National Health Planning and Resources Development Act: Implications for the Academic Medical Center." Washington, D.C.: Association of American Medical Colleges, 1978.

Russell, John M. "New Federal Regional Medical Programs." *New England Journal of Medicine,* 275, 6, 1966.

Salkever, D., and Bice, T. W. *Impact of State Certificate of Need Laws on Health Care Costs and Utilization.* Rockville, Maryland: NCHSR Research Digest Series, HRA 77–3163, 1977.

——————. "Certificate of Need Legislation and Hospital Costs." In Zubkoff, M., Raskin, I., and Hanft, R., Eds., *Hospital Cost Containment: Selected Notes for Future Policy.* New York: PRODIST, 1978.

Shapiro, J. R., and Russell, E. L. "P. L. 93–641: Fundamental Problems." *New England Journal of Medicine,* 295,725, 1976.

Sieverts, S. "Putting P. L. 93–641 Into Proper Perspective." *Hospitals, J.A.H.A.,* June 16, 1976, p. 125.

Sigmond, R. M. "Health Planning." *Milbank Memorial Fund Quarterly,* 46 (Suppl.), 91, 1968.

Simler, S. L. "Certificate-of-Need Data: Much-Questioned Criteria." *Modern Health Care,* 8, 42, 1978.

Spiegel, A. D., and Hyman, H. H. *Basic Health Planning Methods.* Germantown, Maryland: Aspen Systems Corp., 1978.

Stebbins, E. L., and Williams, K. N. "History and Background of Health Planning in the United States." In Rienke, W. A., Ed., *Health Planning: Qualitative*

Aspects and Quantitative Techniques. Chapter 1. Baltimore, Maryland: Johns Hopkins University Press, 1972.

Sullivan, D. F. *Conceptual Problems in Developing an Index of Health*. USDHEW, National Center for Health Statistics, *Vital and Health Statistics*, Ser. 2, No. 17, Washington, D.C. 1966.

Sullivan, P. R., et al. "A Critique of the Massachusetts Determination of Need Program." *New England Journal of Medicine, 14*, 794, 1979.

Susser, M. W., and Watson, W. *Sociology in Medicine*. 2nd Ed. London: Oxford University Press, 1971.

Taylor, C. E. "Stages of the Planning Process." In Rienke, W. A., Ed., *Health Planning: Qualitative Aspects and Quantitative Techniques*. Chapter 2. Baltimore, Maryland: Johns Hopkins University Press, 1972.

U.S. Department of Health, Education and Welfare. *Congressional Hearings Data Book Fiscal Year 1970*. Rockville, Maryland: Health Services and Mental Health Administration, Community Profile Data Center, 1969.

——————. Public Health Service. *Facts About the Hill-Burton Program: 1 July 1947–30 June 1970*. Washington, D.C.: USGPO, 1970.

——————. *Trends Affecting the U.S. Health Care System*. Washington, D.C.: USGPO, 1976.

——————. "Health Planning: National Guidelines." *Federal Register*. March 28, 1978, p. 13040.

——————. *National Guidelines for Health Planning, Draft*. Washington, D.C.: Health Resources Administration. July 6, 1979.

Ward, P. W. "The Curious Odyssey of Regional Medical Programs." *Western Journal of Medicine, 120*, 425, 1974.

Werlin, S. H., et al. "Implementing Formative Health Planning Under P. L. 93–641." *New England Journal of Medicine, 295*, 698, 1976.

West, J. P., and Stevens, M. D. "Comparative Analysis of Community Health Planning: Transition from CHPs to HSAs." *Journal of Health Politics, Policy and Law, 1*, 173, 1976.

Whiting, R. N. "The Debate Continues: Is Health Planning Working?" *Hospitals, J.A.H.A.*, April 1, 1977, p. 47. (This paper has a lengthy bibliography.)

Wildavsky, A. "Can Health Be Planned?" The 1976 Michael M. Davis Lecture. Chicago: The Center for Health Administration Studies, University of Chicago, 1976.

Zola, I. K. "Culture and Symptoms: An Analysis of Patients Presenting Complaints." *American Sociological Review, 31*, 615, 1966.

14

Measurement and Control of the Quality of Health Care*

Steven Jonas

> We have granted the health professions access to the most secret and sensitive places in ourselves and entrusted to them matters that touch on our well-being, happiness, and survival. In return, we have expected the professions to govern themselves so strictly that we need have no fear of exploitation or incompetence. The object of quality assessment is to determine how successful they have been in doing so; and the purpose of quality monitoring is to exercise constant surveillance so that departure from standards can be detected early and corrected.

So stated Avedis Donabedian (1978, p. 111). A number of measures show that health care delivered in the United States varies sharply in quality. There is an extensive literature on the subject of the approaches aimed at ensuring good care, but before beginning to review that literature in some detail, we might address ourselves to the question, "Why be concerned about the quality of health care at all?"

Why Be Concerned with Quality of Care?

First, perhaps, is the principle *primum non nocere:* "Primarily, do no harm." This precept is at least as old as the Hippocratic Oath, of which it is a part. As our consideration below of the results of quality determinations will demonstrate, this is an important consideration in a health care delivery system in which a substantial minority of care delivered is of less than good quality and could be harmful.

Second, as pointed out in Chapter 10, our society devotes a significant and increasing portion of its economic resources to providing health services. Americans have a strong interest in obtaining a good product for the

---

*In this chapter we are concerned primarily with the quality of *medical* care, the subject of the bulk of the literature. However, many of the principles, although not all of the practices, apply to health care in general.

money spent. Further, there are social and humanitarian motivations to see that the large sums of money spent actually help those persons who are receiving the services.

Third, from the providers' point of view, a major motivation for doing good work in health care is professionalism. The concepts of "profession" and "professionalism" are related to quality. A profession is, in part at least, a field of human endeavor in which the practitioners themselves control entry and exit, in which a common body of knowledge exists, and in which the practitioners attempt to expand and develop that body of knowledge to improve the quality of human life and extend the understanding of man's existence. This last aspect of professionalism, aside from personal pecuniary and self-protective interests, adds a strong impetus to the thrust of at least part of the medical profession to regulate and improve the quality of medical care.

Finally, there is a strong social ethic in our culture to value doing a good job in and of itself. This principle has deep historical roots in the Judeo-Christian tradition; its origins probably stem from the individual and species survival value of performing tasks well. In health care, of course, there is a direct link between both individual and species survival and doing a good job in personal and community health services.

Can the Quality of Health Care Be Evaluated?

The extent to which quality of care can be evaluated has been a subject of debate. A former president of the American Medical Association, Russell Roth, said in a presidential address that "good quality in medical care is not something which can be expressed in dollars of cost, hours of time, or for that matter, in decibels of political oratory. Quality of such medical care is not a tangible, qualifiable thing" (*American Medical News*, December 10, 1973). He added there are "immense difficulties" inherent in properly identifying high-quality care. On the other hand, many authorities in the field have thought it possible to measure and regulate the quality of discrete instances of care delivery. E. A. Codman has been recognized as the granddaddy of outcome studies (Brook, 1973b, p. 32; Christoffel, 1976a; Lewis; Moore.) Emphasizing his faith in their efficacy as measures of quality, he said: "While a layman could not authoritatively inquire into the details of the reasons why, he could insist that the end-result system should be used, that someone must see that it is used, and that an efficiency committee be appointed for the purpose" (Lewis).

Lee and Jones wrote a landmark work on quality determination in 1933, which was built around the concept that "good medical care is the kind of medicine practiced and taught by the recognized leaders of the medical profession at a given time or period of social, cultural, and professional development in a community or population group" (p. 6). Thus they felt that quality could be measured against the value judgments of recognized professional leaders. In 1951, E. R. Weinerman, reflecting the 1949 statement made by the Subcommittee on Medical Care of the American Public Health Association, "The Quality of Medical Care in a National Health Program," said: "The quality of medical care is a composite of all the technical, organizational, and financial aspects of any program for personal health service. Good quality can be defined, consciously planned, and evaluated" (Subcommittee on Medical Care; Weinerman). Thus Weinerman introduced the concept of structural criteria (see below). The American Public Health Association's belief in the possibility of measuring quality was amply restated in the second volume of *A Guide to Medical Care Administration: Medical Care Appraisal—Quality and Utilization* (Donabedian, 1969).

In their work describing the "tracer method" of quality measurement, David Kessner and his co-authors said: "The question is no longer whether there will be intervention in health services to assure quality, but who will intervene and what methods they will use" (1973). In a review article, Robert Brook said: "Even though the perfect system for assessment and assurance of quality of care may not yet exist, innumerable simple efforts can be made to improve quality of care. If applied in a systematic manner, many are likely to be successful" (1973a).

It happens, as it so often does, that there is nothing new about all of this. In 1732, Dr. Francis Clifton, an English physician, wrote: "Three or four persons should be employed in the hospitals to set down the cases of the patients from day to day candidly and judiciously without any regard to private opinions and public systems, and at the year's end publish these facts just as they are—leaving everyone to make the best use he could for himself" (Lister, 1977).

Methods of Measuring and Controlling the Quality of Care

The first problem in analyzing quality measurement in health care is to classify and understand the different methodologies. Many review articles (Blum; Brook, 1973b, pp. 7–16; Donabedian, 1966, 1968, 1969, 1978; Sanazaro and Williamson; Sheps) have established schemata for classifying the techniques or methodologies used for measuring the quality of medical care delivered by individuals or institutions, a subject to which we shall return. However, before examining the techniques for evaluating the quality of care, it is useful to understand the approaches to quality measurement and control that are actually in use in the U.S. (see Table 14.1). In the early 1970s, M. I. Roemer, Lewis, and Ellwood et al.) began to take this necessary broader view.

Table 14.1

Approaches, Techniques, and Criteria for Measurement of Quality of Health Care

1. Approaches
   General
       Licensing
       Accreditation
       Certification
   Specific
       Hospital medical staff review committees
       Professional Standards Review Organizations
       Patient satisfaction
       Malpractice litigation

2. Techniques
   Evaluation of structure: evaluation of physical facilities
       and administrative organization
   Evaluation of process: evaluation of activities of physicians
       and other health staff professionals in management of patients
   Evaluation of outcome: evaluation of effects of care on
       the end results in terms of health and satisfaction

3. Criteria
   Explicit — written down
   Implicit — exist only in the mind of the evaluator

The *approaches* are those various methods utilized to ensure quality in the health care delivery system, such as licensing, accreditation, and peer review through hospital medical staff committees. *Techniques* are the ways quality is measured within the various approaches. Techniques are only tools; approaches use the tools to effect control, or at least attempt to do so. Thus techniques are scientific constructs, whereas approaches are political ones.

Approaches

The approaches may be divided into two groups—the general and the specific. The general approaches examine an individual's or an institution's ability to meet established evaluative criteria at a particular time. Individuals are evaluated in terms of experience, education, and knowledge (usually measured by examination). Institutions are evaluated on the basis of physical structure, administrative and staff organization, minimum capabilities and standards for the provision of service, and personnel qualifications. If the criteria are met at the time of evaluation, it is then predicted that the individual or institution will function well either indefinitely, as in the case of the medical license, or for a given period of time, as in the case of the hospital license. The general approaches used in the United States are licensing, accreditation, and certification (Cohen and Miike, 1973; USDHEW, 1971, 1977a).

The specific approaches to quality measurement and control, on the other hand, look at discrete instances of provider-patient interaction and evaluate them using one of several available techniques. The major specific approaches in use in the United States are hospital medical staff review committees; Professional Standards Review Organizations; patient satisfaction, and its subset, malpractice litigation, an extreme product of patient dissatisfaction.

Techniques

Donabedian (1969) has provided the generally accepted classification of the techniques of quality assessment:

> Three major approaches* to the evaluation of quality have been identified. These have been designated as the evaluation of structure, process, and outcome or end results.
>
> Appraisal of structure involves the evaluation of the settings and instrumentalities available and used for the provision of care. While including the physical aspects of facilities and equipment, structural appraisal goes far beyond to encompass the characteristics of the administrative organization and the qualifications of health professionals. . . . Two major assumptions are made when structure is taken as an indicator of quality: First, that better care is more likely to be provided when better qualified staff, improved physical facilities and sounder fiscal and administrative organization are employed. Second, that we know enough to identify what is good in terms of staff, physical structure and formal organization. . . .
>
> Assessment of process is the evaluation of the activities of physicians and other health professionals in the management of patients. The criterion generally used is the degree to which management of patients conforms with the standards and expectations of the respective professions. These standards and expectations may be derived from what is considered to be "ideal," "good," or "acceptable" practice as formulated by recognized leaders in the profession. Such standards may also be inferred from patterns of care observed in actual practice. . . .
>
> When evaluation of process is the basis for judgments concerning quality, a major assumption is that health care is useful in maintaining or promoting health. Furthermore, there is the explicit or implicit assumption that particular elements and aspects of care are known to be specifically related to successful or unsuccessful health outcomes or end results. Assessment of outcomes is the evaluation of end results in terms of health and satisfaction. That this evaluation in many ways provides the final evidence of whether care

*Donabedian uses the word "approaches" in the sense in which the word "techniques" is used in this chapter.

has been good, bad or indifferent is so because of the broad fundamental social and professional agreement on what results are deemed desirable. Furthermore, it is assumed that good results are brought about, at least to a significant degree, by good care. (pp. 2–3)

Thus, the structural approach examines the setting of care; the process approach examines what goes on between the provider(s) and the patient; the outcome approach examines the results of the encounter or lack thereof between the patient and the health care delivery system. In the main, the structural technique is used in the general approaches, while the process and outcome techniques are used in the specific approaches, sometimes in combination with the structural technique as well.

Criteria

Explicit criteria. In all three techniques, criteria are used in the evaluation process. Explicit criteria are written down and the work under study is checked against them. For example, in a process study of physician performance, an explicit criterion might be that in the course of a good physical examination, a blood pressure measurement is taken. If a medical record is being used as the medium of evaluation, the evaluator would then check to see if a blood pressure measurement had been recorded. (Actually, if the evaluation is being made solely on the basis of what is in the medical record, a blood pressure notation can mean either that the pressure was taken and recorded, or that it was not taken and a number put down anyway. The absence of a blood pressure reading in the record can mean either that it was not taken, or that it was taken and not recorded. Of the four possibilities, only the first represents good medical care.)

Implicit criteria. Implicit criteria, on the other hand, exist only in the mind of the evaluator. Nothing specific to look for is written down. Evaluators are picked on the basis of their own credentials and reputations. The assumption is made that since they are "good" physicians (or dentists, nurses, etc.), they will know what "good" and "bad" care are and will be able to make valid and reliable assessments of care as they review it.

Thus, there are two groups of approaches, three sets of techniques, and two categories of criteria. They are organized in various combinations in practice in the United States.

General Approaches to Quality of Care Assessment and Control
Licensing

Licensing systems exist for both individual and institutional providers in the United States. As of 1977, 35 health professions and occupations were licensed by one or more states (National Center for Health Statistics, p. 7;

Pennell and Stewart, p. 1; USDHEW, 1977b); 17 types of health facilities are licensed in one or more states (Hollis, p. 1; National Center for Health Statistics, Appendix A). There are certain similarities between the two types of license as well as several important differences. Both use structural standards of measurement and both scrupulously avoid investigations of particular instances of individual care delivery. Individuals' licensing is usually for an indefinite period, whereas licensure of institutions is usually for a set time period. Both types involve governmental authority and are backed by the force of law. By exclusion, the Constitution grants the "police power" to the states; licensing, having been considered to fall in this category, is thus a state function (Derbyshire, 1969, p. 16).

Licensure of individuals. Individuals' licensing is a complex matter (National Advisory Commission on Health Manpower, Appendix VII; USDHEW, 1971, pp. 1–33; USDHEW, 1977a, 1977b). It represents a compact between defined professional groups and state legislatures in which the profession is granted control over individuals' entrance into, maintenance of good standing in, and exit from the profession. Most professions generally define the content of their own work and thus gain a virtual monopoly over the provision to the public of that body of work. In return, the profession, in theory at least, guarantees to the several state legislatures that the work will be of good quality. The states use the criminal justice system to enforce the agreements. The nature of medicine is such that "practicing without a license" constitutes assault and battery.

Among the health professions and occupations licensed in all or most states are: chiropractic; dental hygiene; dentistry; allopathic, osteopathic, and veterinary medicine; nursing; optometry; pharmacy; physical therapy; podiatry; and psychology (Pennell and Stewart, Table A). There are a series of controversial issues relating to licensure of individuals (Cohen, 1973, 1974; Cohen and Miike; Derbyshire, 1969; Egelston; Miike; Morton; National Advisory Commission on Health Manpower, Appendix VII; Nolan; Pennell; R. Roemer, 1971a, 1971b; Shryock; Spieler; USDHEW, 1971).

Licensure can, and apparently often does, lead to elements of guildism. The licensed group, having an area fenced off for itself, can become more interested in maintaining the fence than in regulating the work that goes on within its boundaries. The medical profession in particular has argued that a license, rather than being a compact with a state government concerning quality, is a property right; the courts have often upheld this view (Vodicka). As of 1968, the most recent year for which readily available comprehensive data exist, it was clear that the membership of the various state licensing boards for the independent health professions and occupations for the most part are dominated by members of the profession or occupation (Pennell and Stewart). An exception is dental hygiene—most boards licensing dental hygienists are dominated by dentists, and none includes any dental hygienists (Pennell and Stewart, Table 18). There is no reason to believe that the situation has changed significantly since 1968.

Licensure can lead to rigidity in job descriptions. If job descriptions do not change in accordance with changes in preparatory education, in time people will not be properly trained in relation to the licensing laws. The error in this case is usually on the side of overtraining. However, under-training can also occur when the work content and educational require-ments prescribed by licensing laws do not accord with changing health and health care needs.

The rigidities of licensure also limit geographic mobility, because of different laws and requirements in different states; inhibit health profes-sionals from moving up the career ladder, because most health licensure requirements do not allow credit for education and experience in another health profession or occupation; and discourage innovative and creative use of personnel. Furthermore, until the mid-1970s there was virtually no direct public accountability for, or direct public participation in, any health profession or occupation licensing board. By 1980, public members had been added to medical licensing boards in 24 states (Derbyshire, 1980). It remains to be seen what effects these changes will have. The licensure system rests on the unproven premise that the person who has qualified for a license will tend to deliver good health care over a long period of time. Studies of the work of licensed providers that employ process and/or outcome techniques rather than the structural techniques used in licen-sure show a wide variation in quality, demonstrating that licensing has very little validity as either a predictor or a guarantor of performance. (See the section entitled "Research Studies," below.)

One of the more novel proposals for licensing reform is "institutional licensure" (Miike). In this approach, institutions would be responsible for the competence of the people they employ. Such a system might produce beneficial results, according to Forgotson and Roemer (1968):

> Although licensure of personnel and licensure of facilities are completely separate in our current system of licensure, merger of these two systems into a single regulatory system governing individual and institutional providers of service might be a key to better regulation of quality and more freedom for innovation in delegation of patient-care tasks among members of the health manpower matrix. . . . The institutional licensure approach, which might result from such a merger, would provide a framework for developing innovations in the use of existing categories of personnel and for undertaking experimental programs to train and use new categories of health professions. (p. 352)

The principal affected professions, particularly medicine and nursing, have reacted to this proposal like a neighborhood threatened with a drug-treatment program or a halfway house for discharged mental-hospital patients: "It's a great idea, but not on *my* block, thank you very much." As Miike pointed out, for this reason, among others, institutional licensure must be considered still very much in the experimental stage. In fact, by 1980 no further developments in institutional licensure had occurred.

Ruth Roemer (1971a) considered most of the issues of licensure reform in some detail, as have others (Cohen, 1973, 1974; Cohen and Miike, 1973, 1974; National Advisory Commission on Health Manpower; Spieler). Roemer's most important point is that fundamental reform of the licensure system cannot take place apart from fundamental reform of the health care delivery system. Obviously, neither is a simple task.

Licensing and physician dominance. A prime issue in licensure is the degree to which medical licensing laws assure physician dominance of the health care delivery system. Medicine can be defined as that body of knowledge which concerns the processes by which the human body maintains normal functioning, the mechanisms of health maintenance, the processes of human disease, and the mechanisms of disease prevention, treatment, and rehabilitation. The practice of medicine is the delivery to people of the benefits of that body of knowledge called "medicine." Health care delivery systems are not solely concerned with medical practice. They provide for payment for care, construct and operate institutions, provide employment, and carry out educational and research activities; however, the major purpose of all these activities is to make it possible for medical practice to be carried on. Thus, medical practice is the focus, the *raison d'être* of any health care delivery system.

Whoever controls medical practice, therefore, controls the keystone upon which all the rest depends. For example, insurance companies generally determine their own policies regarding benefits, coverage, premiums, and the like (subject to government regulation in certain instances), but they cannot sell health insurance policies if there is no medical practice to buy. The boards of directors of voluntary hospitals determine hospital size, location, and facilities (again subject to government regulation), but if medical practice is not carried out on their premises, their powers come to nothing. Finally, a local government agency may decide what kind of medical service it wants to offer, but it is dependent upon medical practitioners to supply that service.

In the United States, because of the way the medical licensing laws are written, the physicians have a virtual hammerlock on medical practice. In each state the licensing laws are implemented by medical boards, to which the state legislatures delegate the powers of examination, licensing, and discipline. There is little evidence of accountability, to either the public or the legislature. In most states, physicians dominate the medical boards (Derbyshire, 1980, Chapter 3; Pennell and Stewart, Table 81). Derbyshire studied the backgrounds of the physician members of the boards in 1967 and developed this revealing composite picture of a medical board member:

> He is a Caucasian man, a little over 58 years of age (only one woman serves on a board, that of New Hampshire); most likely a general practitioner; if not, a general surgeon or an internist. He is a leader in the medical community and well known to the members of his state medical society. He possesses no singular attributes which qualify him to judge the academic attainments of applicants for licensure, but he is sincere in carrying out his duties and may seek help in formulating his examination questions. He is a graduate of an approved American medical school and is better qualified to carry out the disciplinary duties of his office than the educational and examining functions. (1969, p. 44)

As of 1980, Derbyshire saw little evidence to indicate that his composite picture was not still accurate.

As of 1967, in about one-half of the states, the medical societies had a direct voice in the appointment of medical board members (Derbyshire, 1969, p. 33). There was no indication that in other states physicians of whom medical societies would disapprove were appointed (Derbyshire, 1969, pp. 34–35). In a few states, such as New York and California, this situation had changed by 1980, and non-medical-society-approved physicians were being appointed.

A medical license is generally granted once and is retained for life, barring practice of extremely poor quality, "moral turpitude," or some similar offense. Physicians in the United States rarely lose their licenses (Derbyshire, 1969, Chapter 6), although the incidence of this occurrence is increasing (American Medical Association, 1980). In the period 1963–1967, Derbyshire found that nationally 938 disciplinary actions were undertaken by state medical boards, about 187 per year. Of these, 334 involved revocation of license, while the rest involved probation, suspension, and reprimand. Nearly 50% of these actions were related to narcotics addiction; only seven involved "gross malpractice." For the eight-year period 1969–1976, there were 2,503 actions taken, about 313 per year. Of these, 594 resulted in revocation of license (Derbyshire, 1980). Narcotics addiction was still the most common cause for action, accounting for 46% of the total. The number of disciplinary actions increased sharply in 1977 (to 685) and again in 1978 (to 1,476), with 216 revocations (American Medical Association, 1980). By 1978, 20 states had enacted all or part of the AMA's model legislation on medical discipline, while 31 states had adopted all or part of the AMA's Disabled Physician Act, a mechanism under which a physician can voluntarily surrender his/her license for reasons of physical or mental disability, without prejudice.

Discounting the possibility that the few disciplinary actions taken were all the disciplinary actions needed, there are several reasons to account for the level of activity (which is still relatively low, considering the fact that there were about 300,000 actively practicing physicians at the end of the 1970s). One reason is the professional dominance of medical licensing boards, noted above, and the possible "reluctance to enforce sanctions against fellow practitioners (perhaps in part because of close professional and social interrelationships)" (Ellwood et al., pp. 30–31). A lack of graduated means of discipline has been another problem: as of 1972 only 19 states provided for probation and only six for reprimand, while all states gave their medical boards revocation authority and 48 gave suspension authority (Ellwood et al., p. 31). By 1978, more states were adding more graded sanctions to the list available to boards: voluntary surrender, suspension, or probation; revocation of narcotics permit; requirement for care and/or counseling; requirement for supervision of practice; requirement for continuing medical education (American Medical Association, 1980). Some medical boards may be reluctant to act because they do not want to get involved in litigation. Physicians who have had their licenses revoked or suspended have been known to successfully sue medical boards on the grounds of deprivation of livelihood without due process—taking the position that the license is a property right (Derbyshire, 1969, Chapter 7.) Other boards would like very much to act more vigorously than they do, but find themselves hamstrung by lack of funds, lack of staff, and lack of enough readily available, qualified legal counsel. Some boards do not have their own legal staffs but must rely on their state attorney general's office, which itself is often overworked and staffed by lawyers who are generally getting paid much less than those that medical defendants can afford to hire. This pay differential may mean that the prosecution has counsel who is young or inexperienced or incompetent, or some combination of these characteristics. Finally, many instances of gross medical misconduct are simply not reported to state boards, even in those states in which the act of not reporting in itself is a violation for the respective licensed health professions.

Through the licensing laws, physicians independently control medical practice, the core of the health care delivery system. In addition, of course, they exert control through the mechanism of fee-for-service private practice, under which they function as independent contractors to their patients, regardless of what relationships patients may have to other components of the system, be they hospitals or third-party payors. Because of the power it gives physicians, medical licensure, far from being an obscure influence on the health care delivery system, is in fact an extremely important determinant of the shape of that system.

Licensure of institutions. As of 1977, 17 types of medical or residential-care facilities were subject to licensure in the U.S. (Hollis, pp. 1–20; National Center for Health Statistics, Appendix C).* All or most states required licensing of psychiatric hospitals, short- and long-stay hospitals, hospitals and homes for the mentally retarded, nursing homes, and other homes for the aged, and homes for unwed mothers and for dependent children (National Center for Health Statistics, Table 323). Among nonhospital services requiring licensure in 21 or more states are ambulance services, clinical laboratories, home health services, and pharmacies. State health departments were most commonly responsible, with social welfare, mental health, and occasionally other departments involved as well (Hollis, Table B; National Center for Health Statistics, p. 299). Licensing of major health care facilities did not become common until the 1940s (Hollis, Table C). The evaluation techniques are almost entirely structural (Hollis, pp. 7–8). Licenses are usually granted on an annual or biennial basis. Although the statutory boards involved in institutional licensing usually include representatives from the health care field, they are much less likely to be completely dominated by providers from the type of institution being regulated than are statutory boards in individual licensing (Hollis, Table H). However, in institutional licensing, unlike individual licensing, the state departments usually have more control over the actual licensing process than do the statutory boards.

Accreditation

Accreditation is another popular general approach to quality measurement and control in the United States (USDHEW, 1971, pp. 9–15). Unlike licensing, accreditation is a voluntary system used only in institutions. Groups of like institutions or organizations with mutual interests get together, set up an organization, establish standards and an examination program, and proceed to inspect and "accredit" (or not accredit) themselves, or the institutions in which they have an interest, on a periodic basis. Certain types of institutions that deliver care, and most of those that educate health care personnel, are subject to accreditation. There is a

---

*In 1977, the Bureau of Health Planning of the USDHEW published a detailed review of health facility licensure. The 10-volume publication is *Characteristics of State Health Facility Licensing Practices*, Washington, D.C., USDHEW Pub. No. (HRA) 231-77-0084, USGPO, 1977.

national voluntary agency, the Council on Postsecondary Accreditation, which recognizes accrediting bodies for educational institutions. In cases in which such accreditation is necessary to qualify for federal funds, the accrediting body must be recognized by the Department of Education as well.

In general, accreditation involves the use of structural techniques of quality assessment. Institutions are evaluated on the basis of their physical and organizational structures and the qualifications of their personnel, who themselves are evaluated, mostly by structural techniques. For example, in accrediting health personnel educational institutions, curricula are closely examined for organization and content on paper. However, the teaching process is rarely, if ever, evaluated.

The basic principles of accreditation are similar to those of licensure in that it is assumed that if the institution meets certain standards of physical and organizational structure at one point in time, then: (1) good quality health care, or health personnel education, is being delivered at that point in time; and (2) it can be predicted that the care will continue to be of good quality for a discrete period of time. The latter provision applies to most institutional licensing.

Accreditation is not a legal procedure, but there are strong legal incentives for accrediting certain kinds of institutions. For example, the Medicare law restricts payments that may be made to unaccredited hospitals, and state medical boards will not grant licenses to graduates of unaccredited medical schools without requiring such persons (that is, most foreign medical graduates) to meet conditions not required for graduates of accredited medical schools.

One organization that carries out institutional accreditation is the Joint Commission on the Accreditation of Hospitals (JCAH). It had its origins in a program for hospital evaluation established by the American College of Surgeons in 1918 (Joint Commission on Accreditation of Hospitals, p. ix; Schlicke). In 1951, the JCAH was formed under the joint sponsorship of the American College of Surgeons, the American College of Physicians, the American Hospital Association, the American Medical Association, and the Canadian Medical Association. In 1959, the Canadians set up their own hospital accreditation program. By 1978, 5,246 of the 7,015 hospitals registered with the American Hospital Association were accredited (American Hospital Association, Table 10A). Osteopathic hospitals are accredited separately, by the American Osteopathic Association, as are rehabilitation facilities, by the Commission on Accreditation of Rehabilitation Facilities.

The JCAH uses structural standards in its evaluations and avoids evaluations using the process and/or outcome methods, which do concern themselves with physicians' actions. It sets one or more standards to be achieved for the governing body and management; for medical staff organization and functioning; for the various hospital services—nursing, anesthesia, outpatients, medical records, laboratory, radiology, and the like—and for physical plant design, structure, and functioning. These standards are published in an *Accreditation Manual*, which is updated periodically. Rather than dealing with discrete instances of care delivery, the standards focus on organization, equipment, quality of staff (as determined by criteria for education and experience), quantity of staff, and the like (Joint Commission on the Accreditation of Hospitals, pp. 3–195). Hospitals desiring accreditation by JCAH are subject to biennial assessments by review teams consisting of JCAH staff and professionals from other hospitals (Joint Commission on the Accreditation of Hospitals, pp. xvii–xxviii).

In the 1980 edition of the *Manual*, the JCAH does require hospitals to have a comprehensive quality-assurance program. For the standard(s) to be achieved in each part of the hospital program, the *Accreditation Manual* states a principle. For quality assurance it is:

> The hospital shall demonstrate a consistent endeavor to deliver patient care that is optimal within available resources and consistent with achievable goals. A major component in the application of this principle is the operation of a quality-assurance program. (p. 151)

The single standard for this principle is:

> There shall be evidence of a well-defined, organized program designed to enhance patient care through the ongoing objective assessment of important aspects of patient care and the correction of identified problems.

The interpretation of the principle and standard then goes on to state some fairly explicit criteria to be used by the assessment team in evaluating the quality-assurance program itself. Specific patient care problems must be identified; objective assessment, including written criteria for the evaluation of patient care, must be used in analysis of those problems; there must be a mechanism for solving identified problems, with follow-up; documentation must be appropriate. Whether or not a hospital has met these criteria is left to the subjective judgment of the assessment team, but the criteria themselves are fairly explicit and should help hospitals significantly in improving their quality assurance programs.

There has been criticism of the JCAH's use of structural standards only in its overall evaluation of a hospital. However, it should be pointed out that for the hospital's quality assurance program itself, the JCAH does require that the hospital have in place a system that at least in part uses explicit criteria in some kind of process and/or outcome evaluation mechanism. Nevertheless, in terms of overall approach of JCAH to the evaluation of a hospital, the structural technique is considered to have limitations. In fact, the structural technique has fallen into such disfavor that it is not even considered by several prominent contemporary academic investigators of methodological problems in medical care evaluation (Brook, 1973a, 1973b; Kessner et al., 1973), who concern themselves with the evaluation of process and outcome techniques only. The evaluation of structure is considered too indefinite to be useful (Donabedian, 1969, 1978); however, such evaluation is not entirely worthless: "While the presence of various input measures in no way assures good care, the converse—good care is unlikely where such inputs are lacking—probably makes sense" (Christoffel, 1976b).

There has also been criticism of the fact that JCAH, a voluntary agency supported by the institutions it inspects, performs semi-public and sometimes public functions (Consumer Commission on the Accreditation of Health Services, 1974a, 1974b, 1975a, 1977; Rubin). The Consumer Commission considers that there are serious potential and sometimes realized conflicts of interest in this situation and would substitute a national inspection program under the DHHS for what JCAH now does.

Accreditation of health sciences educational institutions operates in a different fashion. There are 47 accrediting agencies operating in cooperation with national professional associations representing specific health occupations (National Center for Health Statistics, Appendix D). Additionally, there are 29 organizations that collaborate with the AMA in its Committee on Allied Health Accreditation and Education. This broad array of accrediting bodies, which are sanctioned by the (private) Council on Postsecondary Education and/or the Department of Education, "serve to establish criteria for professional education and . . . set standards for certification, for state licensure, and for the improvement of educational courses and programs . . ." (National Center for Health Statistics, p. 483). In some instances they accredit entire institutions; in others, they accredit specialized programs within institutions. Among the accrediting agencies are the Commission on Accreditation of Dental and Dental Auxiliary Educational Programs, the American Osteopathic Association, the American Council on Pharmaceutical Education, the Council on Education of the American Veterinary Medical Association, and five in nursing, including the two leading nurse organizations, the National League for Nursing, and the American Nurses Association.

Medical schools are accredited by the Liaison Committee on Medical Education (LCME), on which the AMA and the Association of American Medical Colleges (AAMC) are equally represented (Liaison Committee on Medical Education, 1973; National Commission on Accrediting). Schools are generally accredited for seven-year periods, based primarily on a self-study performed to LCME requirements and a three- to four-day visit by a four-person team. The standards to be met are stated in a 3,000-word document entitled "Functions and Structure of a Medical School" (Liaison Committee on Medical Education, 1973). Compared with the lengthy and detailed JCAH standards, the LCME standards seem vague, general, and incredibly brief, although the self-study manual for medical schools undergoing accreditation is quite lengthy. The requirements for new medical schools seem much more rigorous than those for existing, previously accredited schools (Liaison Committee on Medical Education, 1972, 1974). In any event, medical school accreditation shows an extreme reliance on structural standards. There are no examinations of instances of patient care or even of the educational process. The JCAH *Accreditation Manual* is full of explicit criteria. The LCME consciously shies away from them for the most part, being content with setting some general guidelines for use by surveyors in applying their own implicit criteria.

Medical school accreditation in the United States receives virtually no publicity, even though it may well be more critical for the development of American medicine as a whole than hospital accreditation or physician licensing, because of the commanding position of the physicians, who happen to be selected exclusively by medical school admissions committees (Jonas, 1979). There is no trace of public accountability in medical school accreditation. It is invisible, and totally under the control of the largest organizations of physicians and the medical schools. From the time of the Flexner Report (1910) until the mid-1960s, the medical school accreditation process was a principal weapon used by the American Medical Association in its struggle to keep down the number of physicians (Rayack). Because of its isolation from public scrutiny and its total reliance on structural criteria, serious questions must be raised about the validity and reliability of accreditation as a measure of the quality and relevance of medical education in the United States.

Certification*

Certification is the third general approach to quality control found in the United States health care delivery system (Bureau of Health Manpower Education; Pennell, pp. 70–76; National Center for Health Statistics,

---

*Confusion may arise in the terminology here. Some occupations use "registration" in the sense in which we use "certification," while some states use the term "registration" instead of "licensing" in dealing with certain health occupations. In studying a particular state, one should determine exactly how that state uses the various terms. In nursing, "registration" always means licensing.

Appendix B; USDHEW, 1971, pp. 15–20; 1977a). Certification combines features of licensing and accreditation. Applied to individuals, it uses standards of education, experience, and achievement on examination to determine qualification. However, it is a voluntary system undertaken by health care provider professions and occupations and is neither directly sanctioned nor backed up by the force of law. Nevertheless, as with accreditation, there are incentives for individuals to become certified. For example, speech therapy is a health profession licensed in some, but not all, states. The American Speech and Hearing Association (AHSA) has a national certification program, however, and many school districts will hire only speech therapists who are certified by ASHA. There are over 65 professional health agencies at the National Commission for Health Certifying Agencies (National Center for Health Statistics, p. 6, Appendix B). A rapid proliferation of certifying agencies has taken place in the past 25 years, paralleling the large increase in the number of differentiated health professions and occupations.

One variety of certification is used to designate specialists among physicians.* By the 1950s, the majority of medical school graduates in the United States were choosing to become specialists—that is, to devote themselves to one particular field of medical work like orthopedics, dermatology, or psychiatry. The average length of training beyond the B.A. or B.S. degree (ordinarily a prerequisite for admission to medical school) was around eight years: four years of medical school, a first postgraduate year of hospital work called the "internship," and then subsequent postgraduate years of hospital work in specialty training called "residencies," followed in certain specialties by additional "fellowship" time, ranging in all from two to five years or even more in such technically demanding subspecialties as neurosurgery.

One is eligible for licensing by a state medical board after the internship. However, a physician is not designated competent in a specialty until after he or she has completed the residency/fellowship and passed additional examinations. More than 20 "specialty boards"—private voluntary certifying authorities, originally self-appointed—are in charge of these designations. Specialty boards derive their power from the fact that many hospitals will not appoint a physician to their staffs with admitting privileges (the authority to admit and take care of their own patients in the hospital) in a particular specialty unless he is certified by the appropriate board. (The most frequent exceptions to this rule are found in smaller hospitals, which

*The history of medical specialization in the United States has been treated by Stevens (1971), and its status in the mid-1970s was discussed in great detail by Herbert Lerner (1974).

still allow general practitioners to practice adult and pediatric medicine, surgery, and obstetrics. In certain cases, hospitals limit this sort of privilege to grandfathers.) The specialty boards themselves are approved by the American Medical Association through its Council on Medical Education, and the organization of the boards themselves, the Advisory (now American) Board of Medical Specialties.

Medical specialty boards rely entirely on structural techniques of evaluation. Most specialty boards, like licensing boards, certify once, for life. As of 1980, only the American Board of Family Practice required periodic recertification (every six years) for all of its diplomates (recipients of diplomas). The American Boards of Surgery and Thoracic Surgery were planning to introduce such a requirement for new applicants by the mid-1980s (Leymaster). Six other boards had voluntary recertification programs. As with all approaches that use structural techniques, data are lacking relating level of quality at the time of certification with the quality of the individual's output at later times; thus the utility and validity of specialty certification as it is now carried out must be carefully questioned.

Specific Approaches to Quality of Care Assessment and Control Techniques

As pointed out above (p. 402), Donabedian has provided the generally accepted definitions of the process and outcome techniques that are used in the specific approaches to quality of care assessment and control. Ordinarily, it is either one or the other of these methods that is used. However, in the early 1970s, a new approach to quality evaluation called the "tracer method" emerged (Kessner et al., 1973; Kessner and Kalk). According to the researchers, "The tracer method measures both process and outcome of care, which we consider important in any evaluation scheme. It is impossible to pinpoint the strengths and weaknesses without knowing the outcome, but outcome alone can be misleading if the patient receives unnecessary diagnostic tests or inappropriate therapy" (Kessner et al., 1973, p. 190). A tracer is a particular disease process with the following characteristics (Kessner et al., 1973):

1. A tracer should have a definite functional impact. . . .
2. A tracer should be relatively well-defined and easy to diagnose. . . .
3. Prevalence rates should be high enough to permit the collection of adequate data from a limited population sample. . . .
4. The natural history of the condition should vary with utilization and effectiveness of medical care. . . .
5. The technics of medical management of the condition should be

well-defined for at least one of the following processes: prevention, diagnosis, treatment or rehabilitation. . . .

6.   The effects of nonmedical factors on the tracer should be understood. . . . (p. 15–16)

On paper, this technique looked very good and aroused a great deal of interest in the quality assurance community. It has not yet been widely utilized, but it is quite sound theoretically and further attempts at its use ought to be made.

In 1976, Rutstein et al. described an approach to quality evaluation based on epidemiology. They called it the "sentinel method," summarizing it as follows:

> We outline the implementation of a new method of measuring the quality of medical care that counts cases of unnecessary disease and disability and unnecessary untimely deaths. First of all, conditions are listed in which the occurrence of a single case of disease or disability or a single untimely death would justify asking, "Why did it happen?" Secondly, we have selected conditions in which critical increases in rates of disease, disability, or untimely death could serve as indexes of the quality of care. Finally, broad categories of illness are noted in which redefinition and intensive study might reveal characteristics that could serve as indexes of health. . . . These indexes of outcome can be used to determine the level of health of the general population and the effects of economic, political, and other environmental factors upon it, and to evaluate the quality of medical care provided both within and without the hospital to maintain health and to prevent and treat disease. (p. 582)

This approach (not entirely as new as the authors claim [Last; Peterson]) uses an outcome technique to look at discrete instances of patient care. Virtually every disease in the Eighth Revision, *International Classification of Diseases Adapted for Use in the United States* (ICDA) was analyzed. The criteria for unnecessary disease, unnecessary disability, and unnecessary untimely death were derived from state-of-the-art epidemiological knowledge. If for any listed disease, an event deemed unnecessary in the light of current knowledge occurs, attention is called to it. The unnecessary event becomes the sentinel. The circumstances surrounding the unnecessary event can then be examined in detail. This approach represents a marriage between clinical medicine and epidemiology, and thus should hold great promise for useful future development.

There have been a number of studies evaluating the same instances of medical care using both process and outcome techniques. They have found little if any relationship between the ratings arrived at by the two. For example, this was the result of a study by Hulka and colleagues (Hulka et al. 1979; Hulka, 1980) of care for hypertension, diabetes mellitus, dysuria, and the general medical examination. McAuliffe reviewed a number of such studies and found them wanting methodologically. He cited several other studies which show at least a modest relationship between the two methods. Among them is one by Kane et al. (1977), which concluded that: "Those cases [studied] with good outcomes had better process scores than those with bad outcomes."

One of the problems in studying the linkage or lack thereof between process and outcome in medical care is that one must be sure that the medical activity to which process standards are being applied has a clear relationship to outcomes. This is not always the case and is one of the reasons why there have been problems in applying the tracer method, which consciously links the two techniques. Furthermore, it is more likely through the use of process criteria that omissions in care will be discovered. This is especially true when those omissions deal with patient risk factors (the presence of a problem only increases the patient's chance of contracting a certain illness but does not guarantee it, as in cigarette smoking, overweight, and certain occupational exposures), and/or with patient problems which will lead to a bad outcome only many years later, as in hypertension and chronic exposure to asbestos dust. Thus, in these instances only the application of process criteria will demonstrate poor care: failure to take and/or record a smoking history; failure to take and/or record patient weight; failure to take and/or record blood pressure; failure to take and/or record occupational history. Outcome evaluation would appear to be more useful when an active intervention is being undertaken for which there is a clear outcome to be measured, such as many kinds of surgery, many kinds of antibiotic use, a weight-reduction program, or a hypertension control program. Among the more recent of Brook's many contributions to the quality-assessment literature is a large-scale outcome study in which active interventions were used (Brook et al., 1977). Williamson has pointed out that to effectively apply either technique, the setting must be chosen carefully and priorities must be formulated (1978).

But perhaps the most important issue in the discussion of techniques is what is done with the information obtained, regardless of technique used. As Brook (1977) pointed out:

> The literature on quality of care is replete with studies showing deficiencies in medical care no matter what standard or method is used. Clearly, simple process or outcome criteria can identify such problems. Efforts should be concentrated on ameliorating these obvious problems. . . .

But Jessee (1977) lamented that ". . . few can name instances in which lasting changes in physician behavior or organization performance have resulted."

A long-range solution to the problem of deficiencies in the quality of medical care is continuing medical education (CME) to correct identified physician faults. However, conventional CME, which consists of sitting in a classroom being lectured at, has been shown to have little if any positive effect (Egdahl and Gertman). Linkage of nonlecture CME methods with individually identified physician problems would seem to hold much more promise for a positive result (Bloom). The Health Care Financing Administration of HHS, the parent of PSRO, has shown official interest in this approach (Administrator, Health Care Financing Administration). However, as of 1980, they had not supported their interest with money.

Research Studies

Over the years, a large number of research studies have been carried out in the problem area of measuring and controlling the quality of particular instances of medical care delivery using the process and/or outcome techniques. They have generally shown deficits in the quality of care, regardless of the methods used.* Certain studies can be considered landmarks. In 1953–1954, a study of general practice in North Carolina used both structural and process techniques and explicit criteria, in a direct observation method. It was found that: "Many physicians were performing at a high level of professional competence. Of greater importance is the fact that other physicians were performing at a lower level . . ." (Peterson et al., p. 143). Of the various parameters measured, only the length of postgraduate hospital training in internal medicine was consistently related to the quality of a physician's clinical work. Academic performance, for example, was related to quality of clinical work only for physicians aged 35 and less (Peterson et al., p. 55). Paul Lembcke was one of the pioneers in developing the hospital medical audit, using analysis of clinical records. As an example, he evaluated major female pelvic surgery in several hospitals and found that the introduction of auditing techniques reduced both the

---

*There have been a number of reviews of the literature. Mindel Sheps considered a large series of primarily clinical evaluations. Her review included one of the earliest attempts to categorize the techniques of quality evaluation. Anderson and Altman produced an annotated bibliography covering the period 1955–1961. Avedis Donabedian produced three major reviews in the late 1960s (1966, 1968, 1969). In the early 1970s, a large literature review was undertaken by Brook (1973b, Chapter III), and again by Brook and colleagues in 1977. A major review of the state of the art in the early 1970s was held under the aegis of the Graduate Program in Hospital Administration of the University of Chicago in 1973 (Scheye). Christoffel published a comprehensive bibliography in the mid-1970s (1976c), as did the Institute of Medicine (1976). Christoffel and Lowenthal reviewed the literature on ambulatory care quality assessment in 1977.

population hysterectomy rate and the proportion of unnecessary hysterectomies.

In the period 1957–1961, a study of 406 admissions of members of the Teamsters Unions and their families to hospitals in New York City used review of medical records, process and outcome techniques, and implicit criteria (Trussell et al.). The study found that 88% of admissions were justifiable (Trussell et al., p. 21). However, only 57% of the patients received "good or excellent medical care," while a fifth received fair care, a fifth poor care (Trussell et al., p. 25). A second study by this group in 1962, using a slightly different evaluation technique, arrived at similar conclusions (Morehead et al., 1964). Some observers consider that implicit criteria have limited applicability since they rely entirely on the internal judgments of the evaluators (Koran).

In the late 1960s and early 1970s, a series of studies of quality of medical care in Neighborhood Health Centers, primarily using process techniques (Morehead; Morehead et al., 1971; Morehead and Donaldson), showed that such auditing methods could be widely applied; the quality of care in Neighborhood Health Centers was found to be reasonably good compared to that found in other organized ambulatory care settings.

Applying the tracer method to two different pediatric population groups in Washington, D.C., Kessner and colleagues found that: "Inappropriate or ineffective treatment for specific tracer conditions was documented in a large proportion of the children" (Kessner and Kalk, pp. 15–17; Kessner et al., 1974, p. 4).

At the same time that Kessner was breaking new ground in developing a quality measurement method combining the process and outcome techniques, Brook was carrying out another landmark study, comparing five different types of process and outcome evaluations of the same medical care episodes (Brook, 1973b; Brook and Appel). Brook and Appel summarized the work as follows:

> The care of 296 patients with urinary-tract infection, hypertension or ulcerated gastric or duodenal lesions was reviewed with use of the five methods. Depending on the method, from 1.4 to 63.2 percent of patients were judged to have received adequate care. Judgment of process using explicit criteria yielded the fewest acceptable cases (1.4 percent). The largest differences found were between methods using different sources of data. Thus, medical care, judged with implicit criteria, was rated adequate for 23.3 percent of patients when process, and 63.2 percent when outcome was used. (p. 1,323)

In his major publication on his study, Brook (1973b, p. 60) concluded that although serious methodologic problems remain in quality-of-care assessment, it is still nevertheless true that as many as 25% of the patients would have had better outcomes if the medical processes had been better.

"It is, therefore, recommended that simple routine assessments of quality of care which employ carefully selected outcomes and processes should begin even while awaiting definitive methodologic research. Such studies using outcome measurements as a means to identify high priority areas could have a major impact on the health of the American people without dramatically increasing the cost of such care," Brook noted (1973b).

Some more recent studies of the quality of medical care may be summarized as follows:

- In a national quiz of physician volunteers, on knowledge of the use of antibiotics, the average score was 68% (Neu and Howrey).
- In the New Mexico Medicaid program, a peer review program was designed to correct deficiencies. The use of injections, of which half were antibiotics, was considered by the peer reviewers to be inappropriate in 40% of cases. The peer review program did achieve a drop in the use of injections from 41 per 100 ambulatory visits to 16 per 100 ambulatory visits (Brook and Williams, 1976).
- Fewer than 10% of patients admitted to a university hospital had a routine serologic test for syphilis performed, yet in those tested the response was positive in 6% of cases. Effective therapy was not given in one-third of them and in two-thirds of them, syphilis was not listed as a discharge diagnosis (Tomecki and Plaut). Whether or not any of the detected cases was reported to the local health department, a measure essential to control of the disease in the population, was not recorded in the study.
- In an evaluation of burn care in Florida, it could not be shown that, adjusting for case severity, hospitals with burn units did better than those without, and "many records were poor, admissions were inappropriate, patients with minor burns stayed too long, and burn shock was too frequent" (Linn et al.).
- A study of the work of over 1,300 physicians in 22 Maryland and Pennsylvania hospitals used one of the classic process tools, the Physician Performance Index developed by Beverly Payne and colleagues at the University of Michigan. The average score was about 70% (Saywell et al.).

Thus, research in quality assessment marches on. There really are quite a few useful techniques for measurement. The problem remains: What to do with the information? To quote Jessee again: "[We] have not adequately explored methods to effect organizational change in hospitals" (1977). As Brook says, "the central failing of quality assessment is that it has rarely been used to change behavior" (1977). By the end of the 1970s, however, there was some evidence that PSROs could positively affect the quality of patient care (Health Care Financing Administration, p. xiv, Chapter 5).

Hospital Medical Staff Review Committees

The most common specific approach to quality assessment and assurance in the United States is the institution of hospital medical staff review committees. The JCAH requires that the hospital medical staff be organized to provide for review of at least the following: the quality of physician care; the utilization of hospital services, in particular the length of patient stay; the products of surgery; the use of therapeutic agents, specifically including antibiotics, and the pharmacy; medical records; blood and blood products; infection control; disaster plans; and hospital safety (Joint Commission on Accreditation of Hospitals, pp. 105–108, 151–154, 193–194).

Committees dealing directly with physician services all evaluate individual instances of care delivery. They are usually concerned with physician performance in a particular case, although they may become involved with the work of other hospital staff as well.

A Tissue Committee is concerned with the products of surgery and deals with such issues as the technique and necessity of surgical operations. A Medical Records Committee may look at the quality of the records themselves as an indication of the quality of the work, or it can evaluate the work itself, as it is reflected in the record. Usually it does both.

Utilization review was mandated by the original Medicare law as a cost-control measure. Norms were supposed to be established for acceptable lengths of hospital stay for most common conditions. If a patient stayed longer than the norm, the case was to be reviewed and the admitting physician was to justify the excess. If the committee decided that the excess stay was not medically justified, Medicare would not pay for the extra days. Little is known in detail about how the system functioned nationally (Ellwood et al., p. 31). However, it seemed not to work well as originally designed, and it was recast in the 1972 amendments to the Social Security Act as part of the responsibilities of the Professional Standards Review Organizations (see below).

Although hospital medical staff review committees, being required for accreditation, are the most prevalent specific approach to quality measurement and control, little is actually known about how they work or what they do. They have never been comprehensively studied.

An important aid to the work of many hospital medical staff review committees is the Professional Activity Study (PAS) of the Commission on Professional and Hospital Activities (Kuehn; Commission on Professional and Hospital Activities), a process-oriented, computerized system providing information useful in medical auditing. It is carried on by an outside firm, under contract, from data collected by the hospital. A variety of medical staff committees can use the material in their work. As of 1979, PAS served about 2,000 hospitals in the United States, Canada, and several other countries.

Professional Standards Review Organizations

Historically, the general approaches to quality control in the United States have been widely used, formalized, and institutionalized. The specific approaches, on the other hand, have been used to a very limited extent, and moves to formalize and institutionalize them have been slow to develop. The JCAH in the mid-1970s began requiring hospitals to perform process and outcome reviews and, as described above, now requires a rather elaborate and sophisticated quality assurance system (although it does not evaluate the system's output). However, the sector in which the bulk of the health care action takes place—private office practice—remained virtually unregulated except for financial audits of high-earning physicians under Medicare/Medicaid. Thus the advent of the so-called Professional Standards Review Organization could be considered a notable event, marking a major step on the part of the federal government toward the institutionalization of specific approaches. For the first time a law—with some fairly sharp teeth in it—required peer review of individual instances of physician delivery of medical care (Goran et al.). Although in the beginning evaluations were to be confined to hospital care, the law did provide the framework for eventual expansion to ancillary services, long-term care, and ambulatory care. Furthermore, PSRO could be viewed as a prototype system for future use under National Health Insurance.

Professional Standards Review Organizations were established by the 1972 amendments to the Social Security Act (P. L. 92–603; Health Standards and Quality Bureau, 1978, 1979). An excellent summary of the basic structure and functions of the system was offered by the original Program Manual (Office of Professional Standards Review, pp. 1–5).*

---

*As of 1980, at the federal level the PSRO system was supervised by the Health Standards and Quality Bureau of the Health Care Financing Administration, Department of Health and Human Services. The bureau periodically publishes useful descriptions, summaries, and bibliographies, including an *Annual Report*, an *Annual Bibliography*, an annual *Project Directory*, and such publications as *PSRO in Perspective* (1979), and *Legislative History of PSRO* (1978), in part through the National Health Standards and Quality Information Clearinghouse.

102   Information on the PSRO Program
. . . [PSROs are] designed to involve local practicing physicians in the ongoing review and evaluation of health care services covered under the Medicare, Medicaid, and the Maternal and Child Health programs [of the U.S. Department of Health and Human Services]. The legislation is based on the concepts that health professionals are the most appropriate individuals to evaluate the quality of medical services and that effective peer review at the local level is the soundest method for assuring the appropriate use of health care resources and facilities. . . .

The PSRO is responsible for assuring that health care paid for under Medicare, Medicaid, and Maternal and Child Health Programs is medically necessary and consistent with professionally recognized [quality] standards of care. It must also seek to encourage the use of less costly sites and modes of treatment where medically appropriate. . . .

The internal review activities of hospitals and other health care institutions are to be utilized by the PSRO in carrying out its functions to the extent these activities are determined to be effective by the PSRO. . . . Fiscal agents are required to abide by the PSRO's determination as to the medical necessity and appropriateness of services in paying Medicare and Medicaid claims. . . .

106   Summary of PSRO Review Responsibilities
. . . For review in short-stay general hospitals, the PSRO will at a minimum perform (a) admission certification concurrent with the patient's admission, (b) continued stay review, and (c) medical care evaluation studies. . . . As the capability progresses in its area [it has the responsibility] to develop criteria and standards and select norms for each type of review which it performs.* . . .

110   Hearings, Review and Sanctions . . .
110.20   On the basis of its investigations of situations of possible abuse identified in its reviews, the PSRO may (after reasonable notice and opportunity for discussion with the provider or practitioner) recommend to the Secretary appropriate action against persons responsible for gross or continued overuse of services or for inadequate quality of services. . . .

*Definitions, as provided in Chapter VII, Sec. 709 of the PSRO Program Manual, are:
Norms—Medical care appraisal norms are numerical or statistical measures of usual observed performance.
Criteria—Medical care criteria are predetermined elements against which aspects of the quality of medical service may be compared. They are developed by professionals relying on professional expertise and on the professional literature.
Standards—Standards are professionally developed expressions of the range of acceptable variation from a norm or criterion.

PSROs, established nationally in 195 geographic areas designated by the Secretary of the DHHS, obviously represented a new game in town. Not only were individual instances of care to be examined, but penalties could be invoked against transgressors of the law and regulations, although it was not made precisely clear what transgressions were.

The reaction to PSROs clearly demonstrates that one man's meat is another man's poison. For example, the American Medical Association (1974) felt that the penalties for poor performance by a physician were much too strong, whereas the consumer advocate organization Health-PAC felt that they were much too weak (Lander). The literature on the controversy quickly grew to rather large proportions (Aland and Walter; Bennett; Brian; Colock; Davidson; Fishbein; Flashner et al.; Fulchiero et al.; Greenberg; Jessee et al.; McMahon; *Medical World News*, 1974a, 1974b; Sanazaro; Sanazaro and Worth; Simmons; Welch, 1973, 1974). See also bibliographies in Goran et al. (1975) and Goran (1979). An early comprehensive discussion of PSROs is contained in a book by Decker and Bonner. We can outline below a few of the major points discussed in the extensive literature on the subject.

Peer review itself has certain problems in terms of its efficacy: even with HEW looking over their shoulders, can physicians resist guild protectionism any more effectively than they have to date? (Freidson, pp. 178–183, 363–382). Furthermore, one wonders if peer review can effectively deal with patients' complaints about provider-patient communications. For example, the "my-doctor-won't-talk-to-me" syndrome, which seems to concern patients as much as or more than problems with the technical content of care (Birch and Wolfe), is not recognized as a problem by most doctors. Finally, PSRO may quickly succumb to what would be a natural tendency to concentrate on economizing rather than on quality control, a matter that clearly concerned one of the early directors of the program, Michael Goran (M. J. Bernstein).

Many representatives of organized medicine argued that PSROs represent "government interference in the practice of medicine" (American Medical Association, 1974; *American Medical News*, January 14, 1974, February 25, 1975; Fishbein). This argument has a certain logical fallacy when it comes from organized medicine, as the classification of approaches to quality outlined above indicates. History demonstrates that the medical profession does not like specific approaches to quality control, while it has always lent support to general approaches to quality control, licensing in particular. However, licensing certainly constitutes not only government interference in the practice of medicine, but outright suppression of the rights of the unlicensed. Government, through the force of law and the criminal justice system, gives the medical profession a monopoly over that which it defines as the practice of medicine and prevents anyone else from competing. In return, the profession provides a structure-based approach to quality, operated independently. The highest form of governmental interference—a refusal to allow those who have not met organized medicine's requirements to practice—receives the profession's strongest support; that being true, the profession cannot logically attack PSROs simply on the grounds of "government interference in the practice of medicine."

As the program entered the 1980s, its three principal goals remained as follows (Goran):

> The elimination of inappropriate and unnecessary health care services (freeing up scarce resources to alleviate unmet needs); (2) the improvement in the quality of health services (making quality services more uniformly available as well as raising the overall level of performance); and (3) providing assistance in the identification and, where possible, correction of the small minority of practitioners and providers whose practices are harmful to the health and safety of patients (and making necessary referrals of such individuals and facilities to the appropriate agencies for investigation and needed disciplinary actions). (p. 3)

Goran saw the following as problems to be solved in PSRO development:

1. Limitations of the state of the art of quality assessment.
2. Lack of expertise among program staff, not to mention practicing physicians and the medical schools which generally do not provide training in quality assurance.
3. Problems with data.
4. Lack of uniformity among PSROs.
5. Difficulties in changing physician practice behavior.
6. Lack of time needed to accomplish change and unrealistic expectations. (Because PSROs are funded in part by annual appropriations rather than, as originally planned, entirely out of Medicaid/Medicare reimbursements, each year survival of the entire program is called into question.)
7. Lack of agreed-upon measures of success.
8. Lack of adequate funding, which can very easily lead to the self-fulfilling prophecy of failure.
9. An uncertain continuation of the willingness of the medical profession to support the program and make it work. (pp. 30–32)

PSRO, a distinct departure from the American tradition of quality control, has no natural constituency. Annually, there are reports claiming at least modest success for the program, usually from the HHS (see Health Care Financing Administration, 1980); others claim that the positive reports are incorrect or overstated, for example, reports from the Congressional Budget Office or the General Accounting Office (Demkovich). These evaluations were usually in terms of number of dollars saved or not saved, not, until the late 1970s, in terms of the possible effects of PSRO on medical practice (Health Care Financing Administration, Chapters 5 and 6). However, there are no public groups beating the drums for PSRO. On the other hand, there is plenty of opposition. Following the 1980 elections, the AMA reversed field and came out for the abolition of the PSRO system. There is also a great deal of continuing private resistance in the medical profession to PSRO, on the grounds of "government interference in the practice of medicine" (even though it is a peer, not a government, review program). This factor may well account for the determined attacks made on PSRO every year in Congress, usually on the basis that "they didn't save enough money." Without a public constituency, and with private enemies, whether or not PSRO can survive the continued political attacks remains to be seen.

Patient Satisfaction and Malpractice Litigation

Patient satisfaction is one specific approach to quality of care measurement and control that has received little attention. A review has pointed out that although little is known about patient satisfaction, in general patients appear to be less critical of the technical content of care than they are of attitudinal and situational components (Lebow), a conclusion confirmed in one of the largest-scale studies of patient satisfaction carried out by the mid-1970s (Birch and Wolfe).

One gauge of patient satisfaction is the extent of medical malpractice litigation. By the mid-1970s, malpractice litigation had become a matter of major concern in the United States. In 1973, a major commission reported on the matter (USDHEW, 1973), and its many findings and recommendations created a great deal of controversy (Welch, 1975). During the 1970s, the volume of suits increased, the magnitude of settlements rose, and insurance premiums threatened to rise out of sight (Curran, 1975a). The problem is not entirely new. As Curran himself pointed out, in the 1940s there had been complaints about "a plague of malpractice suits." Katz refers to physicians' "alarm at the increase in [malpractice] claims" in the 1840s! Nevertheless, by 1975 the situation had seriously worsened (Cooper and Stephens). Insurance companies stopped writing malpractice policies in several states, often after requests for premium increases of 300% or more were denied by state insurance commissioners. In several states, medical societies set up their own insurance companies. Hospitals saw their rates skyrocket: the annual premium for the Massachusetts General Hospital increased 10 times between 1969 and 1975 (Katz). In California, physicians struck in the spring of 1975, seeking to force legislative changes (Phillips), as they did or threatened to do elsewhere (Curran, 1975b).

The wave of legislative remedies became a flood during that summer. Curran (1975b) states: "The thrust of most of the enacted bills can be classified into three major categories: insurance coverage changes; legal-system reforms; and the strengthening of medical disciplinary mechanisms." Most significant legislative changes, however, gored one ox or another, and, as is well known, in the United States gored oxen often go to court seeking a remedy. Nevertheless, there were malpractice litigation system changes in a number of states, which led to a leveling off in the number of suits, the average size of awards made in successful ones, and, as a result, the rate of premium increase. In 1979, however, the situation began to deteriorate again (*Medical World News*, November 12, 1979).

It is useful to examine some of the causes of the increase in malpractice litigation (Vaccarino). First of all, some care provided by physicians in this country is of poor or doubtful quality. Some, but not all, of this poor care involves negligence. Second, physicians have not shown themselves to be particularly competent or capable of policing their own ranks (*Medical World News*, March 15, 1974). Third, some observers think that an increasing supply of attorneys, particularly when it occurs in states with no-fault automobile insurance, may be a factor. Fourth, other observers think that the incidence of malpractice litigation is related to the deterioration of the doctor-patient relationship. A medical writer in the *Dallas Morning News* wrote a "Message to Doctors and Hospitals." In part she said: "Most of all, doctors and nurses . . . please listen to me. . . . You treat me like a human being, and I wouldn't sue you even if you sew up a scalpel in my stomach" (*American Medical News*, August 25, 1974). Finally, the rapidly rising cost of medical care may itself be a factor.

The role of the profit-making companies that write malpractice insurance should also be considered. Although companies were getting out of the business right and left in the mid-1970s, it apparently was profitable (*New York Times*, June 11, 1975). After the "crisis" passed, many insurance companies got right back in. Retention of premiums for expenses and profits, after paying out settlements, was running as high as 50% (*Lancet*, February 8, 1975). Companies also make profits by investing premiums while they have them. Apparently, the companies were looking at the rapidly rising level of awards made by the courts, and also, it was reported, were having problems with their own investments. Thus, they were asking for huge rate increases, and, if refused, dropped out. As far as is known, however, no insurance company ever saw fit to try to institute reform of quality control and the whole malpractice problem.

Patients, faced with either a true disaster, like total paralysis resulting from negligence during anesthesia, or a medical profession unresponsible to complaints of a not-so-catastrophic nature, have, as a last resort, only the malpractice suit route. The contingency fee system, whereby a lawyer takes on a case on the basis that he will get a percentage of any settlement and nothing if the suit fails, makes access to legal assistance relatively easy.

The problems, then, are evident; solutions, involving as they do the interests of both the legal and medical professions, health care institutions, the commercial insurance industry, state governments, and aggrieved and injured patients (Consumer Commission on the Accreditation of Health Services, 1975b; *Consumer Reports*), are difficult to find. Among proposed measures are: changes in tort (negligence) law; modification of the contingency fee system for lawyers; no-fault insurance; shorter statutes of limitations; upper limits on judgments for "pain and suffering"; voluntary arbitration; better regulation and improved quality control of physicians and hospitals; and better controls over elective surgery (Special Advisory Panel on Medical Malpractice).

In looking for solutions that will work, however, it is necessary to confront and resolve the basic contradiction presently facing the system. Originally, the medical malpractice system was established to protect patients from and indemnify them for acts of medical *negligence*. To this end, the malpractice insurance system paid damages to victims of negligence and protected the assets of physicians, other health care providers, and hospitals should they happen to commit a negligent act. To win a suit under these conditions, a plaintiff has to clearly demonstrate not only a bad outcome from a medical encounter, but that that bad outcome was due to negligence, that is a wrongful act of commission or omission, not merely bad luck or a non-negligent error of judgment that any physician in the same circumstance might make. In recent years, however, some courts and juries have been viewing the system more as one which should provide *compensation* to victims of medical accidents, defining medical negligence more broadly, almost to the point of expecting perfection from every physician. By creating the *medical mystique* (Belsky and Gross), which projects an image not only of "doctor knows best," but also of "doctor knows all," the profession may well have contributed significantly to this problem. This contradiction between a *negligence* approach and a *compensation* approach lies at the heart of the current malpractice problem.

Replacing the present tort/liability negligence system with a no-fault compensation system has aroused considerable interest in this country (A. H. Bernstein, 1978a; Institute of Medicine, 1978) and is in place in at least two foreign countries (A. H. Bernstein, 1978b, 1978c; Cooper; Special Advisory Panel on Medical Malpractice). However, no-fault is considered to have serious limitations (A. H. Bernstein, 1978a). For one thing, the "deterrence signal" to potential medical wrongdoers would be attenuated by a no-fault system (Schwartz and Komesar). In fact, the latter authors would strengthen the present negligence system by applying individual experience ratings to physicians' malpractice insurance premiums, much the way that automobile liability insurance premiums are calculated, something which is not now done. In 1979, the British court system decided that the malpractice insurance system should clearly remain based on the negligence concept and not convert to the compensation concept (Lister, 1980). It remains obvious, however, that there are no easy solutions in sight for the problem in this country.

Some Remaining Problems in Quality Assurance

A number of serious problems remain in quality measurement and control. One encounters methodologic problems in both process and outcome techniques (Brook, 1973a; Brook and Appel). Physicians cannot be sure that their clinical assessments are valid, even when undertaken (Koran). Moreover, any evaluation of the quality of care that relates to health must take into account that health care is only one factor in the determination of health status (Blum; Brook and Williams, 1975; Lewis). (See also Chapters 2 and 15).

Regardless of the direction of the academic discussion of process versus outcome, the structural technique for quality measurement and control is the only one widely and consistently applied in the United States. It is the basis for licensing, accreditation, and certification, the only approaches that meet with broad provider acceptance. As noted above, experts in the field reject structural techniques as ineffective, but the governmental and medical establishments continue to rely on them. The structure-process outcome gap leads one to recognize the chasm that exists between the academic researchers in the quality field and those professionals who are charged with implementing the quality control measures on the books. Not only do they generally not talk to each other, but they sometimes don't even speak the same language. In a study of the work of the New York State Health Department in implementing quality control programs enacted by law, it was found that certain high officials involved were unfamiliar even with the "structure-process outcome" vocabulary, much less the literature (Jonas, 1977). At one time the Health Department had a Bureau of Medical Review, which was supposed to concern itself with broad methodological problems, but it was closed down in an economy drive. It is not known what the bureau did, but as one measure of its level of success and influence, the Health Department had no summary material on its work available (Jonas, 1977, p. 114). At the same time, there is a noticeable lack in the academic literature of any consideration of the real problems encountered by professionals in the field, whether they are with governmental or voluntary agencies, when they attempt to implement quality control measures. The two groups virtually ignore each other, with sad results.

The limitations of peer review must be carefully considered (Ellwood et al., p. 54; McCarthy, pp. 11 ff.). Peer review is central to most approaches, both general and specific, in regular use today, with the possible exception of the licensing of institutions. Consumer involvement is a possible option (Lewis, 1974); the Consumer Commission on the Accreditation of Health Services thinks that quality measurement and control without consumer involvement is virtually worthless (1973).

Finally, one must recognize that the public at large is generally not concerned with quality measurement and control. Most people never seem to question the technical competence of their physicians, although they are concerned with other aspects of their performance (Birch and Wolfe). Patient complaints about health services are more likely to focus on provider attitudes, waiting time, the physical environment of care, availability and accessibility, and, of course, costs. Creating public awareness of the technical failings of medical care, and then translating such awareness into action, is the greatest challenge faced by those concerned with the quality of health care.

References

Administrator, Health Care Financing Administration. *Draft Memorandum, The Role of Continuing Medical Education in Professional Standards Review Organizations, 1979.* (n.d.)

Aland, K. M., and Walter, B. A. "Hospitals in Utah Reduce Costs, Improve Use of Facilities." *Hospitals, J.A.H.A.*, 52, March 16, 1978, p. 85.

American Hospital Association. *Hospital Statistics, 1979 Edition.* Chicago, 1979.

American Medical Association. *PSRO Deleterious Effects: Information Kit.* Chicago, May 1974.

————. "Disciplinary Actions Against Physicians Continue Upward Trend." *News Release,* Chicago, Illinois, February 11, 1980.

American Medical News. "Peers' Role Stressed by AMA President." December 10, 1973, p. 3.

————. "PSRO Prompts Surgeon to Retire." January 14, 1974.

————. "In the Hospital, I Am a Bundle of Fears." August 25, 1974.

————. "PSRO Law Assailed by Indiana Legislature." February 25, 1975.

Anderson, A. J., and Altman, I. *Methodology in Evaluating the Quality of Medical Care.* Pittsburgh: University of Pittsburgh Press, 1962.

Belsky, M. S., and Gross, L. *Beyond the Medical Mystique: How to Choose and Use Your Doctor*. New York: Arbor House, 1975.

Bennett, W. F. "Education Is PSRO Goal." *Hospitals, J.A.H.A.*, March 1, 1974, p. 53.

Bernstein, A. H. "Will No-Fault Insurance End the Medical Malpractice Crisis?" *Hospitals, J.A.H.A.*, 52, p. 40, June 1, 1978a.

————. "Paying for Medical Injury: No-Fault in Sweden and New Zealand." *Hospitals, J.A.H.A.*, 52, p. 42, July 1, 1978b.

————. "Defining the Compensable Event in No-Fault: New Zealand's Experience." *Hospitals, J.A.H.A.*, 52, p. 48, August 1, 1978c.

Bernstein, M. J. "Outgoing PSRO Head Sees Solid Future for Peer Review." *Hospitals, J.A.H.A.*, December 1, 1978, p. 103.

Birch, J. S., and Wolfe, S. "Consumers Assess Alternative Kinds of Health Service." Delivered at Annual Meeting, American Public Health Association, November 20, 1975, Chicago, Illinois.

Bloom, M. "Second Thoughts on CME." *Medical World News*, November 12, 1979.

Blum, H. L. "Evaluating Health Care." *Medical Care*, 12, 999, 1974.

Brian, E. "Foundation for Medical Care Control of Hospital Utilization: CHAP—A PSRO Prototype." *New England Journal of Medicine*, 288, 878, 1973.

Brook, R. H. "Critical Issues in the Assessment of Quality of Care and Their Relationship to HMO's." *Journal of Medical Education*, 48, 114, April 1973a. Part 2.

————. *Quality of Care Assessment: A Comparison of Five Methods of Peer Review*. National Center for Health Services Research and Development. Washington, D.C.: USDHEW, 1973b.

————. "Quality—Can We Measure It?" *New England Journal of Medicine*, 296, 170, 1977.

Brook, R. H., and Appel, F. A. "Quality of Care Assessment: Choosing a Method for Peer Review." *New England Journal of Medicine*, 288, 1323, 1973.

Brook, R. H., and Williams, K. N. "Quality of Health Care for the Disadvantaged." *Journal of Community Health*, 1, 132, 1975.

Brook, R. H., and Williams, K. N. "Effect of Medical Care Review on the Use of Injections." *Annals of Internal Medicine*, 85, 509, 1976.

Brook, R. H., et al. "Assessing the Quality of Medical Care Using Outcome Measures: An Overview of the Method." *Medical Care*, 15, No. 9, Supp., September 1977.

Bureau of Health Manpower Education. *Certification in Allied Health Professions: 1971 Conference Proceedings*. Bethesda, Maryland: USDHEW 1973, Pub. No. (NIH) 73–246.

Christoffel, T. "Medical Care Evaluation: An Old New Idea." *Journal of Medical Education*, 51, 83, 1976a.

————. Personal communication, March 15, 1976b.

————. "A Selected Bibliography of Literature of Quality Patient Care." *Quality Review Bulletin*, Jan./Feb. 1976c, p. 30.

Christoffel, T., and Lowenthal, M. "Evaluating the Quality of Ambulatory Health Care: A Review of Emerging Methods." *Medical Care*, *15*, 877, 1977.

Cohen, H. S. "Professional Licensure, Organization Behavior and the Public Interest." *Health and Society*, *51*, 73, 1973.

──────. "Manpower and Social Controls." *Hospitals, J.A.H.A.*, April 1974, p. 105.

Cohen, H. S., and Miike, L. H. *Developments in Health Manpower Licensure*. Washington, D. C.: USDHEW, Pub. No. (HRA) 74–3101, 1973.

Cohen, H. S., and Miike, L. H. "Toward a More Responsive System of Professional Licensure." *International Journal of Health Services*, *4*, 265, 1974.

Colock, B. P. "PSRO's." *New England Journal of Medicine*, *290*, 1318, 1974.

Commission on Professional and Hospital Activities. *PAS: Meeting Your Changing Needs*. Ann Arbor, Michigan: 1978.

Consumer Commission on the Accreditation of Health Services. "A Message About the Commission." *Health Perspectives*, *1*, April 1973.

──────. "Consumer Experiences in Hospital Accreditation." *Quarterly*, Spring 1974a.

──────. "JCAH Accreditation—The Lincoln Experience." *Quarterly*, Summer 1974b.

──────. "Hospital Accreditation—Where Do We Go From Here?" *Health Perspectives*, March–April 1975a.

──────. "Malpractice! A Consumer View." *Health Perspectives*, May–June 1975b.

──────. "Hospital Licensure by Private Accreditation." *Quarterly*, Summer 1977.

Consumer Reports. "Medical Malpractice." Parts I, II, III, September, October, November 1977, pp. 544, 598, 674.

Cooper, J. K. "No-Fault Malpractice Insurance: Swedish Plan Shows Us the Way." *Hospitals, J.A.H.A.*, *52*, p. 115, December 16, 1978.

Cooper, J. K., and Stephens, S. K. "The Malpractice Crisis—What Was It All About?" *Inquiry*, *14*, 240, 1977.

Curran, W. J. "Malpractice Insurance: A Genuine National Crisis." *New England Journal of Medicine*, *292*, 1223, 1975a.

──────. "Malpractice Crisis: The Flood of Legislation." *New England Journal of Medicine*, *293*, 1182, 1975b.

Davidson, S. M. "Professional Standards Review Organizations: A Critique." *Journal of the American Medical Association*, *226*, 1106, 1973.

Decker, B., and Bonner, P. *PSRO: Organization for Regional Peer Review*. Cambridge, Massachusetts: Ballinger, 1973.

Demkovich, L. E. "The Physicians' Peer Review Program—Does It Cost More Than It Saves?" *National Journal*, May 3, 1980, p. 733.

Derbyshire, R. C. *Medical Licensure and Discipline in the United States*. Baltimore, Maryland: Johns Hopkins Press, 1969.

──────. Personal communications, January 14, February 19, 1980.

Donabedian, A. "Evaluating the Quality of Medical Care." *Milbank Memorial Fund Quarterly*, *44*, 166, 1966.

—————. "Promoting Quality through Evaluating the Process of Patient Care." *Medical Care, 6,* 181, 1968.

—————. *A Guide to Medical Care Administration. II: Medical Care Appraisal—Quality and Utilization.* New York: American Public Health Association, 1969.

—————. "The Quality of Medical Care." Chapter VI in Office of the Assistant Secretary for Health, *Health: United States, 1978,* Hyattsville, Maryland: DHEW Pub. No. (PHS) 78–1232, USGPO, December 1978.

Egdahl, R. H., and Gertman, P. M., Eds. *Quality Health Care: The Role of Continuing Medical Education.* Germantown, Maryland: Aspen Systems Corp., 1977.

Egelston, E. M. "Licensure—Effects on Career Mobility." *American Journal of Public Health, 62,* 50, 1972.

Ellwood, P. M., Jr., et al. "Assessing the Quality of Health Services." In *Assuring the Quality of Health Care.* Chapter 3. Minneapolis: Interstudy, 1973.

Fishbein, M. "On PSRO's and Government Interference with Medicine." *Medical World News,* February 8, 1974, p. 88.

Flashner, B. A., et al. "Professional Standards Review Organizations." *Journal of the American Medical Association, 223,* 1473, 1973.

Forgotson, E. H., and Roemer, R. "Government Licensure and Voluntary Standards for Health Personnel and Facilities: Their Power and Limitation Is Assuring High Quality Care." *Medical Care, 6,* 345, 1968.

Freidson, E. *Profession of Medicine.* New York: Dodd, Mead, 1975.

Fulchiero, A., et al. "Can the PSROs Be Cost Effective?" *New England Journal of Medicine, 299,* 574, 1978.

Goran, M. J. "The Evolution of the PSRO Hospital Review System." *Medical Care, 17,* No. 5, Supp., May 1979.

Goran, M. J., et al. "The PSRO Hospital Review System." *Medical Care, 13,* No. 4, Supp., April 1975.

Greenberg, D. S. "Medicine and Public Affairs." *New England Journal of Medicine, 290,* 1493, 1974.

Health Care Financing Administration. *Professional Standards Review Organization 1979 Program Evaluation.* Washington, D.C.: USGPO, 1980.

Health Standards and Quality Bureau. *Legislative History of Professional Standards Review Organizations.* Washington, D.C.: USDHEW, USGPO, 1978.

—————. *PSRO in Perspective.* Washington, D.C.: USDHEW, USGPO, 1979.

Hollis, G. *State Licensing of Health Facilities.* Washington, D.C.: National Center for Health Statistics, USDHEW, 1968.

Hulka, B. S. "Quality of Ambulatory Care: An Exploration of the Discrepancy Between Explicit Process Criteria and Performance." Hyattsville, Maryland: DHEW Pub. No. (PHS) 80–3244, USGPO, April 1980.

Hulka, B. S., et al. "Peer Review in Ambulatory Care: Use of Explicit Criteria and Implicit Judgments." *Medical Care, 17,* No. 3, Supp., March 1979.

Institute of Medicine. *Assessing Quality in Health Care: An Evaluation*. Washington, D.C.: National Academy of Sciences, 1976.

————. "Beyond Malpractice: Compensation for Medical Injuries." Washington, D.C.: National Academy of Sciences, March 1978.

Jessee, W. F. "Quality Assurance Systems: Why Aren't There Any?" *Quality Review Bulletin*, 3, 16, 1977, cited in Fiter, W. R. "Quality Assurance." *Hospitals*, *J.A.H.A.*, April 1, 1979, p. 163.

Jessee, W. F., et al. "PSRO: An Educational Force for Improving Quality of Care." *New England Journal of Medicine*, 292, 668, 1975.

Joint Commission on Accreditation of Hospitals. *Accreditation Manual for Hospitals, 1980*, Chicago, 1979.

Jonas, S. *Quality Control of Ambulatory Care: A Task for Health Departments*. New York: Springer, 1977.

————. *Medical Mystery: The Training of Doctors in the United States*. New York: Norton, 1979.

Kane, R. L., et al. "Relationship Between Process and Outcome in Ambulatory Care." *Medical Care*, 15, 961, 1977.

Katz, B. F. "The Medical Malpractice Crisis—Its Cause and Effects." Presented at the Annual Meeting, American Public Health Association, November 19, 1975, Chicago, Illinois.

Kessner, D. M., and Kalk, C. E. *Contrasts in Health Status, 2: A Strategy for Evaluating Health Services*. Washington, D.C.: Institute of Medicine, 1973.

Kessner, D. M., et al. "Assessing Health Quality—The Case for Tracers." *New England Journal of Medicine*, 288, 189, 1973.

Kessner, D. M., et al. *Contrasts in Health Status, 3: Assessment of Medical Care for Children*. Washington, D.C.: Institute of Medicine, 1974.

Koran, L. M. "The Reliability of Clinical Methods, Data and Judgments." *New England Journal of Medicine*, 293, 642, 695, 1975.

Kuehn, H. R. "The Commission on Professional and Hospital Activities." *Bulletin, American College of Surgeons*, October 1973.

Lancet. "Keeping Calm on Malpraxis Insurance." February 8, 1975, p. 325.

Lander, L. "PSRO's: A Little Toe in the Door." *Health/PAC Bulletin*, July/August 1974, p. 1.

Last, J. M. "The Iceberg." *The Lancet*, July 6, 1963, p. 28.

Lebow, J. L. "Consumer Assessments of the Quality of Medical Care." *Medical Care*, 12, 328, 1974.

Lee, R. I., and Jones, L. W. *The Fundamentals of Good Medical Care*. Chicago: University of Chicago Press, 1933. (Reprinted, Hamden, Connecticut: Archon Books, 1962.)

Lembcke, P. A. "Medical Auditing by Scientific Methods." *Journal of the American Medical Association*, 162, 646, 1956.

Lerner, H. J. *Manpower Issues and Voluntary Regulation in the Medical Specialty System*. New York: Prodist, 1974.

Lewis, C. E. "The State of the Art of Quality Assessment—1973." *Medical Care*, 12, 999, 1974.

Leymaster, G. R. Personal communication, January 31, 1980.

Liaison Committee on Medical Education. *Information to Be Supplied by Developing Medical Schools*. Chicago, 1972.
————. *Functions and Structure of a Medical School*. Chicago, 1973.
————. *Provisions Leading to Provisional Accreditation of New Medical Schools*. Chicago, 1974.
Linn, B. S., et al. "Evaluation of Burn Care in Florida." *New England Journal of Medicine*, 296, 311, 1977.
Lister, J. "By the London Post." *New England Journal of Medicine*, 296, 436, 1977.
————. "By the London Post." *New England Journal of Medicine*, 302, 733, 1980.
McAuliffe, W. E. "Studies of Process-Outcome Correlations in Medical Care Evaluations: A Critique." *Medical Care*, 16, 907, 1978.
McCarthy, C. M. "Public Policy and Peer Review: A Study of the Implications of the PSRO Amendment and Its Impact in Nassau and Suffolk Counties in New York." M. S. thesis, State University of New York at Stony Brook, 1974.
McMahon, J. A. "PSRO's—Implications for Hospitals." *Hospitals, J.A.H.A.*, January 1, 1974, p. 53.
Medical World News. "How Well Does Medicine Police Itself?" March 15, 1974a, p. 62.
————. "NMA Blasts PSRO as Discriminatory." September 6, 1974b, p. 16.
————. "Malpractice Demon Stirring Again." November 12, 1979, p. 11.
Miike, L. H. "Institutional Licensure: An Experimental Model, Not a Solution." *Medical Care*, 12, 214, 1974.
Moore, F. D. "Surgical Biology and Applied Sociology: Cannon and Codman Fifty Years Later." *Harvard Medical Alumni Bulletin*, January–February, 1975, p. 12.
Morehead, M. A. "Evaluating Quality of Medical Care in the Neighborhood Health Center Program of the Office of Economic Opportunity." *Medical Care*, 8, 118, 1970.
Morehead, M. A., and Donaldson, R. "Quality of Clinical Management of Disease in Comprehensive Neighborhood Health Centers." *Medical Care*, 12, 301, 1974.
Morehead, M. A., et al. *A Study of the Quality of Hospital Care Secured by a Sample of Teamster Family Members in New York City*. New York: Columbia University School of Public Health and Administrative Medicine, 1964.
Morehead, M. A., et al. "Comparisons between OEO Neighborhood Health Centers and Other Health Care Providers of Ratings of the Quality of Health Care." *American Journal of Public Health*, 61, 1294, 1971.
Morton, J. H. "Licensure and Certification in the United States: Present Development and Future Plans." *Journal of the American Medical Association*, 237, 47, 1977.
National Advisory Commission on Health Manpower. *Report*, Vol. II. Washington, D.C.: USGPO. November 1967.
National Center for Health Statistics. *Health Resources Statistics*. DHEW Pub. No. (PHS) 79–1509, Hyattsville, Maryland: USGPO, 1979.
National Commission on Accrediting. *Accreditation in Medicine*. Washington, D.C., November 1970.

Neu, H. C., and Howrey, S. P. "Testing the Physician's Knowledge of Antibiotic Use." *New England Journal of Medicine*, 293, 1291, 1975.

New York Times. "State Malpractice Insurers Found to Be Profit-Making." June 11, 1975.

Nolan, P. "A Matter of License." *Physicians Forum*, Fall 1975, p. 1.

Office of Professional Standards Review. *PSRO Program Manual*. Washington, D.C.: USDHEW, 1974. (Updated periodically)

Pennell, M. Y. "Accreditation, Certification and Licensure." In McTernan, E. T., and Hawkins, R. O., Eds., *Educating Personnel for the Allied Health Professions and Services*. Chapter 7. St. Louis, Missouri: Mosby, 1972.

Pennell, M. Y., and Stewart, P. A. *State Licensing of Health Occupations*. USDHEW, Washington, D.C.: USGPO, 1968.

Peterson, O. L. "Medical Care: Its Social and Organizational Aspects." *New England Journal of Medicine*, 269, 1238, 1963.

Peterson, O. L., et al. "An Analytical Study of North Carolina General Practice." *The Journal of Medical Education*, 31, December 1956, Part 2.

Phillips, D. F. "The California Physicians' Strike." *Hospitals, J.A.H.A.*, August 1, 1975, p. 49.

P. L. 92–603. Amendments to the Social Security Act.

Rayack, E. "The American Medical Association and the Supply of Physicians: A Study of the Internal Contradictions in the Concept of Professionalism." *Medical Care*, 2, 244, 1964; and 3, 17, 1965.

Roemer, M. I. "Controlling and Promoting Quality in Medical Care." In Havighurst, C. C., and Weistart, J. C., Eds. *Health Care from the Library of Law and Contemporary Problems*. Dobbs Ferry, New York: Oceania Publications, 1972.

Roemer, R. "Legal Regulation of Health Manpower in the 1970's." *HSMA Health Reports*, 86, 1053, 1971a.

——————. "Licensing and Regulation of Medical and Medical-Related Practitioners in Health Service Teams." *Medical Care*, 9, 42, 1971b.

Rubin, D. "The Accreditation of Hospitals—What Does It Promise?" *Health Law Project Library Bulletin*, 5, 90, 1980.

Rutstein, D. D., et al. "Measuring the Quality of Medical Care: A Clincal Method." *New England Journal of Medicine*, 294, 582, 1976.

Sanazaro, P. J. "Private Initiative in PSRO." *New England Journal of Medicine*, 293, 1023, 1975.

Sanazaro, P. J., and Williamson, J. W. "End Results of Patient Care: A Provisional Classification Based on Reports by Internists." *Medical Care*, 6, 123, 1968.

Sanazaro, P. J., and Worth, R. M. "Concurrent Quality Assurance in Hospital Care." *New England Journal of Medicine*, 298, 1171, 1978.

Saywell, R. M., et al. "A Performance Comparison: USMG–FMG Physicians." *American Journal of Public Health*, 69, 57, 1979.

Scheye, E., ed. "The Hospital's Role in Assessing the Quality of Medical Care." Proceedings of the Fifteenth Annual Symposium on Hospital Affairs, May 1973, Graduate Program in Hospital Administration and Center for Health Administration Studies, Graduate School of Business, University of Chicago.

Schlicke, C. P. "American Surgery's Noblest Experiment." *Archives of Surgery,* *106,* 379, 1973.

Schwartz, W. B., and Komesar, N. K. "Doctors, Damages and Deterrence." *New England Journal of Medicine, 298,* 1282, 1978.

Sheps, M. "Approaches to the Quality of Hospital Care." *Public Health Reports, 70,* 877, 1955.

Shryock, R. H. *Medical Licensing in America, 1650–1965.* Baltimore, Maryland: Johns Hopkins Press, 1967.

Simmons, H. E. "PSRO Today: The Program's Viewpoint." *New England Journal of Medicine, 292,* 365, 1975.

Special Advisory Panel on Medical Malpractice. State of New York, *Report.* Albany, New York, January 1976.

Spieler, E. "Division of Laborers." *Health/PAC Bulletin,* November 1972, p. 3.

Stevens, R. *American Medicine and the Public Interest.* New Haven, Connecticut: Yale University Press, 1971.

Subcommittee on Medical Care, American Public Health Association. "The Quality of Medical Care in National Health Program." *American Journal of Public Health, 39,* 898, 1949.

Tomecki, S. J., and Plaut, M. E. "Syphilis Surveillance." *Journal of the American Medical Association, 236,* 2641, 1976.

Trussell, R. E., et al. *The Quantity, Quality and Costs of Medical and Hospital Care Secured by a Sample of Teamster Families in the New York Area.* New York: Columbia University School of Public Health and Administrative Medicine, 1962.

USDHEW. *Secretary's Report on Licensure and Related Health Personnel Credentialing,* Pub. No. (HSM) 72–11, Washington, D.C.: USGPO, 1971.

————. *Report of the Secretary's Commission on Medical Malpractice.* Washington, D.C.: USGPO, 1973.

————. *Credentialing Health Manpower.* Pub. No. (OS) 77–50057, Washington, D.C.: USGPO, 1977a.

————. *State Regulation of Health Manpower.* Pub. No. (HRA) 77–49, Washington, D.C., USGPO, 1977b.

Vaccarino, J. M. "Malpractice: The Problem in Perspective." *Journal of the American Medical Association, 238,* 861, 1977.

Vodicka, B. E. "Medical Discipline. Part VI. The Offenses." *Journal of the American Medical Association, 235,* 302, 1976.

Weinerman, E. R. "The Quality of Medical Care." *The Annals of the American Academy of Political and Social Science,* January 1, 1951, p. 185.

Welch, C. E. "Professional Standards Review Organization—Problems and Prospects." *New England Journal of Medicine, 289,* 291, 1973.

————. "PSRO's—Pros and Cons." *New England Journal of Medicine, 290,* 1319, 1974.

————. "Medical Malpractice." *New England Journal of Medicine, 292,* 1372, 1975.

Williamson, J. W. "Formulating Priorities for Quality Assurance Activity." *Journal of the American Medical Association, 239,* 631, 1978.

15

National Health Insurance

Steven Jonas

Introduction

The issue of National Health Insurance (NHI) has provoked debate and controversy in the United States since the beginning of the 20th century.* Since no enacted plan will satisfy everyone, the debate is bound to continue far into the future, even after the first act is finally legislated. If the United States experience follows that of other countries, any NHI program will be amended many times, and each time the legislative debate will be fierce. Some might be distressed to learn that—if the past is any guide—both the content and form of the arguments used by the several sides will remain largely fixed over time, regardless of changed circumstances or new information.

In this chapter, we will consider the history of NHI in the United States and the status of NHI in the early 1980s.

Historical Background

Otto von Bismarck was known as the "Iron Chancellor," first of Prussia, then, after 1871, of the unified German state. Shortly after the bourgeois revolution of 1848, he said: "The social insecurity of the worker is the real cause of their being a peril to the state" (Sigerist, p. 127). In 1881, Kaiser Wilhelm I, in a speech written by Bismarck, said: ". . . the healing of social

---

*The "insurance principle" has been discussed in Chapter 11. "Health insurance" is a misnomer, since the various plans are not "insurance" in the conventional sense, but rather prepayment for health services, spreading the costs over a population at large. Furthermore, almost all "health insurance" does not pay for health, but rather covers costs of care during sickness. Nevertheless, as the term is used by convention, so shall it be used in this chapter.

evils cannot be sought in the repression of social-democratic excesses exclusively but must equally be sought in the positive promotion of the workers' welfare" (Sigerist, p. 129). Various fragmented accident, workmen's compensation, and sickness schemes, both compulsory and voluntary, had come into existence over the previous half-century. Building on them, Bismarck in 1883 succeeded in ushering a Sickness Insurance Act through the German Reichstag or Parliament (Sigerist, pp. 121–131). Bismarck had wanted a uniform, national system, excluding the private, profit-making insurance companies. However, he settled for one that used the existing network of "sickness societies" (private "health" insurance companies, some profit-making, some not) to establish a program that paid for medical care and provided cash support during periods of sickness and accidental injury for certain categories of workers. Two-thirds of the premiums were to be paid by the employee, one-third by the employer. Thus the first national health insurance scheme was created—not by a radical government, but by a conservative monarchy. By the 1920s, most European industrialized countries, as well as Japan, had some kind of national health insurance system, usually partial and/or voluntary at first, then progressing to comprehensive and compulsory (Fry and Farndale, Chapters 2, 3; Douglas-Wilson and McLachlan, pp. 1–123, 211–230; Fulcher; Glaser; Jonas, 1975). The non-European English-speaking British Commonwealth countries gradually followed suit after World War II (Lynch and Raphael, Chapters 16–20; Fry and Farndale, Chapters 5, 8; Le Clair). By the early 1980s, the United States had not yet done so.

The first campaign for a national health insurance program in the United States was undertaken by the American Associaton for Labor Legislation (AALL), a middle-class, liberal, reform-minded group, founded in 1906 (Anderson, Part 2; Burrow, 1963, Chapter 7; Burrow, 1977, pp. 138–153). Proposals for a broad social insurance plan had been included in Teddy Roosevelt's Bull Moose Party platform in 1912 (Burrow, 1963, p. 135). In 1916, the AALL put forward a standard bill for compulsory medical care and sickness benefits insurance, which it proposed that the several states adopt independently. The program would have covered persons earning below a certain income level and would have used existing insurance carriers, with costs to be shared by employers, employees, and the states (Anderson, pp. 62–65; Burrow, 1963, p. 136). At first, support was fairly widespread, extending to the American Medical Association and even the National Association of Manufacturers (Burrow, 1963, pp. 138–145). Beginning in 1917, however—when the U.S. entry into World War I was deflating the Reform Movement generally—opposition began to surface from several quarters, including the American Federation of Labor and the commercial insurance industry (Anderson, p. 67; Burrow, 1977, pp. 148–153).

Within the AMA, a battle ensued on the issue (Anderson, Chapter 7; Burrow, 1963, pp. 146–151), but, as part of the general takeover of power by the practitioner wing from the academic wing, the conservative faction won out (Harris, July 2, 1966, p. 30).* In 1920, the AMA House of Delegates passed the following resolution (Burrow, 1963):

> Resolved, that the American Medical Association declares its opposition to the institution of any plan embodying the system of compulsory contributory insurance against illness, or any other plan of compulsory insurance which provides for medical service to be rendered contributors or their dependents, provided, controlled, or regulated by any state or the Federal government. (p. 150)

That remained in toto the AMA position until the late 1960s (Harris). Even in the mid-1970s, by which time the AMA had adopted an NHI proposal of its own that ran counter to the bulk of the 1920 resolution, the "noncompulsory" principle was retained (H. R. 6222).

Serious consideration was next given to national health insurance during the development of the Social Security Act of 1935. This consideration was stimulated in part by the final report of the Committee on the Costs of Medical Care. Although it did not recommend NHI per se, concentrating instead on proposals for group practice and health insurance that could be either private or government-operated, compulsory or voluntary, it did use hard data to show the need for action (Anderson, Chapter 10; Stevens, pp. 183–187). In 1934, President Franklin Roosevelt created the Committee on Economic Security to consider the whole question of social insurance. NHI did not last long on the agenda. The Committee's Executive Director, Edwin E. Witte, wrote (Anderson):

> When in 1934 the Committee on Economic Security announced that it was studying health insurance, it was at once subjected to misrepresentation and vilification. In the original social security bill there was one line to the effect that the Social Security Board should study the problem and make a report thereon to Congress. That little line was responsible for so many telegrams to the members of Congress that the entire social security program seemed

*Both Burrow's books and the Harris articles contain detailed histories and analyses of the AMA's involvement in legislative battles over NHI, the 1963 Burrow book detailing them through the 1950s and the Harris articles covering the Medicare struggles. An excellent overall historical perspective is provided by Falk (1977).

endangered until the Ways and Means Committee unanimously struck it out of the bill. (p. 108)

The principal opposition came from the American Medical Association (Burrow, 1963, p. 193). The President wanted the basic Social Security Act, one of the cornerstones of the New Deal. It was passed with no reference to NHI.*

The next major legislative foray was made by Senator Robert F. Wagner, Sr., of New York State, whose landmark Wagner Act of 1938 had established the right to collective bargaining for all nonpublic employees in the United States. In 1939, he introduced S. 1620 "to provide for the general welfare by enabling the several states to make more adequate provision for public health, prevention and control of disease, maternal and child health services, construction, and maintenance of needed hospitals and health centers, care of the sick, disability insurance, and training of personnel" (Sigerist, pp. 189–190). The bill proposed to subsidize state public health programs (this later became federal policy through a series of acts); the construction of hospitals (enacted in 1946 as the Hill-Burton Act); and state programs for medical care for the poor (eventually enacted in part in 1960 as the Kerr/Mills Medical Assistance for the Aged, then expanded as Title XIX of the Social Security Act—Medicaid—in 1965). The bill also offered cash sickness benefits (a standard feature of the European/Japanese approach to NHI that has never made headway in the United States) and a program of federal subsidies to those states enacting comprehensive health insurance programs (Sigerist, pp. 190–191; Harris, July 2, 1966, pp. 31–32). The bill died in committee, after being vigorously attacked by the AMA (Harris, July 2, 1966, pp. 38–40).

Senator Wagner tried again in 1943, this time in concert with Senator Murray and Congressman Dingell. Their S. 1161 "advocated a national (i.e., federal) compulsory system of health insurance, financed from payroll taxes and providing comprehensive health and medical benefits through entitlement to specified medical service (service benefits) . . ." (Stevens, p. 272). This was the first major legislative proposal for a federal rather than a state-based system. Once again, the AMA responded with vigor (Harris, July 2, 1966, pp. 40–42). The bill was reintroduced in several successive Congresses, as S. 1606 in 1945 and S. 1320 in 1947 (Anderson, pp. 112–113). That year, Senator Robert Taft, Sr., also introduced a proposal (S. 545) for federal subsidies to the states to pay for medical care for the poor (Stevens, p. 273).

---

*The details of all major NHI proposals made between 1935 and 1957 have been summarized by A. W. Brewster, *Health Insurance and Related Proposals for Financing Personal Health Services* (Washington, D.C.: USDHEW, USGPO, 1958).

In 1949, the newly reelected President, Harry Truman, having Democratic majorities in both houses of Congress, decided to make NHI a major goal of his Administration. He proposed a national, compulsory system, to be paid for by a combination of Social Security and general taxation, based upon the following principles, which he had originally enunciated in 1945 (Truman):

> Everyone should have ready access to all necessary medical, hospital, and related services. . . . A system of required prepayment would not only spread the costs of medical care, it would also prevent much serious disease. . . . Such a system of prepayment should cover medical, hospital, nursing, and laboratory services. It should cover dental care—[as far as] resources of the system permit . . . the nation-wide system must be highly decentralized in administration. . . . Subject to national standards, methods and rates of paying doctors and hospitals should be adjusted locally. . . . People should remain free to choose their own physicians and hospitals. . . . Likewise physicians should remain free to accept or reject patients. . . . Our voluntary hospitals and our city, county, and state general hospitals, in the same way, must be free to participate in the system to whatever extent they wish . . . what I am recommending is not socialized medicine. Socialized medicine means that all doctors work as employees of government. . . . No such system is here proposed. . . . (pp. 629–630)

The AMA mounted a furious attack on the plan, based primarily on the thesis that it was indeed "socialized medicine" (Harris, July 2, 1966, pp. 40–62). Using a major public relations firm and a war chest of over $2,000,000, a very substantial sum in those days, the AMA, with allies from the drug and insurance industries (Stevens, pp. 273–274), was successful that year and in succeeding years through 1952. With the election of a Republican government, that year, the AMA was able to breathe easily (Burrow, 1963, pp. 361, 385).

A number of factors contributed to the success of the AMA and other opponents of NHI. The nation's economy was relatively prosperous following World War II, particularly with "rearmament" underway, beginning in 1948. A Republican majority controlled both houses of Congress during 1946–1948. Voluntary health insurance, given a major stimulus by wartime wage-stabilization policies which had allowed more expansion of fringe benefits than of wages, was providing increasing numbers of employed workers with at least partial coverage of their medical bills (Stevens, p. 271). The AMA did engineer a remarkable, if not entirely straightforward, public relations campaign.

Finally, the Cold War was a decisive influence. Although President Truman was a moderate opponent of the most virulent forms of McCarthyite anti-Communism at home, he is frequently considered to have been one of the coldest of Cold Warriors abroad (Freeland). In a climate of domestic and foreign anti-Communism, it was difficult for Truman to win support at home for a program consistently attacked as "Communist," or at least "socialist," but in any case "red" (Harris, July 2, 1966, p. 50). Thus; in 1951, on the recommendation of Oscar Ewing, the Federal Security Administrator, the Truman Administration withdrew its support for NHI and began the campaign that led to the passage of Medicare, limited health insurance for the aged, in 1965 (Harris, July 2, 1966, pp. 58–60; Stevens, p. 274).

Medicare and Medicaid

The campaign for what is now called Medicare* was long and arduous (Stevens, pp. 432–443; Harris, July 9, 16, 23, 1966). The AMA, ever-vigilant, in 1952 opposed and defeated a proposal to expand the Old Age and Survivors Insurance Program of the Social Security Act. Part of that proposal would have provided pensions to persons under 65 who were permanently and totally disabled. The AMA opposed it because the Social Security Administration would have had the authority to hire physicians to determine whether applicants were indeed permanently and totally disabled (Anderson, p. 133). The AMA apparently saw this provision as the tip of the iceberg. With Medicare, the threat was evident; the AMA fought hard, but in the end lost. (Or did it? In fact, physicians have done rather well financially under Medicare. They would probably do well financially under NHI too, as they have done in Canada [Le Clair, p. 69].) In any case, Medicare and its companion, Medicaid, did indeed represent a step on the road to NHI. The major operational aspects of both programs are described in Chapter 10.†

Both programs, of course, had their historical antecedents. In almost every country in which the central government has undertaken some responsibility for providing or supervising the provision of health insurance on a national scale, the plan started by taking care of only part of the population. This part was ordinarily segregated by income. This is the basic principle of Medicaid, although Medicaid cannot strictly be considered an

*Before the passage of Title XVIII of the Social Security Act in 1965, "Medicare" referred to a medical care program for dependents of armed forces personnel (Somers and Somers, p. 528).

†The provisions of both Medicare and Medicaid as they stood in the late 1970s are presented in detail by Wilson and Neuhauser in their descriptive outline of the United States health care delivery system (*Health Services in the United States*, Cambridge, Massachusetts: Ballinger, 1976, pp. 141–160).

insurance program, since the beneficiaries make no direct contributions at all. The concept first appeared in the United States in the earliest AALL proposals, although they were aimed at the working poor, whereas Medicaid covers the nonworking poor. Medicaid-like proposals appeared in Senator Wagner's prewar bill and Senator Taft's postwar bills. Segregation of an eligible population by age, was, however, a new twist, going back only to 1950.

Although they were passed together, Medicare and Medicaid are in principle quite different measures, aside from the different population groups at which they were aimed (Committee on Finance, 1970). Medicare is a uniform federal program, based in the Health Care Financing Administration, financed primarily by Social Security taxes, available to all persons 65 and over regardless of income (persons ineligible for Social Security may buy into the program). It has co-payment and deductible features, offers a limited range of benefits and separate plans for in-hospital and out-of-hospital services, uses fiscal intermediaries (insurance companies) to make payments to providers, and pays hospitals on a cost-reimbursement basis and individual providers on a "usual and customary fee" basis. Medicaid is under the general supervision of HCFA but is in fact 49 different state programs run by 49 different state agencies—recall that Arizona has no Medicaid program (HCFA). It embodies the means-test principle, has, in theory, unlimited benefits, but in reality limited ones because of chronic money shortages, is financed from general taxation, rarely provides for co-insurance, may or may not use fiscal intermediaries, pays hospitals on a cost-reimbursement basis and individual providers on a fee schedule.

The experience with Medicare and Medicaid has been mixed (Stevens, Chapters 19, 20; Davis, 1975a, pp. 41–55; Burney; Gornick; Friedman; Lander, pp. 4–35).* Some persons in both the 65-and-over age group and the medically indigent group have undoubtedly benefited. However, both programs lack stringent cost-controls and are thought to have contributed significantly to the acceleration in the rise of health care costs experienced since 1965 (Lander, pp. 20–25; Davis, 1973; Committee on Finance, 1970, Chapters 2, 3). Medicaid, in particular, has suffered from uneven implementation and is especially sensitive to expenditure-cutting when states find themselves short of funds (Lander, p. 28; Stevens, pp. 479–482; *New York Times*, Sept. 30, 1971; Dec. 27, 1975 *Health/PAC*). Medicare too, although intended as a uniform program, has suffered from some uneven-

---

*The legislative and programmatic history of Medicaid has been documented in great detail by Stevens and Stevens, *Welfare Medicine in America* (New York: The Free Press, 1974).

ness in implementation, benefiting higher-income and white people and lower-income and nonwhite people differentially (Davis, 1975b).

Since serious attempts to create some kind of *national* health insurance program had been under way since 1912, there was no reason to expect that they would stop with the passage of Medicaid and Medicare. Thus, after a short respite, the struggle started anew (Falk, 1973).

National Health Insurance in the 1970s

More legislative proposals for NHI than we have room to describe have been made since the late 1960s. The original group, made in the 1969–1971 period, have been widely discussed (Falk, 1973, 1977; Bills; Burns; New York Academy of Medicine; Eilers; Eilers and Moyerman). Since that time, the major proposals have been summarized periodically by the Ways and Means Committee of the House of Representatives, as in a 1974 publication (Committee on Ways and Means) and the Senate Finance Committee (Committee on Finance, 1979). The American Hospital Association or AHA, the Committee for National Health Insurance or CNHI, of Washington, D.C., and other major interest groups publish summaries of the details of current NHI legislative proposals periodically. It is interesting to note that in the wide-ranging debate on NHI, the basic arguments of the several sides have changed little since mid-century (Boas; Falk, 1973; McKittrick; Schwartz).

As of 1975, a time when the passage of some sort of NHI seemed imminent to many observers, there were five major proposals before Congress.* The principal sponsors were: Senator Kennedy for organized labor; Congressman Ullman for the American Hospital Association; Senator McIntyre and Congressman Burleson for the Health Insurance Association of America (HIAA); Congressmen Fulton and Duncan for the AMA; and Senators Long and Ribicoff. In brief, these bills may be summarized as follows (*Health Security News*, 1975):

- The Kennedy "Health Security Act" (Kennedy; S. 3) would have established a single, national, federally operated compulsory plan with a very broad benefit package, financed in part by general taxation and in part by employer-employee taxes, with no deductibles or co-insurance. Special features included funds for improving health services and rigorous cost and quality controls.

*An excellent review of the situation in the mid-1970s, covering all of the major legislative proposals with the exception of that of the AMA, is contained in a book by Karen Davis, *National Health Insurance: Benefits, Costs, and Consequences* (Washington, D.C.: The Brookings Institution, 1975b).

- The AHA plan (H. R. 1; McMahon) would have established a comprehensive private compulsory insurance system regulated primarily at the state level and operated by the insurance companies, with separate plans for the employed, the self-employed, and the poor, with a broad benefit package, financed by taxation and employer-employee contributions, with limited deductibles and co-insurance. A special feature was the Health Care Corporation concept, which provided for voluntary or governmental agencies to coordinate delivery of health services within designated geographic areas. State Health Commissions would have been responsible for planning, regulation, and cost control.
- The HIAA plan (S. 1438) would have established a voluntary health insurance system operated by the insurance companies and regulated primarily by state insurance departments, from which individuals could "opt out," continuing Medicare and Medicaid as independent entities, with a moderately broad benefit package, financed primarily by premiums and tax deductions, with deductibles and co-insurance. Special features included support for HMO development and the strengthening of state health planning capabilities.
- The AMA plan (H. R. 6222) would have required employers to offer private health insurance plans to employees who could choose to participate, regulated by state insurance departments, continuing Medicare and Medicaid as independent entities, with a moderately broad benefit package, financed primarily by employer-employee contributions and federal tax credits, with deductibles and co-insurance. Special features included no provision for cost-control and a weakening of the PSRO system for quality-assurance.
- Long-Ribicoff was a combination of so-called catastrophic health insurance (see p. 451) operated by private insurance companies for the Social Security Administration, continuing Medicare and federalizing Medicaid, with a limited benefit package made available only after a certain out-of-pocket payment threshold had been reached, financed by Social Security and general federal taxes. It would also have established minimum guidelines for "national certification" of voluntary insurance which could be offered by nonprofit and commercial companies to persons not otherwise covered.

Since all of the major actors were on stage, surely one of these proposals or some compromise among them would find its way through Congress. And in the 1976 Presidential campaign, Candidate Jimmy Carter said, in his only speech on health policy (*The Nation's Health*):

We must have a comprehensive program of national health insurance. . . .
The coverage must be universal and mandatory. We must lower the present
barriers, in insurance coverage and otherwise, to preventive and primary
care—and thus reduce the need for hospitalization. We must have strong
cost and quality controls, and . . . rates . . . should be set in advance. . . . We
must phase in the program as rapidly as revenues permit, helping first those
who need help, and achieving a comprehensive program well-defined in the
end. (p. 7)

However, by 1980, no NHI program had even been voted out of a health
subcommittee in Congress, much less been passed by both Houses and
signed into law by the President; the number of major contending proposals had been reduced. Senator Kennedy had markedly changed his position and President Carter had entered the list with a proposal based on
rather different principles than those he stated in his campaign. Only
Senator Long had not changed his basic stance, although he appeared to be
willing to compromise down to virtually nothing as a first step in order to
get something on the books (*American Medical News*, May 30, 1980).

NHI Proposals in 1980

According to the Congressional Research Service of the Library of Congress (Cavalier), the major policy issues that ought to be addressed in
designing an NHI program are:

1.   The rising costs of health care;
2.   The gaps in present health insurance coverage, in terms of both
     services and populations;
3.   Geographic maldistribution of personnel and facilities;
4.   Access to service by ability to pay, social class, age group, and
     geography;
5.   The impact or lack thereof of NHI on the population's health status.

Not all of the several proposals current in 1980 addressed all of these
policy issues. The major contenders were "The Health Care for All Americans Act" (HCAAA), sponsored by Senator Kennedy and Congressman
Waxman (Chairman of the Health Subcommittee of the House of Representatives Commerce Committee) with the backing of the AFL-CIO;
HealthCare, proposed by the Carter Administration; and several variants
of Senator Long's "Catastrophic Health Insurance Plan," the only intact
leftover from the mid-1970s contest. These three proposals will be presented in some detail below. (For further information, see Committee on

Finance, 1979; Kimble; Subcommittee on Health; S. 1720; and S. 1812). We will then present three other proposals, which did not have major political support in 1980 but have some interesting features that might someday find their way into an NHI program: the concept of a National Health Service; the so-called Consumer Choice Plan; and NHI-by-contract. We also will consider the potential impact of the six above listed proposals on the major policy issues as outlined by the Congressional Research Service. In addition, the alternative that has been around for the longest time and has consistently beaten back all comers, "No Plan," will be considered.

The Health Care for All Americans Act (Kennedy/Waxman)

HCAAA would provide financial coverage for a broad set of health care services for all Americans. There would be unlimited hospital and physician, laboratory, X-ray, and ambulance services. There would be limited psychiatric, home health, outpatient physical and speech therapy, skilled nursing home and pharmaceutical services, and certain other benefits. Excluded would be long-term nursing home care, cosmetic surgery, and certain other services. There would be two major plans. One would be an expanded Medicare system, which could cover all of the elderly, whether presently under Medicare or not, plus many persons not now covered, in some states at least, by Medicaid. It would be paid for by a combination of Social Security taxes, Medicare premiums, and federal and state general taxes. The other would be a new, mandatory, private health insurance program covering employed workers and their families. It would be paid for through employer-employee premiums. Employees could be required to pay no more than 35% of their total premium, and their payments would be income-related. The self-employed and persons living on unearned income would be required to join when they used health services and their premiums would be income-related.

Employers would be required to offer at least two different plans to employees. At least one would be a conventional private doctor, private hospital type plan, and at least one would be a Health-Maintenance-Organization-type plan, of either the Group Practice or so-called Independent Practice Association variety. Medicare and Defense Department beneficiaries would each have one plan.

Patients would be guaranteed confidentiality and freedom of choice of provider, but participation would be required for anyone using the health care delivery system. Institutional providers and physicians could choose whether or not to participate, as could eligible insurance companies.

The program would be administered at the top by a National Health Board (NHB), reporting directly to the President. Below the NHB would be 50 State Health Boards. Insurance companies and HMOs would deal with employers as they do now in the voluntary health insurance system, and would act as "fiscal intermediaries" between the federal government and the providers as they do now under the Medicare program. However, the National and State Health Boards would have a great deal of power in regulating the insurance companies, and they would be called upon to do things in quality-assurance and cost-control that they have not previously done.

A major objective of HCAAA would be to establish in advance for each year a health services budget, applying to all providers. The national health services budget would be related to the Gross National Product. The national budget would be allocated on a proportional basis to each state. There would be negotiations to establish: (1) the total national budget, (2) the allocations to each state, and (3) the rates at which the institutional and individual providers would be paid. The negotiations would be three-cornered and highly complex, involving the national and state boards, provider representatives, and the insurance companies. The insurance companies would be represented by four "consortia," one each for the not-for-profit companies, the commercials, the HMOs, and the IPAs.

Institutional providers, such as hospitals, nursing homes, home health agencies, and neighborhood health centers would be paid on the basis of item-of-service rates tied to annual budgets negotiated in advance, that is prospective reimbursement, a significant departure from the retrospective reimbursement system presently used in most localities (see Chapter 11). Payments to physicians and other fee-for-service providers would be on the basis of negotiated fee schedules, subject to the annual, budget-related maximum. Thus, for the first time in this country, there would be annual limits on physicians' incomes. The mechanism of using an annually budgeted sum, from which physicians could draw payments on a fee-for-service basis, but which could not be exceeded even if it were to run out before the year is up, is in other countries called the "pool system." This seemingly radical idea was first introduced in the German Empire in the late 19th century.

Prospective budgeting, the complex negotiating system, and shared federal-state administrative responsibilities in a completely new set of agencies represent innovations beyond anything that exists or is proposed in other plans. Yet it is another innovation which has the most far-reaching implications for the development of the U.S. health care delivery system. In a section entitled "Health Care Improvement," the proposed Act spells out a series of provisions that would gradually develop a system to tie reimbursement to quality-control; to the evaluation of technical and mechanical medical and surgical diagnostic and therapeutic interventions (usually lumped together under the term "technology assessment"); and to planning for health manpower and facility requirements. Thus, under HCAAA there would or at least could be direct intervention in the content of the health care delivery and indeed in medical, surgical, and hospital practice. The intent is to use the payment system to directly influence such things as the supply and distribution of hospital beds, the balance of physicians among the various specialties, and the use of therapies of less than proven value.

In essence, HCAAA combines compulsory participation and active intervention in the health care delivery system, features of Senator Kennedy's Health Security Act, with the multiple plan system, providing a major role for the insurance companies, which was featured by most of its mid-1970s competitors.

National Health Plan

The Carter Administration's National Health Plan, or NHP, has two prongs. The package is similar in some ways to the Long-Ribicoff proposal of the mid-1970s. However, it is envisioned as the first step toward a comprehensive NHI program, each piece to be legislated separately. The first part of the NHP is called HealthCare, a merging and broadening of Medicare and Medicaid into a single, national program. The 24 million present Medicare beneficiaries would be joined by the 16 million low-income Medicaid beneficiaries plus 10 million not-quite-so-low-income persons. Private individuals and employers could also purchase Health-Care if they so chose. The benefit package would be similar to that of HCAAA, with a particular stress on maternal and infant care. However, HealthCare would call for beneficiary cost-sharing for the nonpoor of up to $1,250 per year. Thus, for former Medicare beneficiaries and the not-so-poor covered by the Act, co-insurance payments could be levied, up to $1,250. However, unlike the present system, no one could pay more than that, thus protecting persons against "catastrophic illness." Maternal and infant care services would have no cost-sharing requirements.

HealthCare would be administered by the Department of Health and Human Services, as Medicare and Medicaid are now. It would be financed by Social Security taxes, Medicare and direct-pay premiums, and state and federal general revenues. Physicians would be paid on a fee schedule and would not be allowed to bill patients extra. Hospitals would be reimbursed much as they are now, but would be subject to strict cost-controls. Cost-control would be achieved by limiting annual percentage increases in hospital's revenues, the so-called cap approach, plus direct controls on capital expenditures. System reforms would also be encouraged by further stimulation of HMO growth and of preventive health services."

The second part of NHP would be an "Employer-Guaranteed Plan (EGP). Employers would be required to provide a basic health insurance package for any person, and his or her family, who worked for more than 25 hours per week for 10 consecutive weeks. The basic benefit package would have to be the same as under HealthCare. However, these private plans could require an annual deductible of up to $2,500 per year, per family. Employer-employee negotiations could reduce or eliminate the deductible, and in many major industries whose workers are covered by existing bargained-for health insurance plans, that would surely happen. However, for many workers not so covered, the new insurance would primarily provide protection against catastrophic illness. Employer premiums would pay for at least 75% of the costs. The insurance policies would be purchased from private companies and they would administer them as they do now. Hospitals would be paid by the cost-reimbursement system as they are now, and would be under HealthCare, but would be subject to "cap" type cost controls. For physicians, the HealthCare fee schedule would be advisory and they could charge patients covered by EGP more if they chose to do so.

NHP takes some steps toward NHI. It establishes a fully paid system for the poor. It limits the potential expenditures of the nonpoor elderly. It provides at least catastrophic illness protection for almost everyone else. It puts an external "cap" on hospital expenditures. It stiffens controls over hospital capital expenditures and encourages the growth of HMOs. Unlike HCAAA, it studiously avoids any interference with the way doctors and hospitals do business, except for imposing a fee schedule on doctors for some of their work.

The Long Plan

Throughout the 96th Congress (1979–1980), Senator Long offered several variations on the theme of catastrophic health insurance. Having no success for a number of reasons, including a very tight federal budget, by mid-1980, he was offering a very watered-down version of his own limited proposal—and still not having success (*American Medical News*, May 30, 1980). His original proposal, however, was similar in many ways to NHP and thus to the earlier Long-Ribicoff plan (*Washington Report on Medicine and Health*, 1979). It would require that all employers provide catastrophic illness cost-protection for all employed persons and their families. Insurance would be provided by private companies for the fully employed and by a federal program created for the self-employed and the partially employed and unemployed. Financial assistance in meeting the bill's requirements would be provided to small employers. The deductible amount to be paid before the insurance would be triggered would be in the

$2,500–$3,500 range. Plans would have to be approved by the Secretary of Health and Human Services. Under different versions of the plan, financing could be either by a 1% payroll tax or left to employer-employee negotiations, and a tax-credit system. Benefits would be roughly comparable to those presently provided under Medicare.

Under the second part of Senator Long's proposal, the "Medical Assistance Plan for Low-Income People," Medicaid would be federalized and its beneficiaries provided with a fairly broad benefit package. Beneficiaries would be subject to a means test. It would be financed by federal and state general tax revenues.

Under the third part of the Long package, DHHS would set a minimum-standards certification program for private insurance policies, similar to the Good Housekeeping Seal of Approval. There would be no requirement to do so, but only companies that did would be eligible to participate in Medicare, which would be continued as is, and the federalized Medicaid program.

Administration of the whole program would rest primarily with the DHHS. Provider payment would generally follow the present Medicare system of retrospective reimbursement for hospitals and "usual and customary fees" for physicians, although details are lacking in this area (Committee on Finance, 1979, p. 23). There are no significant health care delivery system reform provisions in the Long proposal.

Catastrophic health insurance is the central feature of Senator Long's plan, the starting point for President Carter's plan (with hoped-for expansion later), and at one time even Senator Kennedy said that he would agree to begin with catastrophic health insurance if a whole package that would eventually be phased in to comprehensive health insurance were legislated at the beginning. Catastrophic health insurance pays what economists call "last-dollar" costs. After an individual pays X thousand dollars, either out of pocket or via other insurance, catastrophic health insurance picks up the rest. It is major medical insurance with no upper limit. It is attractive to the general public because of the pervasive fear of the medical "wipeout," that is, the illness whose costs are so great that they eat up all of the family's assets. However, that kind of event is relatively rare, although certainly it is catastrophic for the afflicted. Most present observers agree that people should be protected against its occurrence, but critics of catastrophic insurance claim that to provide that kind of coverage alone would have catastrophic effects on the health care delivery system as a whole (*Health Security News*, 1974, p. 1).

Critics claim that catastrophic insurance creates provider incentives to offer expensive care. It would "take the heat off" enactment of a comprehensive program. It would create an incentive to raise prices, so that it

would be "easier" for families to get up under the "catastrophic umbrella."
It would make the high-income specialties even more attractive for physicians. Most important, the critics say, it would intensify the hospital
system's focus on high-cost, acute-care services, and away from prevention, ambulatory care, and reasonable-cost long-term care services in
institutions or at home.

In a study of high-cost patients in 17 acute-care hospitals in the San
Francisco Bay area, Steven Schroeder et al. (1979) found that:

> The percentage of patients whose yearly hospital charges exceeded $4,000 in
> 1976 ranged from 4 at a community hospital to 24 at a referral hospital.
> Hospital costs charged to these patients ranged from 20 to 68 percent of total
> billings, with the highest percentages generally occurring at large referral
> hospitals. 47 percent of adult high-cost patients had chronic medical condi-
> tions, and only one in 6 suffered from an acute medical "catastrophe." In
> addition, more than 13 percent of high-cost patients died in the hospital.
> National catastrophic health insurance is likely to pay for much chronic
> illness and terminal care (which could be dealt with better and cheaper in
> long-term care institutions) and divert resources toward acute-care hospitals.

No-Plan

Except in 1965 when Medicare/Medicaid was passed, No-Plan has always
been the strongest contender in the Congressional NHI Sweepstakes.
No-Plan, of course, has no features to distinguish it from the present
situation. Therefore, there is little to say about it, except that if their
silence or negative comments concerning the three major contenders of
1980 meant anything, the major provider interest groups, the hospitals,
the physicians, and the insurance companies really did like the idea, a
marked change from their (public) posture in the mid-1970s.

National Health Service

Beginning in the early 1970s, several different proposals for a national
health service were advanced by such groups as the Medical Committee
for Human Rights (Bodenheimer; Bodenheimer et al.; Kotelchuk and
Levy; Jonas, 1974; Lander, pp. 58–61) and the Committee for a National
Health Service (1976). Draft legislation to create a "community-controlled"
National Community Health Service was put forward by the Institute for
Policy Studies (1976). The Committee for a National Health Service, or
CNHS, had developed a somewhat different approach. Although based on
the concept of "community control," it emphasized national coordination
of policy in quality control, health sciences education, occupational safety
and health, use of drugs, health rights, and finance and planning (Commit-

tee for a National Health Service; 1976). A national health service would bypass the insurance mechanism entirely, providing services directly to patients. It could do this in one of two ways: by owning and operating all health care facilities and employing all health workers itself, or by contracting with institutional and individual providers to supply health services and reimbursing them on a basis other than payment for item of service. Financing would be either from general taxation or through a special, progressive health care tax. By 1979, most support for an American NHS had coalesced around a bill introduced by Congressman Dellums (H. R. 2969) and supported by the re-formed Coalition for a National Health Service (1980).

Under the Dellums proposal (Dellums; *Health Law Newsletter*), a U.S. Health Service would provide a very broad range of services in facilities that it would own and operate. There would be no deductibles or co-insurance. All health services personnel would be salaried. The Service would be operated by four levels of Health Boards: community (25,000–50,000 population); district (100,000–500,000); region (500,000–3,000,000); and nation. Community health board members would be directly elected and then each level of board would choose the membership of the boards at the next level. Two-thirds of the membership of each board would represent users of the service; one-third, health services personnel. Health services funds would be distributed on a population basis, with extra funds going to presently underserved geographic areas and populations. There would be a detailed Health Bill of Rights, quality assurance would be a basic responsibility of the Health Boards, occupational and preventive health services would receive strong support, geographic and specialty maldistribution would be directly addressed, and all health personnel education and health research would be Board responsibilities. The Service would be financed by employer and graduated individual taxes.

The "Consumer-Choice Plan"

In the late 1970s, Alain Enthoven, a Stanford economist, developed a concept of health care financing that he described as "Consumer-Choice" (Enthoven, 1978a, 1978b; Brazda).* In 1979–1980, several legislative versions of his concept, also described as the "Competitive Model," were introduced in Congress. Among them were bills sponsored by Senator Durenberger (S. 1485 and S. 1968); Senator Schweiker (S. 1590); and Representative Ullman (H. R. 5740). The "Competitive Model" has re-

---

*The bulk of this section is based on a paper by Brazda (1980), "Special Report: Competition, the New Model of Health Care Financing Plans." *Washington Report on Medicine and Health*, March 17, 1980.

ceived strong support from Paul Ellwood, creator of the HMO concept (HMO at its simplest being a euphemism for prepaid group practice), and his InterStudy consulting firm, and two conservative organizations, the Institute for Contemporary Studies and the American Enterprise Institute.

The Consumer-Choice Model assumes that cost-containment is the most pressing need facing the American health care delivery system. It concludes that regulation is either the wrong or an innately ineffective approach to cost-containment. It proposes to introduce competition as a means to hold down costs, the competition to be created by providing consumers with a choice of health care plans, some more expensive, some less expensive. Presumably, there would be price competition among the various plans to register members.

There are variations in detail among the various legislative proposals based on these principles. Some require that HMOs be included as an option; others do not. Some include catastrophic and Medicaid/Medicare reform; others do not. All involve some sort of limit on the amount of health insurance premium paid for on behalf of employees that employers can deduct from their taxable income as a business expense, the assumption being that the present system of allowing unlimited deductions for health insurance premiums is a spur to inflation. Furthermore, to achieve the allowable tax deductions, employers would have to offer plans meeting minimum standards. The amount of employer contribution to all health insurance premiums would have to meet certain minima, but employees choosing less expensive options would get cash rebates. All of the proposals would leave more or less intact present systems of provider reimbursement, health planning, quality assurance, and resource allocation. All would have some provision for co-payment.

The theory behind all of this is that consumers of health care make the major choices controlling the allocation of resources in the system and that they have enough information about the product being purchased to ensure that it will be of high quality and reasonable cost. There happens to be a great deal of evidence that neither of these assumptions is correct. Physicians, in fact, control the bulk of decision-making on resource utilization (Reinhardt; Worthington), and few patients have at their command the information needed to assess quality and relative cost. Furthermore, demand for medical care is intermittent, most people hurt when they are sick, most people simply want to be healed when they hurt, and many people believe that "doctor knows best."

The concept that competition among providers in response to individual consumer choices made on the basis of price will truly control costs while even maintaining, much less improving quality, thus has some serious problems and remains to be proved. The problem is not with the concept of competition itself as one of several necessary modalities in the effort to control costs and improve quality. The problem concerns the level within the system at which competition is to be introduced, who will be making the choices among competitors, and who will be monitoring the outcomes. Creating competition among providers happens to be a major feature of the Kennedy and Carter proposals, as well as of NHI-by-contract (see next section). The difference between them and Consumer-Choice is that in the former the competition among providers will be for the trade of groups of purchasers, in one form or another, armed with information sufficient to make effective choices, and the collective power to require the behavioral changes on the part of providers necessary to achieve cost-control.

NHI-by-Contract

NHI-by-Contract (Jonas, 1981) is a plan that has not yet been put into legislative language. It would maintain the present pattern of ownership of health facilities, probably but not necessarily result in a change in the employment patterns of presently fee-for-service personnel, provide for the continued existence of the insurance companies in reduced size, place government at arm's length from the direct operation of health services, and provide a significant role for consumers of services in their evaluation, by outcomes.

Using epidemiological methods in health services planning, it would carry out needs assessments on an ongoing basis, set priorities on the basis of those needs assessments, and, within the limits of available resources, make continual program adjustments to meet identified needs. The approach would allow for the direct application of planning information to health services system operation, so that the focus on meeting identified needs could always be maintained, without direct government operation. The assumption is made that the numerous health care providers are incapable of doing rational planning on their own and that government action in this area is necessary. It is also assumed, as it is in most other NHI proposals, that government will play an increasingly important role in the financing of health services, whether through taxes or the imposition and collection of uniform employer-employee contributions to pay for the cost of health services.

A classical approach to the achievement of stated goals and objectives is the contract mechanism. The buyer and seller of a product agree on product or service specifications and cost written down in a contract. The contract usually contains means of enforcement of its terms. A small-scale, partial prototype of such an approach to the financing, planning, and evaluation of health services existed in New York City during the 1970s (Jonas, 1977b, Chapters 5–7). It was colloquially called "Ghetto Medicine."

Under NHI-by-Contract, government would raise the funds necessary to pay for health services. It would then negotiate a series of contracts with providers, under which they would agree to offer a set of services to the population for a given dollar amount. The composition of the service packages would be determined by health planning mechanisms. There would be free competition among the providers for the contracts, bidders offering to provide the specified services at varying prices. Much as group practice and independent practice association health maintenance organizations do now, all contractors would then market their services to consumers.

All persons would be covered for a benefit package that would be determined nationally. Consumers would have free choice of contractor, but once having made their choice, as in present dual-choice situations, would have to stay with the selected provider for a minimum period of time. Advisory boards consisting of patients served by each contractor would be formed. The boards would be party to contract negotiation and enforcement. There would be graded financial penalties for failure to meet contract specifications and rewards for excellent performance. Private ownership of the health services sector would be maintained, but the people, through both the government and the advisory boards, would have a strong voice in deciding how their money is being spent.

Government would have three principal roles: raiser of funds, negotiator of contracts, and enforcer of contracts in concert with the advisory boards. Government responsibilities would be distributed among the national, state, and local jurisdictions. The existing HSA and PSRO systems would be strengthened and used to plan, set priorities, and assure quality. The system would be supported by a combination of employer-employee contributions and general tax revenues. Technology assessment, carried out at the federal level, would provide important data for health planning and priority-setting. Insurance companies could be used as fiscal intermediaries.

The consumer role would focus on the evaluation of outcomes, that is the extent to which contractors met their contract specifications. Most existing providers, whether institutional or individual, would be eligible to become either primary contractors or subcontractors. In this, NHI-by-Contract has much in common with the Health Care Corporation concept of the mid-1970s AHA plan. Primary contractors would be paid on a global budget basis. Private medical practice could be maintained, primarily in a subcontractor role.

NHI-by-Contract provides the opportunity to deal directly with the three principal problems presently facing the U.S. health care delivery system: cost-control, quality-improvement, and implementing a compre-

hensive health promotion and disease-prevention program. It enables the
direct focusing of effort and expenditure. A fair degree of fine-tuning can be
accomplished. It leaves behind the present reliance on regulation and
prayer to achieve program goals and objectives. It does not begin with
benefit packages and decisions on co-payment, which so many other
approaches to NHI do. It does begin with the establishment of planning
principles and assumes that benefit packages will be developed and decisions on co-payment made *after* needs are assessed, goals and objectives
are set, and the amount of available funds is determined. Then the contract
specifications will be written, balancing needs, priorities, and available
funds.

The system would probably be quite cumbersome, especially for the
first few years. Negotiations would be extremely complex. Long lead
times, to which few Americans are accustomed, would be required for
their conclusion. The providers would be called upon to make functional
and psychological changes, although not of the same magnitude as would
be required under the national health service approach. Behavioral change
would be required among patients as well, although recent experience
with HMOs indicates that patient behavioral change would come more
easily than provider behavioral change. From the perspective of most
patients, NHI-by-Contract would look a great deal like a vastly expanded
HMO system. There would be a large redundant staff in the health
insurance industry as individual claims processing became a thing of the
past. However, there would be many positions in negotiating bodies at
many levels and in inspectorates.

Analysis of Impact of Proposals Upon Problems

As pointed out above, the Congressional Research Service outlined five
policy issues to be considered in evaluating NHI proposals: cost and
cost-containment; coverage and gaps therein; geographic maldistribution
of facilities and personnel; access; and impact of NHI on health status
(Cavalier). To the list we shall add quality-assurance and consumer participation and we shall analyze the impact upon them of the Kennedy,
Carter, Long, NHS, Consumer-Choice, and NHI-by-Contract proposals,
along with that of the ever-popular No-Plan.

Cost, Cost-Sharing, the Insurance Companies,
and Reimbursement

One way to look at the cost of NHI is to determine how much the plan itself
would cost. Obviously, plans that cover more services will cost more in
terms of dollars spent through the plan than those that cover fewer services. Thus, less-comprehensive plans appear to be more "economical.

However, a more useful approach is to examine the effect various plans would have on total expenditures for health services. Under NHI, total expenditures could go up, go down, or remain the same. The magnitude of the outlay made through the plan does not necessarily indicate what effect it would have on total expenditures. It must be remembered that ultimately all dollars spent for health services come from the pockets of the consumers of care, whether as direct payments, as taxes, as insurance premiums, or as parts of the payments for goods and services sold by companies that pay taxes and insurance premiums. A plan that funnels a majority of the total expenditure for health service through itself looks very expensive on paper. Yet it might conceivably lead to a reduction of total expenditures if it were able to increase the use of ambulatory services, particularly for prevention; decrease rates of hospitalization (the most expensive service); better regulate the incomes of physicians and dentists; and generally address itself to improving the efficiency of the delivery system. Conversely, a limited benefits plan with no regulatory mechanisms for physician reimbursement and little control over physician use of the delivery system's resources, particularly hospitals, could ultimately be more expensive than a comprehensive plan with comprehensive controls.

The Kennedy approach would attempt to meet the cost problem head on by relating total expenditures to the GNP, providing for annual budgeting rather than reimbursement by item of service for hospitals, requiring careful evaluation before introducing new and costly technologies, making fee-for-service the least favored mechanism for paying doctors, and encouraging HMOs. The Carter plan would "cap" expenditures on an annual allowable increase basis, would encourage prospective reimbursement, would limit hospital capital expenditures, would stimulate HMO development, and would institute physician fee-schedules for care for the poor. The several Long plans would appear to do little for cost-containment and, if its critics are correct, would actually increase overall costs by encouraging the utilization of expensive care.

A National Health Service would operate with a single national budget. Its supporters claim extensive cost-savings through the elimination of fee-for-service, the substitution of global budgeting for all hospitals, and the elimination of many claims-processing and eligibility-determination costs. Consumer-Choice claims to be a cost-containment mechanism. It could be, if consumers were very well-informed about the services they buy. NHI-by-Contract would have cost-control features similar to those of the Kennedy plan plus the capability to clearly set priorities related to health and health-care needs. No-Plan would leave the present situation unchanged.

A critical and sometimes emotionally charged issue is "cost-sharing," wherein the user of services pays some of the cost directly out of pocket. This is featured in the Carter, Long, Consumer-Choice, and No-Plan approaches. It might be present in NHI-by-Contract, depending upon available funds and priorities. It would be eliminated in the Kennedy and NHS proposals.

The arguments on this issue have raged hot and heavy over the years (Davis, 1975b, pp. 59–67). Proponents of user co-payments usually cite two arguments in their favor, not always at the same time. First, they say they are needed to hold down the amount of tax funds and employer-employee contributions necessary to finance NHI. Second, they say that co-payments are required to control utilization of services, on the theory that patients will "overutilize" and "abuse" entirely free services.

The theory of patient abuse of services that are free at the time of service has a long history. It is based on the supposition that health services are like any other commodity of service; people will use all that they can get their hands on. However, there is little, if any, evidence in support of this point, and logic argues against it, since health services are associated with sickness, an unpleasant event, rather than with health. Furthermore, though a frequent user of health services may not be "sick" in the eyes of the average provider, such a user may actually have an illness characterized by the need to seek care, in the basic sense of the word, frequently. In addition, there is a great deal of concern that co-payments can easily constitute a serious barrier to the utilization of needed services (as need is defined by providers, not patients; Roemer et al.). Those who worry about patient abuse of services also assume that patients make most or all decisions regarding utilization, which, as has been pointed out several times, is not the case.

Major advocates of co-payments have been concerned that an NHI plan without significant co-payments would result in so much overutilization, particularly of ambulatory services, that the delivery system would be "wrecked" (Newhouse et al.). Research has been done in the field and in the literature to support their premises (Newhouse et al.; Brian and Gibbens), but the work has been criticized on methodological and theoretical grounds (Greenlick; Hopkins et al., 1975a, 1975b; Jonas, 1977a; Kasten; Myers; Roemer et al.). Furthermore, experience in other countries that have introduced NHI programs providing care free at the time of service indicates that the "swamping" effect predicted by proponents of co-payments does not occur (Jonas, 1977a).

All of the proposals except NHS would maintain a role for the insurance companies, although it would be somewhat limited under the Kennedy plan and markedly reduced and altered under NHI-by-Contract. Under Kennedy, Carter, Long, and Consumer-Choice, in one way or another, for most beneficiaries, policies meeting federal/state standards would be purchased from private insurance companies, either by employers for employed workers, or by state or federal government for nonworking persons, with Medicare being retained for persons 65 and older. No proposals distinguish between the for-profit and the not-for-profit insurance companies. Regulation would be shared by the federal and state governments, with the federal role most prominent in the Kennedy plan. The concept of involving private insurance companies in NHI is historically newer in the United States than is not involving them; it arose only as private companies began to become a significant factor in health insurance after World War II. The first legislative proposals for NHI based on private insurance companies did not appear until the late 1940s (Davenport). Fee-for-service private medical practice would disappear under NHS, be limited under Kennedy and NHI-by-Contract, and be strengthened by Carter, Long, and Consumer Choice.

Quality-Assurance and Consumer Participation

The previous chapter illustrated the problems that exist with the level of the quality of health and medical care delivered in the United States. The Kennedy plan would strengthen existing quality-assurance mechanisms, establishing a National Commission on Quality, and relate quality-assessment results to planning and budgeting. There would be a prominent consumer role in planning, and "ombudsmen" and "advocates" would be available to investigate complaints and assist consumers in negotiating the system. The Carter, Long, Consumer-Choice, and No-Plan approaches would generally continue the present quality-assurance system. The NHS and NHI-by-Contract plans would introduce consumer participation into quality-assessment, the former at the process and outcome levels, the latter at the outcome level only. NHS would, of course, be "run" by consumer-majority boards, which would "control" all aspects of the service. Under NHI-by-Contract, consumers would focus on needs, priorities, and results, participating in contract negotiations and enforcement. The whole issue of consumer participation in NHI has been considered at some length by Kindig and Sidel (pp. 15–22, 38–43).

Gaps in Coverage

Gaps in coverage currently exist. There are limitations in benefits for many persons who already have some form of insurance: persons 65 and over, most employed workers, some of the poor and self-employed. There is lack of coverage altogether for some employed and self-employed persons and for many of the poor. NHS and NHI-by-Contract would fill all of the gaps, covering everyone under a single health plan. The choices consumers make would be among providers, on bases other than price. The Kennedy plan would fill most of the gaps. The Carter plan would fill some of them.

The Long plans, which include federalization of Medicaid, would fill fewer gaps than the Carter plan but more than most of the Consumer-Choice plans, which do not address the issue. No-Plan would leave the present situation unchanged.

Geographic Maldistribution of Personnel and Facilities

The Kennedy and NHS plans would attack these problems with vigor. NHS-by-Contract provides a needs-assessment-related mechanism to do so. The Carter plan would strengthen the existing HSA system and clamp down hard on hospital capital expenditures. Long, Consumer-Choice, and No-Plan do not address these problems.

Access to Care

NHS and NHI-by-Contract would eliminate financial barriers to care. The Kennedy plan would virtually eliminate them. NHS and Kennedy would make strong efforts to eliminate geographic barriers to care, as pointed out in the previous section, and NHI-by-Contract could do so. By having one system of health care for all persons, NHS and NHI-by-Contract would eliminate the current "dual-track" system, one for the poor and one for everyone else (*Health Law Newsletter*). Although the Kennedy plan would maintain Medicaid for financing services for the poor, everyone would have the same insurance card and package of benefits. Thus the effect on the dual-track system would be similar to that of NHS and NHI-by-Contract. The Carter and Long plans would reduce but not eliminate financial barriers to care. Consumer-Choice would have little effect on them and No-Plan would have none. The Carter plan would reduce geographic barriers to care. Long, Consumer-Choice, and No-Plan do not address the issue. Carter, Long, Consumer-Choice, and No-Plan would all maintain the dual-track system.

Impact on Health Status

Because of the huge amounts of money and power involved, the stakes in the outcome of the struggle over the design of an NHI system are higher than in any other major conflict in health care delivery in the United States. The providers, both individual and institutional, as well as the consumers, have major interests in the design of an NHI system, as do the insurance companies. The providers are concerned about their continuing existence in modes acceptable to them; usually, they want little or no change. Consumers want "better" and "cheaper" health services, but often find it difficult to translate those vague desires into feasible, practical proposals. The insurance companies want at least to maintain their present role, if not expand it.

Among these contending forces and complex issues, we often lose sight of the central question: what is the relationship between national health insurance and health? For the consumer, health service is a means to the end of gaining and maintaining health. Providers are concerned both with the health of the population and with protection of their interests. (Although some providers, particularly in the proprietary sectors, appear to be more interested in the latter than the former, most, in their hearts, will put a healthy population first.) The commercial insurance industry, on the other hand, exists primarily to make profits for its shareholders or policyholders and thus that consideration must come first.

In any case, there is a limited relationship between health and NHI as it is currently being discussed in the United States. In Chapter 2 it was pointed out that for the most part, medical care is not responsible for the improvement in the general health level of the population that has occurred in the past 200 years. Most of the major measurable advances have resulted from improved nutrition, pure water supply and sanitary sewage disposal, environmental sanitation, and communicable disease control; outside of the health field, improved housing, education, and workplace safety have been important factors.

NHI deals primarily with the financing of medical care, and could secondarily affect the organization of services, depending upon which plan is chosen. Therefore, it would have a limited relationship to measurable health levels in the population, since medical care deals not with health in the population, but sickness in individuals. Curing sickness is extremely important, of course, to those who are sick with treatable conditions, and it should be done as well as possible. Any NHI plan must ensure excellence in medical care; however, ensuring health in the population requires other measures. Therefore, even supporters of a national health service responsive to consumers cannot be considered to be dealing with anything more than sickness, unless the system is specifically designed to emphasize prevention.

Healthy People: The Surgeon General's Report on Health Promotion and Disease Prevention

The Surgeon General has described a comprehensive set of preventive medicine and public health services which are do-able now. They are aimed squarely at the leading killers of our era: heart disease, cancer, stroke, accidents, pneumonia and influenza, diabetes, cirrhosis of the liver, emphysema, homicide and suicide, as well as certain nonkilling but important and controllable diseases and conditions, such as venereal disease, tuberculosis, hazardous workplaces, and hazardous environments. Included in the program are a number of personal health services such as: immunization; family planning, prenatal and infant care; case-finding and contact investigation; screening for diabetes, hypertension, and cancer;

and interventions using primarily health education and patient education
to deal with problems of lifestyle, including obesity, dietary imbalance,
cigarette smoking, alcohol and drug misuse, exercise and fitness, and
stress-control.

Public health services such as environmental pollution control and
industrial hygiene are important as well. Certain lifestyle problems require
intervention at the community level as well as the personal level, with
measures such as the regulation of cigarette and alcohol advertising, the
elimination of subsidies for growing tobacco, and the required labeling of
food. But in our era, personal preventive services have a great deal of
potential for improving the health of the people.

It is preventive measures, rather than utilization controls or even health
care delivery system reform, that will best effect control: by raising health
levels, they will reduce the need for sickness services. Much of the debate
over NHI in the United States deals with how to rearrange the existing
pieces of the system. Clearly, the delivery of personal health services is
important; reform of the United States health care delivery system is
essential; and the design of an NHI program will have a critical impact on
the future shape of that system. An appropriately structured NHI program
can in fact have a powerful influence on making the health care delivery
system in the United States truly that rather than what it really is presently:
a disease care delivery system. Milton Terris has put it succinctly: ". . . it is
a serious error—unfortunately a common one—to consider a national
health care program as synonymous with a national health program. The
health of a population is determined only in part by the health care system.
. . . Prevention should be made the keystone of the national health program
. . ." (1972).

The NHS proposal places a heavy emphasis on prevention at both the
personal and community levels. Occupational health services are featured.
A broad range of personal preventive services would be reimbursable
under the Kennedy plan. Certain personal preventive services, especially
for children, are featured under the Carter proposal. NHI-by-Contract
could provide a broad range of preventive services, again depending upon
needs-assessment and priority-setting in contract-specifications design.
The Long and Consumer-Choice plans do not address the issue. And, of
course, neither does No-Plan.

The Future of NHI

Predictors of the passage of some sort of NHI plan in the United States do
so at their peril. After all, the leaders of the American Association for Labor
Legislation thought that it was right around the corner in 1913 (Burrow,
1977, p. 139). By 1979, Alan Greenspan, a chairman of the Council of

Economic Advisors under President Ford, was to say that: "A broad, comprehensive national health insurance plan is a program whose time has come and passed" (*Hospitals*, p. 17). On the stock exchange, the bull market usually begins just as the "little guy" turns bearish, and vice-versa. That could well happen in the history of NHI too. When we have stopped looking for it, it might well appear. It is popular in some circles to say that NHI is too expensive, that the nation can't afford to have it. According to proponents of comprehensive plans, whether it be Kennedy, NHS, or NHI-by-Contract, the truth is just the opposite. With the skyrocketing costs, questionable quality, and massive misallocation of resources that occur under the present voluntary, "free" system, the nation cannot afford *not* to have it, they say. However, achieving it is not that easy, as history has taught us again and again. The provider control groups are very powerful and most of them have indicated that they do not want any significant changes in the present system, other than a reduction in government regulation of their business. For example, the American Medical Association (*American Medical News*, 1979), in a modest retreat from its mid-1970s position that would have required employers to offer private insurance, by the end of the 1970s was recommending only that:

1. Private insurance, if offered, must meet minimum standards and must require co-payments;
2. Medicaid be federalized; Medicare be maintained;
3. A catastrophic insurance program be established; and
4. Administration be carried out at the state level.

This policy is very similar to that of Senator Long. Critics would say that it contains a great deal of bad-debt insurance for physicians. The Association of American Medical Colleges (1979) adopted a similar position. In an era of legislation by special interest, such groups have a great deal of influence.

The two most powerful control groups in the health care delivery system are the physicians and the hospitals. In the past, major changes in the system have taken place when the physicians and/or the hospitals wanted or needed those changes, e.g., the reinstitution of medical licensing laws and the reduction in the number of medical schools in the late 19th and early 20th centuries, and the development of voluntary hospital insurance during the Great Depression. NHI will most likely come when one or the other or both of those groups want it or need it. The private hospitals will want it when an increasing number of them go bankrupt in the face of uncontrolled cost increases, as happened in Great Britain just before the institution of the National Health Service. The physicians will want it when their number is so large that they will no longer be able to sell all the

product they can collectively produce, as they can now. If a majority of
them were still private entrepreneurs at that time, the competition would
be chaotic (Consumer Commission). The shelter of a secure, if somewhat
smaller income would be sought. We are likely to encounter this situation
by the middle of the next decade. Thus the U.S. will probably have NHI by
the year 2000, with so-called catastrophic health insurance and the expansion of welfare health insurance as an interim step. Nevertheless, solutions
of the major system problems—cost-containment, the lack of attention to
prevention, geographic and specialty maldistribution, irrationality in the
allocation of resources, and the elimination of barriers to care and the
dual-track system—will likely require a comprehensive national health
program, à la Kennedy plan, NHS, or NHI-by-Contract. The major question is: can the nation afford to wait until the year 2000 to deal with these
problems?

References

American Medical News. "NHI Policy Reaffirmed." August 3/10, 1979.
American Medical News. "Senators Delay Decision on NHI." May 30, 1980.
Anderson, O. W. The Uneasy Equilibrium: Private and Public Financing of Health
    Services in the United States, 1875–1965. New Haven, Connecticut: College
    and University Press, 1968.
Association of American Medical Colleges. "A Position Paper: The Expansion and
    Improvement of Health Insurance in the United States." Washington, D.C.,
    August 1979.
Bills, S. S. "National Health Insurance: The Battle Takes Shape." Hospitals,
    J.A.H.A., April 16, 1975, p. 126.
Boas, F. P. "Why Do We Need National Health Insurance?" Society for Ethical
    Culture, 1945. Reprinted in Committee on Medical Care Teaching of the
    Association of Teachers of Preventive Medicine, Readings in Medical Care,
    p. 655. Chapel Hill: University of North Carolina Press, 1958.
Bodenheimer, T. "The Hoax of National Health Insurance." American Journal of
    Public Health, 62, 1324, 1972.
Bodenheimer, T. et al., Eds. Billions for Band-Aids, An Analysis of the U.S. Health
    Care System and of Proposals for Its Reform. San Francisco: San Francisco
    Bay Area Chapter, Medical Committee for Human Rights, 1972.
Brazda, J. "Special Report: Competition, the New Model of Health Care Financing
    Plans." Washington Report on Medicine and Health, March 17, 1980.
Brewster, A. W. Health Insurance and Related Proposals for Financing Personal
    Health Services. Washington, D.C.: USDHEW, USGPO, 1958.
Brian, E. W., and Gibbens, S. F. "California's Medi-Cal Copayment Experiment."
    Medical Care, 12, Supplement, December 1974.
Burney, I. L. "Geographic Variation in Physicians' Fees." Journal of the American
    Medical Association, 240, 1368, 1978.
Burns, E. M. "Health Insurance: Not If, or When, But What Kind?" American
    Journal of Public Health, 61, 2164, 1971.

Burrow, J. G. AMA: Voice of American Medicine. Baltimore: Johns Hopkins Press, 1963.

——————. Organized Medicine in the Progressive Era. Baltimore: The Johns Hopkins University Press, 1977.

Cavalier, K. "National Health Insurance." Washington, D.C.: Congressional Research Service, Library of Congress, March 27, 1979.

Coalition for a National Health Service. National Health Service Action, Vol. 1, No. 2, May 1980.

Committee for a National Health Service. Summary of a Bill to Create a National Health Service. New York, 1976.

Committee on the Costs of Medical Care. Medical Care for the American People. Chicago: University of Chicago Press, 1932. Reprinted, Washington, D.C.: USDHEW, 1970.

Committee on Finance, United States Senate. Medicare and Medicaid: Problems, Issues and Alternatives. Washington, D.C., February 9, 1970.

——————. Comparison of Major Features of Health Insurance Proposals. Washington, D.C.: USGPO, 1979.

Committee on Ways and Means, House of Representatives. National Health Insurance Resource Book. Washington, D.C.: USGPO, 1974.

Consumer Commission on the Accreditation of Health Services. "National Health Service V: Building a Medical Staff." Consumer Health Perspectives, V, 3, 1, 1978.

Davenport, R. W. "Health Insurance Is Next." Fortune, March 1950, p. 63. Reprinted in Committee on Medical Care Teaching of the Association of Teachers of Preventive Medicine, Readings in Medical Care, p. 640. Chapel Hill: University of North Carolina Press, 1958.

Davis, K. "Hospital Costs and the Medicare Program." Social Security Bulletin, 36, 18, 1973.

——————. "Equal Treatment and Unequal Benefits: The Medicare Program." Health and Society, 53, 449, 1975a.

——————. National Health Insurance: Benefits, Costs, and Consequences. Washington, D.C.: The Brookings Institution, 1975b.

Dellums, R. "The Health Service Act: H. R. 2969." Congressional Record, Vol. 125, No. 33, March 19, 1979.

Douglas-Wilson, I., and McLachlan, G. Health Service Prospects: An International Survey. Boston: Little, Brown, 1973.

Eilers, R. D. "National Health Insurance: What Kind and How Much." Parts 1 and 2. New England Journal of Medicine, 284, 881, 945, 1971.

Eilers, R. D., and Moyerman, S. S. National Health Insurance: Proceedings of the Conference on National Health Insurance. Homewood, Illinois: R. D. Irwin, 1971.

Enthoven, A. C. "Consumer-Choice Health Plan." New England Journal of Medicine (two parts), 298, 650, 709, 1978a.

——————. "Consumer-Choice Health Plan: A Rational Economic Design for National Health Insurance." The 1978 Michael M. Davis Lecture. Chicago, The Center for Health Administration Studies, University of Chicago, 1978b.

Falk, I. S. "Medical Care in the USA—1932–1972. Problems, Proposals and

Programs *from the* Committee on the Costs of Medical Care *to the* Committee for National Health Insurance." *Health and Society, 51,* 1, 1973.

—————. "Proposals of National Health Insurance in the USA: Origins and Evolution, and Some Perceptions for the Future." *Health and Society,* Spring 1977, p. 161.

Freeland, R. M. *The Truman Doctrine and the Origins of McCarthyism.* New York: Knopf, 1975.

Friedman, E. "Medicaid" (Five parts). *Hospitals, J.A.H.A.,* Vol. 51, 1977: August 16, p. 51; September 1, p. 59; September 16, p. 73; October 1, p. 61; November 1, p. 77.

Fry, J., and Farndale, W. A. J., Eds. *International Medical Care.* Oxford, England: MTP, 1972.

Fulcher, D. *Medical Care Systems.* Geneva: International Labour Office, 1974.

Glaser, W. A. *Health Insurance Bargaining.* New York: Gardner Press, 1978.

Gornick, M. "Ten Years of Medicare: Impact on the Covered Population." *Social Security Bulletin,* July 1976, p. 3.

Greenlick, M. R. "California's Medi-Cal Copayment Experiment." *Medical Care,* 12, 1054, 1974.

Harris, R. "Annals of Legislation: Medicare." *The New Yorker,* July 2, July 9, July 16, July 23, 1966.

Health Care Financing Administration. *Data on the Medicaid Program.* Baltimore: USDHEW Pub. No. (HCFA) 79–20005, USGPO, 1980.

Health Law Newsletter. "National Health Insurance and the Poor." Issue No. 102, October 1979.

Health/PAC. "Medicaid: The Fading of a Dream." *Bulletin,* April 1973, p. 13.

Health Security News. "Catastrophic Still a Threat." October–November 1974, p. 1

Health Security News. "A Comparison of Major National Health Insurance Bills in the 94th Congress." Vol. 4, No. 5, July 7, 1975.

Hopkins, C. E., et al. "Cost-Sharing and Prior Authorization Effects on Medicaid Services in California: Part I: The Beneficiaries' Reactions." *Medical Care,* 13, 582, 1975a.

—————. "Cost-Sharing and Prior Authorization Effects on Medicaid Services in California: Part II: The Providers' Reactions." *Medical Care,* 13, 643, 1975b.

Hospitals. "Hospitals Headlines: Symposium Shows Sentiments Stacked Against National Health Insurance Plan." November 16, 1979.

H. R. 1. "The National Health Care Services Reorganization and Financing Act." House of Representatives, Washington, D.C., 1975.

H. R. 6222. "Comprehensive Health Care Insurance Act of 1975." House of Representatives, Washington, D.C., 1975.

H. R. 2969. "Health Services Act." Washington, D.C.: House of Representatives, March 14, 1979.

H. R. 5740. "The Health Cost Restraint Act." Washington, D.C.: House of Representatives, 1980.

Institute for Policy Studies. *Model Legislation for a National Community Health Service.* Washington, D.C.: Community Health Alternatives Project, 1976.

Jonas, S. "Review Article: Billions for Band-Aids." *International Journal of Health Services,* 4, 723, 1974.

——————. "Japan Strains under Complex Health System." *Hospitals, J.A.H.A.*, September 1, 1975.

——————. "Copayment and National Health Insurance in the United States: A Critique of Work by Newhouse, Phelps and Schwartz." *International Journal of Health Services*, 7, (2), 1977a.

——————. *Quality-Control of Ambulatory Care: A Task for Health Departments*. New York: Springer, 1977b.

——————. "Planning for National Health Insurance by Objective: The Contract Mechanism." In Straetz, R., Ed., *Critical Perspectives and Issues in Health Policy*. Lexington, Massachusetts: Lexington Books, 1981.

Kasten, J. "California's Medi-Cal Copayment Experiment." *Medical Care*, 12, 1058, 1974.

Kennedy, E. M. "A Complete Plan of Health Care for All Americans." *Congressional Record*, January 15, 1975.

Kimble, C. "Special Report: Comparing the Carter and Kennedy National Health Insurance Bills." *Washington Report on Medicine and Health*, November 1979.

Kindig, D. A., and Sidel, V. W. "Impact of National Health Insurance Plans on the Consumer." In Eilers, R. D., and Moyerman, S. S., Eds., *National Health Insurance*. Chapter 1. Homewood, Illinois: Richard D. Irwin, 1971.

Kotelchuk, R., and Levy, H. "MCHR: An Organization in Search of an Identity." *Health/PAC Bulletin*, March/April 1975, p. 1

Lander, L. *National Health Insurance: He Who Pays the Piper Lets the Piper Call the Tune*. New York: Health/PAC, 1975.

Le Clair, M. "The Canadian Health Care System." In Andreopoulos, S., Ed., *National Health Insurance: Can We Learn From Canada?* Chapter 1. New York: Wiley, 1975.

Lynch, M. J., and Raphael, S. S. *Medicine and the State*. Springfield, Illinois: Charles C Thomas, 1963.

McKittrick, L. S. "Medical Care for the American People: Is Compulsory Health Insurance the Solution?" *New England Journal of Medicine*, 240, 998, 1949. Reprinted in Committee on Medical Care Teaching of the Association of Teachers of Preventive Medicine, *Readings in Medical Care*, p. 647. Chapel Hill: University of North Carolina Press, 1958.

McMahon, J. A. *Statement of the American Hospital Association on National Health Insurance before the Health Subcommittee of the House Committee on Ways and Means, November 10, 1975*. Washington, D.C.: American Hospital Association.

Myers, B. A. "California's Medi-Cal Copayment Experiment." *Medical Care*, 12, 1051, 1974.

Nation's Health, The. "Carter Addresses Annual Meeting." November 1976.

Newhouse, J. P., et al. "Policy Options and the Impact of National Health Insurance." *New England Journal of Medicine*, 290, 1345, 1974.

New York Academy of Medicine. "Toward a National Health Program." The 1971 Health Conference. *Bulletin of the New York Academy of Medicine*, 48, January 1972.

New York Times, The. "Cuts in Medicaid Put Into Effect." September 30, 1971.

————————. "Fund-Short States Cut Services." December 27, 1975.

Reinhardt, U. E. *Physician Productivity and the Demand for Health Manpower*. Cambridge, Massachusetts: Ballinger, 1975.

Roemer, M. I., et al. "Copayments for Ambulatory Care: Penny-Wise and Pound-Foolish." *Medical Care, 13*, 457, 1975.

S. 1438. "National Healthcare Act of 1975." U.S. Senate, 94th Congress, 1st Session.

S. 3. "The Health Security Act." U.S. Senate, Washington, D.C., 1975.

S. 1720. "Health Care for All Americans Act." Washington, D.C.: U.S. Senate, 96th Congress, September 6, 1979.

S. 1812. "National Health Plan Act." Washington, D.C.: U.S. Senate, 96th Congress, September 25, 1979.

S. 1590. "The Comprehensive Health Care Reform Act." Washington, D.C.: U.S. Senate, 1980.

S. 1968. "The Health Incentives Reform Act." Washington, D.C.: U.S. Senate, 1980.

Schroeder, S., et al. "Frequency and Clinical Description of High-Cost Patients in 17 Acute-Care Hospitals." *New England Journal of Medicine, 300*, 1306, 1979.

Schwartz, H. *The Case for American Medicine: A Realistic Look at Our Health Care System*. New York: David McKay, 1972.

Sigerist, H. E. *On the Sociology of Medicine*. Edited by M. I. Roemer. New York: MD Publications, 1960.

Somers, H. M., and Somers, A. R. *Doctors, Patients, and Health Insurance*. Washington, D.C.: The Brookings Institute, 1961.

Stevens, R. *American Medicine and the Public Interest*. New Haven, Connecticut: Yale University Press, 1971.

Stevens, R., and Stevens, R. *Welfare Medicine in America*. New York: The Free Press, 1974.

Subcommittee on Health, Committee on Ways and Means. *National Health Insurance*. Washington, D.C.: USGPO, November 27, 1979.

Surgeon General of the United States. *Healthy People*. Washington, D.C.: USDHEW Pub. No. (PHS) 79–55071, USGPO, 1979.

Terris, M. "The Need for a National Health Program." *Bulletin of the New York Academy of Medicine*, 2nd Series, *48*, 24, 1972.

Truman, H. S. *Message from the President of the United States, Transmitting His Request for Legislation for Adoption of a National Health Program*. 79th Congress, 1st Session. Washington, D.C.: USGPO, 1945. Reprinted in: Committee on Medical Care Teaching of the Association of Teachers of Preventive Medicine, *Readings in Medical Care*, p. 629. Chapel Hill: University of North Carolina Press, 1958.

Washington Report on Medicine and Health. "Special Report: Catastrophic Health Insurance Bills before the Senate Finance Committee." Vol. 33, No. 14, April 9, 1979.

Worthington, N. L. "Expenditures for Hospital Care and Physicians' Services: Factors Affecting Annual Changes." *Social Security Bulletin*, November 1975, p. 3.

Appendix I

Sources of Data

Introduction

This guide to the principal sources of health and health services data for the United States has two parts. Part A contains descriptions of the major data sources: who publishes them, how frequently they are published as of 1980, from whom they may be ordered, and what categories of data they contain. All of the tables in the text that derive from sources listed here (that is, all tables from recurring sources), are keyed to Part A—for example, source notes to text tables taken from the *Statistical Abstract of the United States* include the phrase "(See Appendix I, A1)" at the end of the relevant bibliographical information.

Part B lists categories of data and indicates in which publications they can be found. Most of the data sources are obviously the same as those described in Part A; they are simply looked at from a different perspective. Each source listed in Part B that appears in Part A is keyed to Part A so that the reader may locate it with ease.

Using this appendix and the keys in those text tables that derive from recurring sources, the reader can keep the book—or at least the tables—up-to-date. He must determine for himself whether the text has become out-of-date in light of new data.

A. Major Sources of Data

1. *Statistical Abstract of the United States*
   Published annually by the Bureau of the Census, U.S. Department of Commerce, Washington, D.C.* The *Statistical Abstract* reproduces a vast selection of tables containing information from

---

*Almost all U.S. government publications are to be purchased from the Superintendent of Documents, United States Government Printing Office (USGPO), Washington, D.C., 20402, rather than directly from the agency producing them.

many different government agencies. They are accumulated under the following headings: Population; Vital Statistics; Immigration and Naturalization; Health and Nutrition; Education; Law Enforcement, Federal Courts, and Prisons; Geography and Environment; Public Lands, Parks, Recreation, and Travel; Federal Government Finances and Employment; State and Local Government Finances and Employment; Social Insurance and Welfare Services; National Defense and Veterans' Affairs; Labor Force, Employment, and Earnings; Income, Expenditure, and Wealth; Prices; Elections; Banking, Finance and Insurance; Business Enterprise; Communications; Energy; Science; Transportation—Land; Transportation—Air and Water; Agriculture; Forests and Forest Products; Fisheries; Mining and Mineral Products; Construction and Housing; Manufactures; Domestic Trade and Services; Foreign Commerce and Aid; Outlying Areas under the Jurisdiction of the United States; and Comparative International Statistics. The *Abstract* also has its own very large "Guide to Sources," for all categories of data.

2. *U.S. Census of Population*

The Bureau of the Census is part of the U.S. Department of Commerce, Washington, D.C., 20233. The Constitution requires that a census be taken every 10 years, at the beginning of each decade. The original purpose was to apportion seats in the House of Representatives and thus in the Electoral College. In modern times, in addition to the simple counts, a great deal of demographic data is collected by the Census Bureau. Hardcover compendia of decennial national census data are published periodically. Also available are special analyses for a wide variety of geographical subdivisions of the country. Many reports on the decennial censuses are published by the Census Bureau, but a good place to begin is in Section 1 of the *Statistical Abstract*.

3. *Current Population Reports*

In addition to reports from the decennial censuses, the Census Bureau publishes seven series of reports on a continuing basis. These include estimates, projections, sample counts, and special studies of selected segments of the population. The seven series each have a "P" number. They are: P–20, Population Characteristics; P–23, Special Studies; P–25, Population Estimates and Projections; P–26, Federal–State Cooperative Program for Population Estimates; P–27, Farm Population; P–28, Special Censuses; P–60, Consumer Income. Information on the content of each series is of course available from the Census Bureau. Subscriptions are not available for individual series but must be taken in two sets. However, single copies of reports from all series except P–28 may be ordered from the USGPO.

4. *Monthly Vital Statistics Report (MVSR)*
    MVSR is published by the National Center for Health Statistics of the Office of Health Research, Statistics, and Technology of the Department of Health and Human Services, 3700 East–West Highway, Hyattsville, Maryland, 20782. It has several sections. *Provisional Statistics*, published monthly, contains the most recent data for the traditional "Vital Statistics"—deaths, births, marriages, and divorces. There are also a series of Supplements, which appear on a semiregular basis. They contain provisional final annual summaries of vital statistics plus technical information on methodology. Another component of MVSR, *Advance Data*, presents data from such ongoing NCHS activities as the National Ambulatory Medical Care Survey (NAMCS) and the Health and Nutrition Examination Survey (HANES). MVSR publications may be ordered by annual subscription; one subscription covers all of the regular reports and the supplements.

5. *Vital Statistics of the United States*
    This is the annual report of the National Center for Health Statistics (NCHS) concerning vital statistics. The address of the NCHS is given above (under MVSR, Number 4).

6. *Vital and Health Statistics*
    This periodic publication of the NCHS appears at irregular intervals. There are 13 series, not numbered consecutively, most of which report data from ongoing studies and surveys that the NCHS carried out. Several series have been dormant for some time. The publication of some data shifts periodically between *Vital and Health Statistics* and *Monthly Vital Statistics Report*. In the late 1970s, a new publication appeared: *Advance Data from Vital and Health Statistics*. Until the late 1970s, the NCHS published a useful guide, *Current Listing and Topical Index to the Vital and Health Statistics Series*. Presently, they are publishing only a semi-annual list of current numbers in the several series. The 13 series in *Vital and Health Statistics* are as follows:

    Series 1. "Programs and Collection Procedures."
    Series 2. "Data Evaluation and Methods Research."
    Series 3. "Analytical Studies." Primarily of mortality, they stress international comparisons.
    Series 4. "Documents and Committee Reports."
    Series 10. "Data from the Health Interview Survey." These

contain patient-perspective health, illness, and
health services utilization data.

Series 11. "Data from the Health Examination Survey and the
Health and Nutrition Examination Survey."

Series 12. "Data from the Health Records Survey." Reports data
from two studies of nursing homes carried out in the
1960s.

Series 13. "Data on Health Resources Utilization." Includes hospitals, nursing homes, and ambulatory care services.

Series 14. "Data on Health Resources: Manpower and Facilities." Health resources data appear also in *Health
Resources Statistics* and *Health, United States* (see 9
below)

Series 20. "Data on Mortality." Reports of time–trends analyses
for the United States.

Series 21. "Data on Natality, Marriage, and Divorce."

Series 22. "Data from the National Natality and Mortality Surveys." This series differs from the one above in that
special studies are reported.

Series 23. "Data from the National Survey of Family Growth."

7. *Morbidity and Mortality Weekly Report (MMWR)*
This is a regular publication of the Center for Disease Control
(CDC) of the USDHHS, and is available on an annual subscription
basis from the CDC, Atlanta, Georgia, 30333. In the past, it has
been concerned primarily with the communicable diseases for
which reporting is required by law. Most of the diseases covered
are no longer of much importance in the United States and, for
many of them, the reporting rates are poor. Nevertheless, it
provides an important perspective on communicable disease in
the United States. Each week, case reports of specific outbreaks of
communicable diseases are reported; there are also occasional
international notes, status reports on communicable disease control programs, and statements of official United States Public
Health Service positions on various issues in communicable disease control. In recent years MMWR has acquired a broader
purview, reporting on CDC and USPHS activities in chronic disease
control. It is thus becoming a publication of increasing value.

8. *Health Resources Statistics*
Health Resources Statistics is a formerly annual, now periodic
publication of the National Center for Health Statistics. It has
three major parts: manpower, inpatient facilities, and outpatient
and nonpatient health services. It is a voluminous work, reporting

numbers, distribution, and some facilities and services utilization data. It is the major source of census data on health manpower and facilities in the United States, although the American Hospital Association and American Medical Association do, of course, report data on hospitals and physicians (respectively).

9. *Health, United States*

The first edition of this work was published in 1976 under the title *Health, United States, 1975*. A combined effort of the National Center for Health Statistics and the National Center for Health Services Research, it appeared annually through the end of the decade and will presumably continue to appear annually. In each issue, there are several review articles on "Selected Health Topics," and then data are presented on "Health Status and Determinants," "Utilization of Health Resources," "Health Care Resources," and "Health Care Costs and Financing." It also contains a useful appendix, "Sources and Limitations of Data." It is a boon to students and researchers in health care delivery because it provides "one-stop shopping" for most important health and health care data.

10. *American Hospital Association Guide to the Health Care Field*.

This publication of the American Hospital Association, 840 North Lake Shore Drive, Chicago, Illinois, 60611, appears on August 1 of each year. It has two parts. The first contains a listing of almost every hospital in the United States by location, and basic data on size, type, ownership, and facilities, as well as a great deal of information on the AHA and the hospital supply industry. The second part, *Hospital Statistics*, contains a great deal of summary utilization and financial data on United States hospitals, by many different cross-tabulations. Some of the data are presented historically. The *"Guide Issue* of *Hospitals* and *Hospital Statistics* together contain the most detailed available data on hospitals in the United States.

11. *Hospitals*—"Hospital Indicators"

Appearing in the biweekly journal *Hospitals*, sponsored by the American Hospital Association, "Hospital Indicators" reports up-to-date summary data on hospital utilization, personnel, and finances and also has periodic special studies of particular aspects of hospital operations. Since late 1979, "Hospital Indicators" have reported most data in terms of percentage changes only, thereby becoming much less useful than they were previously.

12. *Social Security Bulletin*

The *Bulletin* is a monthly publication of the Social Security Administration, USDHHS, 1875 Connecticut Ave., N.W., Washington, D.C., 20009. Until 1979, it was the principal source of basic financial data for the health care delivery system, going back to 1929. Although it has been replaced for this function by new HCFA publications (see item 13), it still occasionally publishes useful health data and health services data.

13. *HCFA Publications*
     In 1979, the Health Care Financing Administration (HCFA) took over the responsibility from the SSA for publishing annual health care financing data. The *Health Care Financing Review* is a quarterly. It now annually publishes "National Health Expenditures" and "Private Health Insurance," which formerly appeared in the *Social Security Bulletin*. These summaries cover total amounts, where the money comes from, and where it goes. HCFA also publishes two related information sources. *Health Care Financing Trends* presents quarterly data on national health expenditures; community hospitals; consumer and medical care prices; employment, hours, and earnings of health workers; and certain national economic indicators. *Health Care Financing Notes* periodically provides descriptive data for various HCFA programs. HCFA publications are available from its Office of Research, Demonstrations, and Statistics, Oak Meadows Building, 6340 Security Boulevard, Baltimore, Maryland 21235.

14. *"Datagrams" of the Association of American Medical Colleges*
     The "Datagrams" appear monthly in the *Journal of Medical Education*. The AAMC is located at 1 DuPont Circle, Washington, D.C., 20036. Together with the annual issue of the *Journal of the American Medical Association* on medical education (usually the last issue of the year), "Datagrams" provide the principal source of data on medical education in the United States: schools, faculty, curricula, admissions, students, and the like.

15. *Center for Health Services Research and Development of the American Medical Association*
     The Center, which is located in AMA national headquarters, 535 North Dearborn Street, Chicago, Illinois, 60610, produces a wide variety of very useful data on physician manpower from its own files. Two annual publications, containing these data as well as secondary source material, are *Profile of Medical Practice* and *Socioeconomic Issues of Health*. The AMA also publishes periodic reports on special studies. Other major professional organizations are good sources of data on their own members.

16. *Selected National Data Sources for Health Planners*
    This work was published by the National Center for Health Statistics in 1976 (Rockville, Maryland: USDHEW Pub. No. (HRA) 76–1236, USGPO) and may be updated from time to time. It was "designed to provide a convenient set of references to the most useful sources of data available from national organizations for meeting the needs of state and local health planners" (p. iii). It is indeed a much more detailed version of this Appendix.

B. Categories of Data: Sources

1. Population Data
a. *Statistical Abstract of the United States*, Section 1 (A1)
b. *U.S. Census of Population* (A2)
c. *Current Population Reports* (A3)
d. State and local governments. Some state and local governments, and/or state and local independent planning agencies, use detailed Census Bureau data on their local areas, which the bureau does not routinely publish, to produce very detailed compendia of local and/or state census data. Local inquiries must be made to determine if such information is available for a particular area.
e. Utility companies. In many parts of the country, utility companies publish, on a regular, periodic basis, estimates of population changes since the most recent census. They also often add other information, particularly concerning economic growth. Local inquiries should be made.
f. *Health, United States* (A9). Some population data are presented in "Health Status and Determinants."

2. Vital Statistics
a. *Monthly Vital Statistics Report* (A4)
b. *Vital Statistics of the United States* (A5)
c. *Vital and Health Statistics* (A6). Summary vital statistics data appear from time to time in Series 3, 20, 21, and 22.
d. Life Tables. These indicators, which are based on mortality data, are published independently and periodically by the National Center for Health Statistics.
e. *Statistical Abstract of the United States* (A1). Selected vital statistics appear annually in Section 2, "Vital Statistics."
f. Health Departments. Some state and local health departments publish compendia of vital statistics for their jurisdictions.
g. *Current Population Reports* (A3). Fertility data, which are re-

garded technically as vital statistics, are collected by the Bureau of the Census and published in Current Population Reports, Series P–20.

h. *Health, United States* (A9). Some vital health data are presented in "Health Status and Determinants."

3. Morbidity

a. *Vital and Health Statistics* (A6). A wide variety of morbidity data from many different sources is published periodically in Series 10, 11, 12, and 13.

b. *Monthly Vital Statistics Report* (A4). Although they are not technically vital statistics, a variety of morbidity data, some of which also appear in *Vital and Health Statistics*, are published on an irregular basis. They include data from the *National Ambulatory Medical Care Survey* and the Health and Nutrition Examination Survey.

c. *Morbidity and Mortality Weekly Report* (A7)

d. *Statistical Abstract of the United States* (A1). Selected morbidity statistics appear annually in Section 2, "Vital Statistics," and in Section 4, "Health and Nutrition."

e. Health Departments. State and local health departments sometimes publish morbidity surveys for their jurisdictions.

f. *Health, United States* (A9). Some morbidity data are presented in "Health Status and Determinants."

4. Utilization of Health Services

a. *Vital and Health Statistics* (A6). Series 10 presents patient-perspective data from the *Health Interview Survey*. Provider-perspective data are provided from the *National Ambulatory Medical Care Survey* (Series 2) and the *Hospital Discharge Survey* (Series 13).

b. *Monthly Vital Statistics Report* (A4). Provider-perspective ambulatory service data are provided from the *National Ambulatory Medical Care Survey*.

c. *Guide to the Health Care Field* (A10)

d. "Hospital Indicators" (A11)

e. *Health, United States* (A9). Patient- and provider-perspective utilization data are both presented.

f. American Medical Association (A15). *Profile of Medical Practice* and *Socioeconomic Issues in Health* present provider-perspective utilization data.

5. Institutions
a. *Statistical Abstract of the United States* (A1). Basic data on health care institutions is contained in Section 4.
b. *Vital and Health Statistics* (A6). Data on institutions appear in Series 12, 13, and 14.
c. *Health Resources Statistics* (A8). Parts II and III.
d. *Health, United States* (A9). Part B.
e. *Guide to the Health Care Field* (A10)
f. "Hospital Indicators" (A11)
g. "Datagrams" (A14)

6. Health Manpower
a. *Statistical Abstract of the United States* (A1). Section 2.
b. *Vital and Health Statistics* (A6). Series 14.
c. *Health Resources Statistics* (A8). Part I.
d. *Health, United States* (A9). Part B.
e. *Center for Health Services Research and Development of the AMA* (A15)

7. Financing
a. *Statistical Abstract of the United States* (A1). Section 4.
b. *Health, United States* (A9). Part B.
c. *Guide to the Health Care Field* (A10). Certain financial data concerning hospitals appear.
d. "Hospital Indicators" (A11). Certain financial data concerning hospitals appear.
e. *Social Security Bulletin* (A12)
f. *Health Care Financing Review* and related publications (A13).
g. "Datagrams" (A14). Certain financial data concerning medical schools appear.
h. Center for Health Services Research Development of the AMA (A15). Certain financial data concerning physicians appear.

Appendix II

Abbreviations

AAA—Area Agencies on Aging
AALL—American Assocation for Labor Legislation
AAMC—Association of American Medical Colleges
ADAMHA—Alcohol, Drug Abuse, and Mental Health Administration
AHA—American Hospital Association
AIP—Annual Implementation Plan
AMA—American Medical Association
ANA—American Nurses Association
APA—American Psychiatric Association
ASTHO—Association of State and Territorial Health Officials
BCHS—Bureau of Community Health Services
CPR—Cardiopulmonary resuscitation
CDC—Center for Disease Control
CDCP—Center for Disease Control and Prevention
CE—Continuing Education
CEU—Continuing Education Unit
CHAMPUS—Civilian Health and Medical Program of the Uniformed Services
CHC—Community Health Center
CHP—Comprehensive Health Planning
CHSS—Cooperative Health Statistics System
CMHC—Community Mental Health Center
CME—Continuing Medical Education
CNHS—Committee for a National Health Service; Coalition for a National Health Service
CON—Certificate of Need
CONUS—Continental United States
CPH—Children's Psychiatric Hospital
DOD—Department of Defense
DHEW—Department of Health, Education and Welfare
DHHS—Department of Health and Human Services

DRG—Diagnostically Related Group
EGP—Employer Guaranteed Plan
EMT—Emergency Medical Technician
EPA—Environmental Protection Administration or Environmental Protection Agency (check the context)
ERs—Emergency rooms
ESP—Economic Stabilization Program
FHA—Federal Housing Authority
FMC—Foundation for Medical Care
FMG—Foreign Medical Graduate
FTE—Full-time equivalent
GAO—General Accounting Office
GMENAC—Graduate Medical Education National Advisory Committee
HANES—Health and Nutrition Examination Survey
HCAAA—Health Care for All Americans Act
HCFA—Health Care Financing Administration
HDS—Hospital Discharge Survey
HHS—Health and Human Services
HIAA—Health Insurance Association of America
HIS—Health Interview Survey
HMO—Health Maintenance Organization
HRA—Health Resources Administration
HRG—Health Research Group
HS—Household Survey
HSA—Health Systems Agencies
HSP—Health Systems Plans
ICDA—International Classification of Diseases, Adapted
IPA—Individual Practice Association
IHS—Indian Health Service
IOM—Institute of Medicine
JCAH—Joint Commission on Accreditation of Hospitals
LCME—Liaison Committee on Medical Education
LHD—Local Health Department
LPN—Licensed Practical Nurse
MCH—Maternal and Child Health
MCHR—Medical Committee for Human Rights
MCEPEN—Midwest Continuing Education Professional Education for Nurses
MVSR—Monthly Vital Statistics Report
NAMCS—National Ambulatory Care Survey
NCA—National Council on Aging
NCHCT—National Center for Health Care Technology
NCHS—National Center for Health Statistics

NCHSR—National Center for Health Services Research
NHC—Neighborhood Health Center
NHI—National Health Insurance
NHP—National Health Plan
NHS—National Health Survey or National Health Service (check the context)
NIH—National Institutes of Health
NIMH—National Institute of Mental Health
NIOSH—National Institute of Occupational Safety and Health
NLN—National League for Nursing
NMA—National Medical Association
NMCUES—National Medical Care Utilization and Expenditures Survey
N.P.—Nurse Practitioner
NPHPRS—National Public Health Program Reporting System
OSHA—Occupational Safety and Health Administration
OASH—Office of the Assistant Secretary for Health
OEO—Office of Economic Opportunity
OHMO—Office of Health Maintenance Organizations
OMB—Office of Management and Budget
P.A.—Physicians' Assistant or Associate
PAC—Political Action Committee
PAS—Professional Activity Study
PPGP—Prepaid Group Practice
PHS—Public Health Service
PSRO—Professional Standards Review Organization
RAG—Regional Advisory Group
RMP—Regional Medical Program
R.N.—Registered Nurse
RTC—Residential Treatment Center
SHA—State Health Agency
SHCC—Statewide Health Coordinating Council
SHPDA—State Health Planning and Development Agency
SMSA—Standard Metropolitan Statistical Area
SMHS—State Medicaid Household Survey
SSA—Social Security Administration
USDA—United States Department of Agriculture
USDHEW—United States Department of Health, Education and Welfare
USDHHS—United States Department of Health and Human Services
USHUD—United States Department of Housing and Urban Development
USGPO—United States Government Printing Office
USPHS—United States Public Health Service
WHO—World Health Organization

Index